Selected Papers from the 3rd International Symposium on Life Science

Selected Papers from the 3rd International Symposium on Life Science

Special Issue Editor

Valentin A. Stonik

MDPI • Basel • Beijing • Wuhan • Barcelona • Belgrade • Manchester • Tokyo • Cluj • Tianjin

Special Issue Editor
Valentin A. Stonik
Far Eastern Branch of Russian
Academy of Sciences
Russia

Editorial Office
MDPI
St. Alban-Anlage 66
4052 Basel, Switzerland

This is a reprint of articles from the Special Issue published online in the open access journal *Marine Drugs* (ISSN 1660-3397) (available at: https://www.mdpi.com/journal/marinedrugs/special_issues/3rd-Int-Symp-on-Life-Science).

For citation purposes, cite each article independently as indicated on the article page online and as indicated below:

LastName, A.A.; LastName, B.B.; LastName, C.C. Article Title. *Journal Name* **Year**, *Article Number*, Page Range.

ISBN 978-3-03928-728-4 (Pbk)
ISBN 978-3-03928-729-1 (PDF)

Cover image courtesy of Boris Grebnev.

Contents

About the Special Issue Editor

Valentin A. Stonik Academician, D.Sc., Professor.
Affiliation: G.B. Elyakov Pacific Institute of Bioorganic Chemistry, Far East Branch of the Russian Academy of Sciences.
Address: 690022, Vladivostok, pr. 100 let Vladivostoku, 159. Russian Federation.
Tel. +7(423)-2311430; Fax: +7(423)-2314050; E-mail: stonik@piboc.dvo.ru, piboc@eastnet.febras.ru.
Position: Research Superviser of PIBOC.
Date of birth: 4 December, 1942.
Education: 1960–1965, Far East State University, Department of Chemistry (Vladivostok, Russia).
Degrees and honors:
1969 - Ph.D. (speciality: organic chemistry. Title of thesis: "Synthesis of Hydroacrydines and Relative Compounds").
1988 - D.Sc. (specialty: bioorganic chemistry, chemistry of natural and physiologically active compounds. Title of thesis: "Biphyllic Physiologically Active Compounds from Echinoderms and Sponges. Structure and Properties").
1995 - The Russian Academy of Sciences M.M. Shemyakin Prize Winner.
1997 - Corresponding Member of the Russian Academy of Sciences.
2003 - Full Mermber of the Russian Academy of Sciences (Academician).
2010 - Dr. causa of Vietnamese Academy of Science and technology.
2010 - Golden Medal of Vietnamese Academy of Science and technology.
2013 - Badge of honor of the Academy of Sciences of Mexico (Invencion, Ingenieria e Investigacion, Academia de Ciencias).

High-qualified expert in natural products chemistry and biochemistry of bioactive compounds (secondary metabolites: alkaloids, unusual lipids, isoprenoids, polyhydroxysteroids, steroidal glycosides of polyhydroxysteroids, triterpenoidal and steroidal oligoglycosides, etc.), their biomedical properties. Citations: more than 8,600, Hirsch Index = 43 (Google Scholar).
Author and co-authors of more than 430 publications in Russian and international journals, 4 monographs, about 40 patents, and 1 university textbook.
Member of the Editorial Board of the Journals: Natural Product Communications, Bioorganic Chemistry, Russin Chemical Bulletin.

Some publications

1. Antonov A.S., Kalinovsky A.I., Afiyatullov Sh.Sh., Leshchenko E.V., Dmitrenok P.S., Yurchenko E.A. Kalinin V.I., Stonik V.A. Erylosides F8, V1–V3 amd W–W2 – new triterpene oligoglycosides from the Carribean sponge Erylus goffrilleri // Carbohydrate Res. 2017. V. 449. P. 153–159.
2. Dyshlovoy S., von Amsberg G., Rast S., Hauschild J., Otte K., Alsdorf W., Madanchi R., Kalinin V.I., Silchenko A.S., Avilov S.A., Dierlamm J., Honecker F., Stonik V.A., Bokemeyer C. Frondoside A induces AIF-associated caspase-independent apoptosis in Burkitt's lymphoma cells // Leukemia and Lymphoma. 2017. V. 58, N 12. P. 2905–2915.
3. Dyshlovoy S.A., Madanchi R., Hauschild J., Otte K., Alsdorf W. H., Schumacher U., Kalinin V.I., Silchenko A.S., Avilov S.A., Honecker F., Stonik V.A., Bokemeyer C., von Amsberg G. The marine

triterpene glycoside frondoside A induces p53-independent apoptosis and inhibits autophagy in urothelial carcinoma cells // BMC Cancer. 2017. V. 17, N 2. P. 93[1–10].
4. Dyshlovoy S.A., Otte K., Venz S., Hauschild J., Junker H., Makarieva T.N., Balabanov S., Alsdorf W.H., Madanchi R., Honecker F., Bokemeyer C., Stonik V.A., von Amsberg G. Proteomic-based investigations on the mode of action of the marine anticancer compound zhizochalinin // Proteomics. 2017. V. 17, N 11. P. 1700048[1–11].
5. Ivanchina N.V., Malyarenko T.V., Kicha A.A., Kalinovsky A.I., Dmitrenok P.S., Stonik V.A. A new steroidal glycoside granulatoside C from the starfish Choriaster granulatus, unexpectedly com-bining structural features of polar steroids from several different marine invertebrate phyla // Nat. Prod. Commun. 2017. V. 12, N 10. P. 1585–1588.
6. Silchenko A.S., Kalinovsky A.I., Avilov S.A., Dmitrenok P.S., Kalinin V.I., Berdyshev D.V., Chingizova E.A., Andryjaschenko P.V., Minin K.V., Stonik V.A. Fallaxosides B1 and D3, triterpene glycosides with novel skeleton types of aglycones from the sea cucumber Cucumaria fallax // Tetrahedron. 2017. V. 73, N .
7. Shubina L.K., Makarieva T.N., Guzii A.G., Denisenko V.A., Popov R.S., Dmitrenok P.S., Stonik V.A. Absolute configuration of the cytotoxic marine alkaloid monanchocidin A // J. Nat. Prod. 2018. V. 81, N 4. P. 1113–1115.
8. Yun S.-H., Sim E.-H., Han S.-H., Kim T.-R., Ju M.-H., Han J.-Y., Jeong J.-S., Kim S.-H., Silchenko A.S., Stonik V.A., Park J.-I. In vitro and in vivo anti-leukemic effects of cladoloside C2 are mediated by activation of Fas/ceramide synthase 6/p38 kinase/c-Jun NH2-terminal kinase/caspase-8 // Oncotarget. 2018. V. 9, N 1. P. 495–511.
9. Malyarenko T.V., Malyarenko O.S., Kicha A.A, Ivanchina N.V., Kalinovsky A.I., Dmitrenok P.S., Ermakova S.P., Stonik V.A. In vitro anticancer and proapoptotic activities of steroidal glycosides from the starfish Anthenea aspera // Mar. Drugs. 2018. V. 16, 420.

Preface to "Selected Papers from the 3rd International Symposium on Life Science"

Studies on marine natural compounds are becoming increasingly interdisciplinary. In obtaining and discussing new valuable scientific data, a wide range of different specialists have become involved, from environmental chemists to hydrobiologists and pharmacologists. Long-term studies at our G.B. Elyakov Pacific Institute of Bioorganic Chemistry (PIBOC), belonging to the Russian Academy of Science, have led to the isolation and structural elucidations of many hundreds of marine natural compounds including low molecular weight bioregulators and biopolymers. A series of marine drugs, food supplements, and functional food products were created on this basis. Some of them have been approved for industrial production and medicinal or other applications in Russia. These studies were conducted in collaboration with scientists from many countries around the world. Fruitful discussions on domestic and international scientific conferences were useful for the development of such studies. The Third International Symposium on Life Science, held 4–8 September, 2019 in Vladivostok, was organized by this Institute. Scientists from several geographic areas of the Russian Federation, from Moscow to Vladivostok, as well as chemists and biologists from Germany, the Republic of Korea, the Peoples Republic of China, and Taiwan, participated in this Symposium and delivered 81 lectures and poster presentations. The regular sub-symposium of the series Korus (Korean–Russian symposiums) was held within the framework of this scientific meeting. This was the third conference of this series, which started with the Symposium in 2012. The aim of the Symposium is to share advanced ideas not only in the field of marine natural products but also in organic and inorganic syntheses, molecular immunology, biotechnology, pharmacology, and molecular genetics to promote the obtaining of new important scientific results in life science. In accordance with invitation and sponsor support of the international scientific journal Marine Drugs, this Special Issue of this journal was published. This Issue focuses its attention on bioactive compounds from sea urchins, particularly quinoid pigments, like echinochrome A and spinochromes. Their diverse biomedicinal properties, stability, and possibility to be obtained using organic synthesis methods have attracted attention to these biologically active compounds. Studies on many other important groups of natural products, including enzymes and lectins, sterol sulfates, and alkaloids, were also discussed as well as the promise of this type investigation with the participation of several neighboring countries.

Valentin A. Stonik
Special Issue Editor

marine drugs

Editorial

Selected Papers from the Third International Symposium on Life Science

Valentin A. Stonik [1,2]

[1] G.B. Elyakov Pacific Institute of Bioorganic Chemistry, Far Eastern Branch, Russian Academy of Sciences, 690022 Vladivostok, Russia; stonik@piboc.dvo.ru

[2] School of Natural Sciences, Far East Federal University, 690001 Vladivostok, Russia

Received: 31 January 2020; Accepted: 11 February 2020; Published: 18 February 2020

The search for and isolation of marine biologically active compounds, as well as relevant studies on their structure and properties are important for the adding knowledge about molecular diversity in nature and creation of medicines and other useful products on this basis. Long-term studies by G. B. Elyakov Pacific Institute of Bioorganic Chemistry (PIBOC) belonging to the Russian Academy of Sciences have led to the isolation and structural elucidation of many hundreds of new marine natural compounds as well as to creation of a series of marine drugs, food additives, and functional food ingredients which were approved for industrial production and medicinal or other applications in Russia. PIBOC actively collaborates with scientists from many countries of the world and performs regular marine expeditions in the North-Western Pacific and other geographic areas using R/V "Academik Oparin". Colleagues from other countries, particularly from Vietnam, also participate in these expeditions. Over the course of its more than 50-year history, our institute has repeatedly organized international scientific conferences.

The Third International Symposium on Life Science, held September 4–8 in Vladivostok, has been also organized by PIBOC. Scientists from several towns of the Russian Federation from Moscow to Vladivostok, as well as chemists and biologists from Germany, the Republic of Korea, the Peoples Republic of China, and Taiwan attended this Symposium and delivered 81 plenary lectures, and oral and poster presentations co-authored by scientists from several other countries. A sub-symposium of the Korus series (Korean-Russian symposiums, started from 2012) was held in the frameworks of this scientific meeting. The aim the Third Symposium on Life Science was to share advanced ideas not only in the field of chemistry of marine natural products, but also in determination of molecular mechanisms of action of new marine metabolites, pharmacology, enzymology, and molecular genetics in order to achieve important new scientific results.

The Special Issue "Selected Papers from the Third International Symposium on Life Science (http:/mdpi.com/journal/marinedrugs/special_issues/Selected Papers from the Third International Symposium on Life Science) in the open access journal Marine Drugs (ISSN 1660-3397) was running from the end of 2018 to the end of 2019. Totally, it comprises 17 articles, concerning with different aspects of Life Science and recent experimental studies, carried out on the basis of marine natural products.

Structures and biological activities of low molecular weight secondary metabolites from marine organisms were discussed in several selected papers. Tabakmakher et al. from PIBOC and colleagues from University Medical Center Hamburg-Eppendorf, Germany, and Institute of Marine Biochemistry, Vietnam, have described seven new polysulfated sterols isolated from the Vietnamese marine sponge *Halichondria vansoesti*. Of particular interest is the fact that compounds similar to some steroids isolated by this group which contain both bromine and chlorine atoms have never been found among marine steroids. The effects of these compounds on human prostate cancer cells, expression of the prostate-specific antigen (PSA), and glucose uptake have been discussed. This was the first report on the ability of marine steroids to suppress PSA expression/androgen receptor signaling in cancer cells [1].

A series of oxysterols including 4 previously unknown compounds has been isolated by Kolesnikova et al. from extracts of a sponge *Inflatella* sp. collected in the Sea of Okhotsk [2]. The influence of isolated compounds on the viability and reactive oxygen species (ROS) formation in neuronal Neuro2a cells using 6-hydroxydopamine-induced cell model of Parkinson's disease was clarified. Some compounds of this series showed the essential neuroprotective activity in these in vitro experiments, probably due ROS scavenging effect.

Yurchenko et al. from PIBOC together with Vietnamese colleagues from Institute of Technology Research and Application (Nhatrang) and Graduate University of Science and Technology (Hanoi) have isolated and studied a new melatonin analogue, 6-hydroxy-*N*-acetyl-β-oxotryptamine, from the marine-derived fungus *Penicillium* sp. KMM 4672 and several other compounds of different chemical nature from *Aspergillus flocculosis* and *Aspergillus* sp. Activities of these metabolites in the 6-hydroxydopamine- and paraquat-induced Parkinson's disease cell models were studied. The new melatonin analogue protects Neuro2a cells more effectively in these experiments in comparison with melatonin itself [3].

Ga-Bin Park et al. from Kosin and Jnje Universities (Republic of Korea) have discussed interesting activities of gliotoxin, a mycotoxin, containing disulfide bond in a piperazine ring and an aromatic amino acid residue and isolated from the marine fungus *Aspergillus fumigatus*. Its action on paclitaxel-resistant ovarian cancer cells has been studied. They have shown that treatment with gliotoxin at nanomolar concentrations inhibits growth and reduces resistance to cytotoxic agents in these cancer cells. Gliotoxin induces apoptotic cell death in an autophagy-dependent manner via the death-associated protein kinase-1 (DAPK1)-TAp63 signaling pathway. The treatment with gliotoxin before paclitaxel treatment inhibited the expression of multidrug resistant-associated proteins and increases expression of DAPK1 and TAp63. The obtained results suggest that DAPK1-mediated TAp63 upregulation is one of the critical pathways inducing apoptosis in chemoresistant cancer cells [4].

The possible microbial origin of some highly active marine metabolites, such as toxins and antitumor agents isolated from invertebrates, has previously been the subject of discussions. Indeed, it has been found that many marine invertebrates contain endo- and epibiotic microorganisms and that some metabolites found in marine invertebrates are structurally related to bacterial natural products. This suggests the microbial origin of some marine invertebrate metabolites [5]. Moreover, microbial origin of bryostatins in bryozoans and some other natural products in lithistid sponges was confirmed by experiments [6].

In this Issue, Makarieva et al. (PIBOC) have reported isolation of more than 20 bacterial strains from the secreted mucus trapping of polychaete *Chaetopterus variopedatus*, and the strain CB-1-14 was recognized as a new species belonging to the genus *Vibrio*. This bacterium was cultured, and 6-*epi*-monanchorin A was obtained from both cells and culture broth using preparative HPLC. This natural compound along with the related guanidine alkaloid monanchorin were earlier found only in marine sponges and the same polychaete species. Thus, the microbial origin of this guanidine alkaloid in marine invertebrates has been established [7].

Venoms of sea anemones are well known as a rich source of peptides acting on different molecular targets such as enzymes, membrane receptors and ion channels. Magnificamide, the major α-amylase inhibitor, comprising of 44 amino acid residues (4770 Da), was isolated from the sea anemone *Heteractis magnifica* mucus. Sintsova and colleagues from PIBOC and University of Lueven, Belgium, have reported that the recombinant magnificamide inhibits porcine and human saliva α-amylases in low nanomolar concentrations and could be considered as a promising drug candidate for the type 2 diabetes treatment [8].

A series of articles has been published by Korean scientists, in majority from National mitochondrial signaling of cardiovascular and metabolic disease center (Pusan, Republic of Korea) and their colleagues from other Korean Universities with participation of Russian co-authors from PIBOC. Professor Jin Park is scientific leader of many such studies. They have investigated molecular mechanisms of action of the Russian medicine Histochrome and active substance of this drug, echinochrome A (Ech A). In its two drug forms, Histochrome has been permitted for clinical application in cardiology and ophthalmology in the Russian Federation. In the published papers, other potential applications of these biopreparations and new peculiarities of their action on cellular and organism levels have been considered.

Ga-Bin Park and co-authors have investigated a possibility to use Ech A as a well-established and non-toxic antioxidant to facilitate ex vivo application of sensitive to oxidative damage hematopoetic stem and progenitor cells (HSPCs), released from the bone morrow. Ech A promoted ex vivo expansion of peripheral blood-derived $CD34^+$ cells by suppressing reactive oxygen species generation and p38 MAPK/JNK phosphorylation in them. Activation of Lyn kinase and p110δ as a mechanism to enhance expansion of $CD34^+$ cells was also shown. An assumption that Ech A initially induces Src/Lyn activation, upregulates p110δ, and finally activate PI3K/Akt pathway was made. More or equal hematopoietic colony forming cells were induced by $CD34^+$ cells expanded in the presence of Ech A in comparison with unexpanded $CD34^+$ cells. Therefore, Ech A is an effective agent for promoting cell proliferation and maintaining the stemness of HSPCs. It is beneficial to maintain self-renewal potential of $CD34^+$ cells during the ex vivo and possibly in vivo expansion of HSPCs [9].

In the related article, Jl Hye Park and collaborators has discussed the results of the studies on cell protective effect of Histochrome under oxidative stress in human cardiac progenitor cells (hCPCs). There are small portions of these stem cells in ischemic hearts, where they participate in repairing the damaged heart tissues. Histochrome does not influence surface expression markers of hCPCs. It reduces cellular and mitochondrial ROS levels in these cells at oxidative stress, induced by H_2O_2, protects hCPCs, and shows anti-apoptotic effects through downregulation of pro-apoptotic signals and upregulation of anti-apoptotic signals. Histochrome delayed the progression of cellular senescence in hCPCs. It was concluded that the use of histochrome as biosafe agent is promising as potential therapeutic strategy at application of patients-derived hCPCs to treat cardiovascular diseases [10].

In confirmation of positive effects of Ech A at cardiovascular problems, Ran Kim and co-authors have reported a significant effect of Ech A on the injured region and behavioral decline at ischemic stroke in a rat middle cerebral artery occlusion model after reperfusion. Ech A alleviated the infarcted brain region and encouraged affirmative behavioral changes after ischemic stroke. It altered the expression levels of cell viability-related factors. It was concluded that the protective role of this natural compound against cell death is connected with its antioxidant effect [11].

In their paper, Su-Jeong Oh and co-authors have discussed a beneficial impact of Ech A on inflammatory bowel disease, using a murine model of experimental colitis. Intravenous injection of this compound prevented subsequent lethality and body weight loss in colitis-induced mice. In in vitro experiments, this preparation stimulated generation of regulatory T cells, suppressed the activation of proinflammatory M1 type macrophages and induced the production of M2 type macrophages. It has been suggested that due to these features of the action, Ech A can correct imbalances in the intestinal immune system, help resolve inflammation and initiate tissue repair [12].

Unexpectedly, the Russian team from PIBOC, G.M. Somov Institute of Epidemiology and Microbiology (Vladivostok), and Institute of Vaccines and Sera (Moscow) has found that Ech A not only exhibits anti-oxidant properties, but also shows anti-viral activities against tick-borne encephalitis virus and herpes simplex virus type 1. A mixture of Ech A, ascorbic acid and tocopherol (5:5:1) showed even higher anti-oxidant and anti-viral effects in comparison with Ech A itself [13].

Not only Ech A, but also some other quinoid pigments from sea urchins, so-called spinochromes, have also been shown to be potential therapeutic agents. In fact, Chang Shin Yoon and co-authors have discussed the results of the studies on protective action of spinochrome D (spD), a structural analogue of Ech A, on cardiomyocytes against doxorubicin (Dox). As it is well known, doxorubicin demonstrates suppressive activity against different cancers, but, being cardiotoxic, it increases ROS level in heart cells. Authors of this article have reported that spD protected the Ac16 human cardiomyocyte cell line against Dox cytotoxicity, but did affect anticancer properties of DOX in relation of MCF-7 human breast tumor cells. As it was established by proteomic and metabolomic analyses, its action led to alterations in glutathione metabolism. The increase of ATP level and oxygen consumption rate, induced by spD, was detected in galactose-treated AC-16 cardiomyocytes. These findings suggested that spD could be considered as a potential cardioprotective agent at Dox therapy of oncological patients [14].

Sokolova and colleagues from PIBOC reported that Ech A is soluble in aqueous solutions of carrageenans from red algae. Its complexes with carrageenans showed the ability to decrease expression of pro-inflammatory cytokines Il-6 and TNFα and increase the expression of anti-inflammatory cytokine Il-10. Thus, carrageenans can modulate biological properties of Ech A [15].

Problems of the studies on biopolymer natural compounds and last results, obtained by participants of the symposium at investigation of the corresponding biopreparations were also discussed and later published as scientific articles involved in this issue. For example, a group of co-authors from PIBOC and Far East Federal University has published the results of mutagenesis studies and structure-function relationship of GalNac/Gal lectin and its mutant forms. This lectin, named CGL, from the mussel *Crenomytilus grayanus* (family Mytilidae, class Bivalvia) is a representative of novel lectin family with β-trefoil fold. The crystal structure of this lection and mutagenesis studies revealed three carbohydrate-binding sites capable to recognize globotriose on the surface of breast cancer cells. In their article, Kovalchuk and colleagues have analyzed how alanine substitution of His 37, His 129, Glu-75, His 85, Asn 27, and Asn 119 in these sites affects mucin-binding capability of CGL. It was shown that this binding is determined by the number of hydrogen bonds in CGL-ligand complexes [16].

The review of Besednova and coauthors "Metabolites of Seaweeds as Potential Agents for the Prevention and Therapy of Influenza Infection" (G.M. Somov Institute of Epidemiology and Microbiology) contains analysis of literature data about anti-influenza effects of algal polysaccharides such as fucoidans, carrageenans, and ulvans as well as other biopolymer substances from algae (lectins and polyphenols). It was concluded that use of recently developed drugs can lead to the selection of resistant viral strains. That is why some metabolites from algae with a broad spectrum of anti-viral activity could be of interest as a potential basis for creation of new drugs [17].

The obtaining of recombinant form of alkaline hosphatase/phosphodiesterase, Cam PhoD, from the marine bacterium *Cobetia amphilecti* KMM 296, expressed in *Escherichia coli* cells, has been described in the article of Noskova et al from PIBOC and Far East Federal University. The enzyme catalyzes the cleavage of diester and phosphate bonds in nucleotides. It was shown that Cam PhoD, exhibiting maximum activity in the presence of Co^{2+} and Fe^{3+} ions, is a new member of PhoD family [18].

Genomic studies on two recently described species of marine bacteria, *Zobellia amuskyensis* and *Zobellia laminariae* from the PIBOC Collection of marine microorganisms (KMM), have been discussed in the paper of Chernysheva et al. Two novel draft genomes were obtained and compared with known genomes of this genus representatives. Pan-genome of this genus is composed of 4853 orthologous clusters. Carbohydrate active enzyme repertoires were highly diverse and biotechnogically promising as biocatalysts for obtaining of oligosacchharides and other products with possible applications in food and pharmaceutical industries [19].

In summary, this issue covers a series of in their majority experimental studies recently carried out in the field of marine bioactive low molecular weight and biopolymer substances. In their publications, scientists from Russia, the Republic of Korea, Vietnam, Germany, and Belgium have discussed new results obtained at the search for new marine natural compounds, their isolation and structure determination, biological activity, interaction with molecular targets, biomedicinal properties, biogenesis, and perspectives of practical application. A wide spectrum of biological activities was reported for these compounds, including antitumor, neuroprotective, anti-inflammatory, antioxidant, antiviral, and other useful properties. In my opinion, the discovered new properties found for echinochrome A, the active substance of the Russian drugs belonging to the Histochrome series, are of particular interest and should open the way to new areas of medical use of this type drugs.

As a guest editor, I am thankful to all scientists from diverse research institutes and universities, who contributed to the success of a special Issue "Selected Papers from the Third International Symposium on Life Science".

Conflicts of Interest: The author declares no conflict of interest.

References

1. Tabakmakher, K.M.; Makarieva, T.N.; Denisenko, V.A.; Popov, R.S.; Dmitrenok, P.S.; Dyshlovoy, S.A.; Grebnev, B.B.; Bokemeyer, C.; von Amsberg, G.; Cuong, N.X.; et al. New Trisulfated Steroids from the Vietnamese Marine Sponge Halichondria vansoesti and Their PSA Expression and Glucose Uptake Inhibitory Activities. *Mar. Drugs* **2019**, *17*, 445. [CrossRef] [PubMed]
2. Kolesnikova, S.A.; Lyakhova, E.G.; Kalinovsky, A.I.; Popov, R.S.; Yurchenko, E.A.; Stonik, V.A. Oxysterols from a Marine Sponge Inflatella sp. and Their Action in 6-Hydroxydopamine-Induced Cell Model of Parkinson's Disease. *Mar. Drugs* **2018**, *16*, 458. [CrossRef] [PubMed]
3. Yurchenko, E.A.; Menchinskaya, E.S.; Pislyagin, E.A.; Trinh, P.T.H.; Ivanets, E.V.; Smetanina, O.F.; Yurchenko, A.N. Neuroprotective Activity of Some Marine Fungal Metabolites in the 6-Hydroxydopamin- and Paraquat-Induced Parkinson's Disease Models. *Mar. Drugs* **2018**, *16*, 457. [CrossRef] [PubMed]
4. Park, G.-B.; Jeong, J.-Y.; Kim, D. Gliotoxin Enhances Autophagic Cell Death via the DAPK1-TAp63 Signaling Pathway in Paclitaxel-Resistant Ovarian Cancer Cells. *Mar. Drugs* **2019**, *17*, 412. [CrossRef] [PubMed]
5. König, G.M.; Kehraus, S.; Seibert, S.F.; Abdel-Lateff, A.; Müller, D. Natural products from marine organisms and their associated microbes. *Chembiochem.* **2006**, *7*, 229–238. [CrossRef] [PubMed]
6. Haygood, M.G.; Davidson, S.K.; Schmidt, E.W.; Faulkner, D.J. Microbial Symbionts of Marine Invertebrates: Opportunities for Microbial Biotechnology. *J. Mol. Microbiol. Biotechnol.* **1999**, *1*, 33–43. [PubMed]
7. Makarieva, T.; Shubina, L.; Kurilenko, V.; Isaeva, M.; Chernysheva, N.; Popov, R.; Bystritskaya, E.; Dmitrenok, P.; Stonik, V. Marine Bacterium Vibrio sp. CB1-14 Produces Guanidine Alkaloid 6-epi-Monanchorin, Previously Isolated from Marine Polychaete and Sponges. *Mar. Drugs* **2019**, *17*, 213. [CrossRef] [PubMed]
8. Sintsova, O.; Gladkikh, I.; Kalinovskii, A.; Zelepuga, E.; Monastyrnaya, M.; Kim, N.; Shevchenko, L.; Peigneur, S.; Tytgat, J.; Kozlovskaya, E.; et al. Magnificamide, a β-Defensin-Like Peptide from the Mucus of the Sea Anemone Heteractis magnifica Is a Strong Inhibitor of Mammalian α-Amylases. *Mar. Drugs* **2019**, *17*, 542. [CrossRef] [PubMed]
9. Park, G.-B.; Kim, M.-J.; Vasileva, E.A.; Mishchenko, N.P.; Fedoreyev, S.A.; Stonik, V.A.; Han, J.; Lee, H.S.; Kim, D.; Jeong, J.-Y. Echinochrome A Promotes Ex Vivo Expansion of Peripheral Blood-Derived CD34+ Cells, Potentially through Downregulation of ROS Production and Activation of the Src-Lyn-p110δ Pathway. *Mar. Drugs* **2019**, *17*, 526. [CrossRef] [PubMed]
10. Park, J.H.; Lee, N.-K.; Lim, H.J.; Mazumder, S.; Rethineswaran, V.K.; Kim, Y.; Jang, W.B.; Ji, S.T.; Kang, S.; Kim, D.Y.; et al. Therapeutic Cell Protective Role of Histochrome under Oxidative Stress in Human Cardiac Progenitor Cells. *Mar. Drugs* **2019**, *17*, 368. [CrossRef] [PubMed]
11. Kim, R.; Hur, D.; Kim, H.K.; Han, J.; Mishchenko, N.P.; Fedoreyev, S.A.; Stonik, V.A.; Chang, W. Echinochrome A Attenuates Cerebral Ischemic Injury through Regulation of Cell Survival after Middle Cerebral Artery Occlusion in Rat. *Mar. Drugs* **2019**, *17*, 501. [CrossRef] [PubMed]
12. Oh, S.-J.; Seo, Y.; Ahn, J.; Shin, Y.Y.; Yang, J.W.; Kim, H.K.; Han, J.; Mishchenko, N.P.; Fedoreyev, S.A.; Stonik, V.A.; et al. Echinochrome A Reduces Colitis in Mice and Induces In Vitro Generation of Regulatory Immune Cells. *Mar. Drugs* **2019**, *17*, 622. [CrossRef] [PubMed]
13. Fedoreyev, S.A.; Krylova, N.V.; Mishchenko, N.P.; Vasileva, E.A.; Pislyagin, E.A.; Iunikhina, O.V.; Lavrov, V.F.; Svitich, O.A.; Ebralidze, L.K.; Leonova, G.N.; et al. Antiviral and Antioxidant Properties of Echinochrome A. *Mar. Drugs* **2018**, *16*, 509. [CrossRef] [PubMed]
14. Yoon, C.S.; Kim, H.K.; Mishchenko, N.P.; Vasileva, E.A.; Fedoreyev, S.A.; Stonik, V.A.; Han, J. Spinochrome D Attenuates Doxorubicin-Induced Cardiomyocyte Death via Improving Glutathione Metabolism and Attenuating Oxidative Stress. *Mar. Drugs* **2019**, *17*, 2. [CrossRef] [PubMed]
15. Sokolova, E.V.; Menzorova, N.I.; Davydova, V.N.; Kuz'mich, A.S.; Kravchenko, A.O.; Mishchenko, N.P.; Yermak, I.M. Effects of Carrageenans on Biological Properties of Echinochrome. *Mar. Drugs* **2018**, *16*, 419. [CrossRef] [PubMed]
16. Kovalchuk, S.N.; Buinovskaya, N.S.; Likhatskaya, G.N.; Rasskazov, V.A.; Son, O.M.; Tekutyeva, L.A.; Balabanova, L.A. Mutagenesis Studies and Structure-function Relationships for GalNAc/Gal-Specific Lectin from the Sea Mussel *Crenomytilus grayanus*. *Mar. Drugs* **2018**, *16*, 471. [CrossRef] [PubMed]

17. Besednova, N.; Zaporozhets, T.; Kuznetsova, T.; Makarenkova, I.; Fedyanina, L.; Kryzhanovsky, S.; Malyarenko, O.; Ermakova, S. Metabolites of Seaweeds as Potential Agents for the Prevention and Therapy of Influenza Infection. *Mar. Drugs* **2019**, *17*, 373. [CrossRef] [PubMed]
18. Noskova, Y.; Likhatskaya, G.; Terentieva, N.; Son, O.; Tekutyeva, L.; Balabanova, L. A Novel Alkaline Phosphatase/Phosphodiesterase, CamPhoD, from Marine Bacterium Cobetia amphilecti KMM 296. *Mar. Drugs* **2019**, *17*, 657. [CrossRef] [PubMed]
19. Chernysheva, N.; Bystritskaya, E.; Stenkova, A.; Golovkin, I.; Nedashkovskaya, O.; Isaeva, M. Comparative Genomics and CAZyme Genome Repertoires of Marine Zobellia amurskyensis KMM 3526T and Zobellia laminariae KMM 3676T. *Mar. Drugs* **2019**, *17*, 661. [CrossRef] [PubMed]

marine drugs

MDPI

Article

New Trisulfated Steroids from the Vietnamese Marine Sponge *Halichondria vansoesti* and Their PSA Expression and Glucose Uptake Inhibitory Activities

Kseniya M. Tabakmakher [1], Tatyana N. Makarieva [1,*], Vladimir A. Denisenko [1], Roman S. Popov [1], Pavel S. Dmitrenok [1], Sergey A. Dyshlovoy [1,2], Boris B. Grebnev [1], Carsten Bokemeyer [2], Gunhild von Amsberg [2,3] and Nguyen X. Cuong [4]

1 G.B. Elyakov Pacific Institute of Bioorganic Chemistry, Far Eastern Branch of the Russian Academy of Sciences, Pr. 100-let Vladivostoku 159, 690022 Vladivostok, Russia
2 Department of Oncology, Hematology and Bone Marrow Transplantation with Section Pneumology, Hubertus Wald-Tumorzentrum, University Medical Center Hamburg-Eppendorf, 20251 Hamburg, Germany
3 Martini-Klinik Prostate Cancer Center, University Hospital Hamburg-Eppendorf, 20251 Hamburg, Germany
4 Institute of Marine Biochemistry, Vietnam Academy of Science and Technology (VAST), Hanoi 100000, Vietnam
* Correspondence: makarieva@piboc.dvo.ru; Tel.: +7-950-295-6625

Received: 26 June 2019; Accepted: 24 July 2019; Published: 27 July 2019

Abstract: Seven new unusual polysulfated steroids—topsentiasterol sulfate G (**1**), topsentiasterol sulfate I (**2**), topsentiasterol sulfate H (**3**), bromotopsentiasterol sulfate D (**4**), dichlorotopsentiasterol sulfate D (**8**), bromochlorotopsentiasterol sulfate D (**9**), and 4β-hydroxyhalistanol sulfate C (**10**), as well as three previously described—topsentiasterol sulfate D (**7**), chlorotopsentiasterol sulfate D (**5**) and iodotopsentiasterol sulfate D (**6**) have been isolated from the marine sponge *Halichondria vansoesti*. Structures of these compounds were determined by detailed analysis of 1D- and 2D-NMR and HRESIMS data, as well as chemical transformations. The effects of the compounds on human prostate cancer cells PC-3 and 22Rv1 were investigated.

Keywords: marine sponge; *Halichondria vansoesti*; trisulfated steroids; topsentiasterol sulfates; halistanol sulfates; anticancer activity; PSA expression; glucose uptake

1. Introduction

Biologically active trisulfated steroids are characteristic secondary metabolites found in some marine sponges. These polar steroids comprise several structural subgroups in the sponges. The first compound, bearing a common 2β,3α,6α-trisulfoxy steroid nucleus, halistanol sulfate, was isolated in 1981 from the Okinawan sponge *Halichondria* cf. *moorei* [1] (Figure S1). The subgroup also includes sokotrasterol sulfate from the sponge *Halichondria* sp. [2], halistanol sulfates A-J and polasterol B, found in the sponges *Epipolasis* sp. [3,4], *Pseudoaxinissa digitata* [5], and *Halichondria* sp. [6], ophirapsranol trisulfate from *Topsentia ophiraphidites* [7], four sterols isolated from the sponges *Trachyopsis halichondroides* and *Cymbastela coralliophila* [8], amaranzoles A-F from *Phorbas amaranthus* [9,10], and topsentinol K trisulfate from the sponge *Topsentia* sp. [11]. Another subgroup of these metabolites consists of ibisterol sulfates and lembesterol A from the sponges *Topsentia* sp. [12], *Xestospongia* sp. [13], and *Petrosia strongilata* [14]. In their steroid nuclei, 2β,3α,6α-trisulfoxy functionality is combined with a C-9(11)-double bond and a methyl group at C-14. One more subgroup includes topsentiasterol sulfates A–E from the sponge *Topsentia* sp. [15], Sch 575867 from the deep-water sponge belonging to the family Astroscleridae [16], spheciosterol sulfates from the sponge *Spheciospongia* sp. [17], as well as chloro- and iodotopsentiasterol sulfates D, isolated from the sponge *Topsentia* sp. in our laboratory [18].

These compounds contain a common $\Delta^{9(11)}$-unsaturated, 4β-hydroxy-14α-methyl, 2β,3α,6α-trisulfated steroid nucleus.

In addition to unusual structural features, trisulfated steroids possess promising biological properties [19]. In fact, a broad range of activities has been described to trisulfate steroids such as antibacterial [1,15,20], antifungal [15,16,21], antiviral (including anti-HIV and anti-HSV effects) [5,12,13,22,23], antiparasitic [21], and antiplatelet activities [24]. In addition, the inhibition of different enzymes [6,11,18], promotion of angiogenesis [25], and antitumor activity against various tumor cell lines [7,15,17,26] have been described. Thus, the search for new trisulfated steroids from sponges, including the analyses of their chemical structures and physiological properties, continues to be a promising area of research. Hopefully, this may lead to the development of a new generation of drugs for a broad spectrum of diseases.

In the course of our ongoing interest in new biologically active secondary metabolites of marine invertebrates, *Halichondria vansoesti* sponge, collected in Vietnamese waters during the 49th scientific cruise aboard the R/V 'Academic Oparin', was investigated. As a result, ten trisulfated steroids **1–10** were isolated (Figure 1). Using NMR spectroscopy, including ^{1}H, ^{13}C, HSQC, COSY, HMBC, and NOESY, as well as high-resolution mass spectrometry and chemical transformations, **1–4** and **8–10** were identified as new, unusual analogues of topsentiasterol sulfates and halistanol sulfates. Compounds **5–7** were previously known as chlorotopsentiasterol sulfate D, iodotopsentiasterol sulfates D [18], and topsentiasterol sulfate D, respectively [15]. Herein, we report the isolation, structural elucidation, proposed biosynthetic pathways, and the study of the biological activities of the isolated compounds.

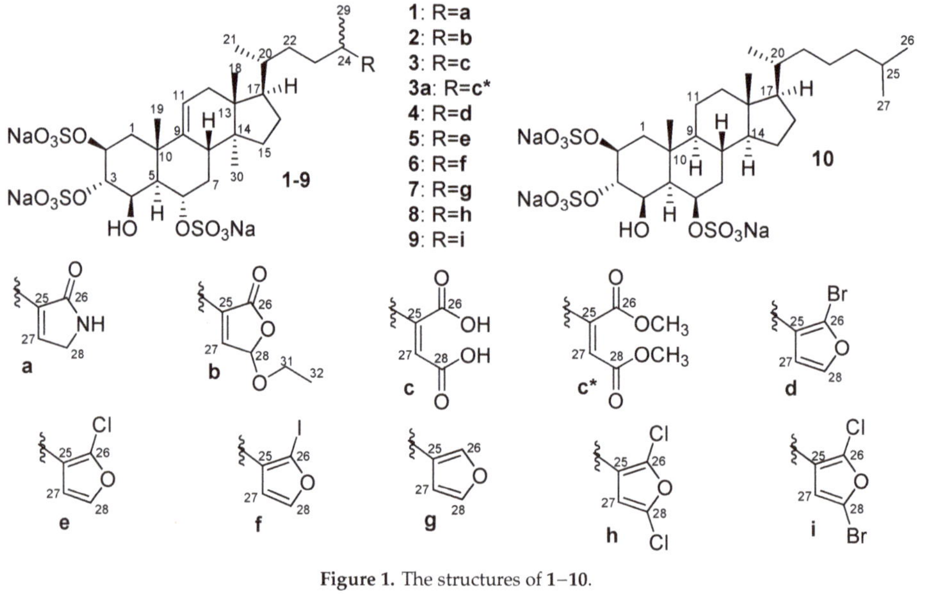

Figure 1. The structures of **1–10**.

2. Results and Discussion

Concentrated EtOH extract of the sponge *Halichondria vansoesti* was partitioned between aqueous EtOH and *n*-hexane. The aqueous EtOH-soluble materials were further applied on a reversed-phase column chromatography (YMC-gel) and eluted successively with H_2O→EtOH:H_2O (3:7)→EtOH:H_2O (2:3)→EtOH:H_2O (1:1)→EtOH:H_2O (3:2) resulting in several subfractions. Subfractions obtained by elution with EtOH:H_2O (3:7) to EtOH:H_2O (6:4) were further purified by a reversed-phase HPLC (YMC-ODS-A) to give **1**, **2** and **4–10**. The subfraction, eluted with H_2O, was further extracted with BuOH, after which the butanol solution was concentrated and subjected to a reversed-phase HPLC (YMC-ODS-A) to obtain 3.

The molecular formula of **1**, $C_{30}H_{44}NNa_3O_{14}S_3$, was established from the $[M_{3Na} - Na]^-$ ion peak at *m/z* 784.1724 in the (−)-HRESIMS. In addition, the peaks at *m/z* 380.5927 and 246.0657, corresponding to doubly-, and triply-charged ions ($[M_{3Na} - 2Na]^{2-}$ and $[M_{3Na} - 3Na]^{3-}$), respectively, were indicated in the (−)-HRESIMS of **1** (Figure S2).

The data of 1D- and 2D-NMR spectra of **1** (Tables 1 and 2, Figures S3–S7) indicated that this compound contained five methyl groups, including three angular methyl groups in the steroid nucleus (δ_H 0.70/δ_C 15.6, δ_H 0.82/δ_C 19.4, δ_H 1.44/δ_C 26.0) and two methyl groups of the side chain (δ_H 0.92/δ_C 19.5, δ_H 1.13/δ_C 20.1), eight methylene groups (including a *N*-substituted methylene), eleven methine groups, including four oxygenated methines (δ_H 4.98/δ_C 76.4, δ_H 4.83/δ_C 76.6, δ_H 4.78/δ_C 77.1, δ_H 4.49/δ_C 69.2), three quaternarysp^3 carbons (δ_C 15.6, δ_C 26.0, δ_C 19.4), two trisubstituted double bonds (δ_H 5.35/δ_C 118.2, 147.1, δ_H 6.85/δ_C 139.4, 144.3), and an amide carbon (δ_C 177.6).

Table 1. ^{1}H NMR data for **1–4**, **8** and **10**.

Position	1 [a] (δ_H, Mult, *J* in Hz)	2 [a] (δ_H, Mult, *J* in Hz)	3 [b] (δ_H, Mult, *J* in Hz)	4 [c] (δ_H, Mult, *J* in Hz)	8 [c] (δ_H, Mult, *J* in Hz)	10 [c] (δ_H, Mult, *J* in Hz)
1a	1.84 dd (3.6, 14.5)	1.84 brd (14.5)	1.87 dd (3.6, 14.6)	1.83 dd (3.7, 14.5)	1.84 brd (14.8)	1.46 dd (3.6, 14.5)
1b	2.39 brd (14.5)	2.41 brd (14.5)	2.37 brd (14.6)	2.40 brd (14.5)	2.38 brd (14.8)	2.29 brd (14.5)
2	4.98 m	4.98 m	4.96 m	4.97 m	4.98 m	4.87 m
3	4.78 m	4.77 m	4.77 m	4.76 m	4.80 m	4.74 m
4	4.49 m	4.49 m	4.48 m	4.49 m	4.48 m	4.45 m
5	1.51 dd (2.5, 11.4)	1.51 dd (2.7, 11.4)	1.52 dd (2.6, 11.4)	1.51 dd (2.9, 11.3)	1.50 dd (2.5, 11.5)	1.48 m
6	4.83 dt (4.5, 11.4)	4.83 dt (4.5, 11.4)	4.83 dt (4.4, 11.4)	4.83 dt (4.4, 11.3)	4.83 dt (4.5, 11.5)	4.60 dt (4.5, 11.3)
7a	1.58 q (11.9)	1.58 q (11.9)	1.57 dt (11.4, 12.9)	1.57 m	1.57 m	1.11 m
7b	2.23 dt (4.6, 11.9)	2.23 dt (4.6, 11.9)	2.22 dt (4.4, 11.8)	2.21 dt (5.0, 12.0)	2.23 dt (4.5, 11.5)	2.32 dt (4.2, 12.1)
8	2.51 m	2.51 m	2.48 m	2.49 m	2.50 m	1.58 m
9						0.71 m
11a	5.35 brd (5.6)	5.35	5.33 brd (5.8)	5.35 dt (2.0, 6.2)	5.35 dt (2.0, 6.2)	1.50 m
11b						1.34 m
12a	2.13 brd (17.6)	2.13 brd (17.3)	2.10 brd (17.1)	2.11 brd (17.5)	2.12 brd (17.5)	1.14 m
12b	1,97 dd (5.5, 17.6)	1.97 dd (5.9, 17.3)	1.95 dd (5.9, 17.1)	1.95 ddd (1.5, 6.1, 17.5)	1.95 dd (6.0, 17.5)	2.01 dt (12.5, 3.4)
14						1.11 m
15a	1.39 m	1.39 m	1.30 m	1.37 m	1.38 m	1.62 m
15b	1.47 m	1.46 m	1.41 m	1.45 m	1.46 m	1.12 m
16a	1.33 m	1.33 m	1.30 m	1.25 m	1.27 m	1.28 m
16b	1.91 m	1.91 m	1.92 m	1.86 m	1.87 m	1.85 m
17	1.66 q (9.4)	1.66 q (9.4)	1.64 q (9.3)	1.63 m	1.63 m	1.13 m
18	0.70 s	0.71 s	0.68 s	0.68 s	0.69 s	0.69 s
19	1.44 s	1.45 s	1.42 s	1.44 s	1.45 s	1.29 s
20	1.42 m	1.43 m	1.38	1.37 m	1.45 s	1.38 m
21	0.92 d (6.5)	0.92 d (6.5)	0.90 d (6.5)	0.90 d (6.5)	0.90 d (6.5)	0.93 d (6.6)
22a	1.09 m	1.09 m	1.08 m	1.04 m	1.05 m	1.01 m
22b	1.49 m	1.43 m	1.40 m	1.45 m	1.46 m	
23a	1.51 m	1.52 m	1.42 m	1.38 m	1.36 m	1.18 m
23b	1.55 m	1.55 m	1.46 m	1.62 m	1.61 m	
24a	2.48 m	2.48 m	2.69 m	2.45 m	2.55 m	1.11 m
24b						1.12 m
25						1.53 m
26						0.87 d (6.6)
27	6.85 br s	6.93 br s	5.92 br s	6.39 d (2.0)	6.31 s	0.87 d (6.6)
28	3.92 br s	5.91 br s		7.48 d (2.0)		
29	1.13 d (6.9)	1.15 d (6.9)	1.10 d (7.0)	1.14 d (7.0)	1.15 d (6.9)	
30	0.82 s	0.82 s	0.82 s	0.81 s	0.81 s	
31a		3.74 m				
31b		3.85 m				
32		1.24 t (7.1)				

[a] Measured in CD_3OD at 500 MHz. [b] Measured in a mixture of $CD_3OD + CDCl_3$ (~10:1) at 700 MHz. [c] Measured in CD_3OD at 700 MHz.

Table 2. ^{13}C NMR Data of **1–4**, **8**, and **10**.

Position	1 [a] (δ_C, Type)	2 [a] (δ_C, Type)	3 [b] (δ_C, Type)	4 [a] (δ_C, Type)	8 [a] (δ_C, Type)	10 [a] (δ_C, Type)
1	37.9, CH_2	37.8, CH_2	37.7, CH_2	37.8, CH_2	38.0, CH_2	39.3, CH_2
2	76.4, CH	76.4, CH	76.3, CH	76.4, CH	76.4, CH	76.3, CH
3	77.1, CH	77.2, CH	76.8, CH	77.1, CH	77.2, CH	77.3, CH
4	69.2, CH	69.2, CH	69.0, CH	69.2, CH	69.2, CH	69.0, CH
5	48.7, CH	48.6, CH	48.3, CH	48.6, CH	48.7, CH	50.8, CH
6	76.6, CH	76.4, CH	76.5, CH	76.6, CH	76.6, CH	76.4, CH
7	36.1, CH_2	36.1, CH_2	35.8, CH_2	36.1, CH_2	36.1, CH_2	40.8, CH_2
8	42.0, CH	42.0, CH	41.7, CH	42.0, CH	42.0, CH	35.9, CH
9	147.1, C	147.2, C	147.1, C	147.1, C	147.2, C	57.1, CH
10	40.1, C	40.2, C	40.1, C	40.2, C	40.1, C	37.6, C
11	118.2, CH	118.2, CH	118.2, CH	118.2, CH	118.2, CH	22.0, CH_2
12	38.9, CH_2	38.9, CH_2	38.7, CH_2	38.9, CH_2	38.9, CH_2	41.7, CH_2
13	46.2, C	46.2, C	46.2, C	46.2, C	46.2, C	44.4, C
14	48.7, C	48.7, C	48.7, C	48.7, C	48.7, C	58.2, CH
15	35.5, CH_2	35.5, CH_2	35.3, CH_2	35.5, CH_2	35.4, CH_2	25.8, CH_2
16	29.5, CH_2	29.5, CH_2	29.3, CH_2	29.4, CH_2	29.5, CH_2	29.8, CH_2
17	52.8, CH	52.8, CH	52.7, CH	52.8, CH	52.8, CH	58.2, CH
18	15.6, CH_3	15.7, CH_3	15.6, CH_3	15.6, CH_3	15.6, CH_3	13.1, CH_3
19	26.0, CH_3	26.0, CH_3	25.8, CH_3	26.0, CH_3	26.0, CH_3	18.0, CH_3
20	37.9, CH	37.8, CH	37.7, CH	38.0, CH	38.0, CH	37.7, CH
21	19.5, CH_3	19.4, CH_3	19.4, CH_3	19.6, CH_3	19.5, CH_3	19.8, CH_3
22	35.3, CH_2	35.2, CH_2	35.4, CH_2	35.8, CH_2	35.7, CH_2	37.9, CH_2
23	33.8, CH_2	33.4, CH_2	34.2, CH_2	35.4, CH_2	35.4, CH_2	25.5, CH_2
24	32.4, CH	32.5, CH	39.7, CH	32.2, CH	32.5, CH	41.3, CH_2
25	144.3, C	144.6, C	157.9, C	133.6, C	129.9, C	29.7, CH
26	177.6, C	173.7, C	171.9, C	126.4, C	132.1, C	23.5, CH_3
27	139.4, CH	144.4, CH	125.9, CH	112.4, CH	109.6, CH	23.8, CH_3
28	48.3, CH_2	104.0, CH	166.8, C	146.0, CH	136.1, C	
29	20.1, CH_3	19.5, CH_3	20.5, CH_3	21.7, CH_3	21.4, CH_3	
30	19.4, CH_3	19.4, CH_3	19.4, CH_3	19.4, CH_3	19.4, CH_3	
31		67.1, CH_2				
32		16.1, CH_3				

[a] Measured in CD_3OD at 175 MHz. [b] Measured in a mixture of CD_3OD + $CDCl_3$ (~10:1) at 175 MHz.

Further analysis of the 1D- and 2D-NMR data of **1**, and the comparison of its NMR data with those in the literature revealed that **1** contains a $\Delta^{9(11)}$-4β-hydroxy-14α-methyl-2β,3α,6α-trisulfated steroid core (Figure 2, substructure I) and the same side chain, containing C-20 (21) to C-24 (29) (Figure 2, substructure III), as that found in the previously described topsentiasterol sulfates A–E [14], Sch 575867 [16], spheciosterol sulfates A–C [17], and chloro- and iodotopsentiasterol sulfates D (**5**,**6**) [18]. The ^1H and ^{13}C NMR spectra of **1** (Tables 1 and 2, Figures S3 and S4) were almost identical to those of topsentiasterol sulfate C [15]. The only exceptions were the signals of the protons linked to C-27 and C-28, which were shifted to lower frequencies (δ_H 6.85/δ_C 139.4, δ_H 3.92/δ_C 48.3) in the spectrum of **1**. Moreover, the HRESIMS (Figure S2) data showed that the molecular mass of **1** was 1 amu less than that of topsentiasterol sulfate C. Based on the above data, and in combination with 2D NMR data (Figures S5–S7), the presence of the 1,5-dihydro-2*H*-pyrrol-2-one portion in the terminal part of the side chain of **1** (Figure 2, substructure III) was proposed. To the best of our knowledge, this is the first report on the 1,5-dihydro-2*H*-pyrrol-2-one moiety found in polysulfated steroids from sponges. Comparison of the NOESY (Figure S8) data of the steroid nucleus of **1** with those of topsentiasterol sulfate C and the related analogs [15–18] suggests that all the stereogenic centers of these compounds have the same relative configurations. Key NOESY correlations of the steroid core of **1** are shown in Figure 3. Thus, **1** is a new analogue of the topsentiasterol sulfate C [15], containing a unique structural element with a nitrogen atom in the side chain. Therefore, it was named topsentiasterol sulfate G.

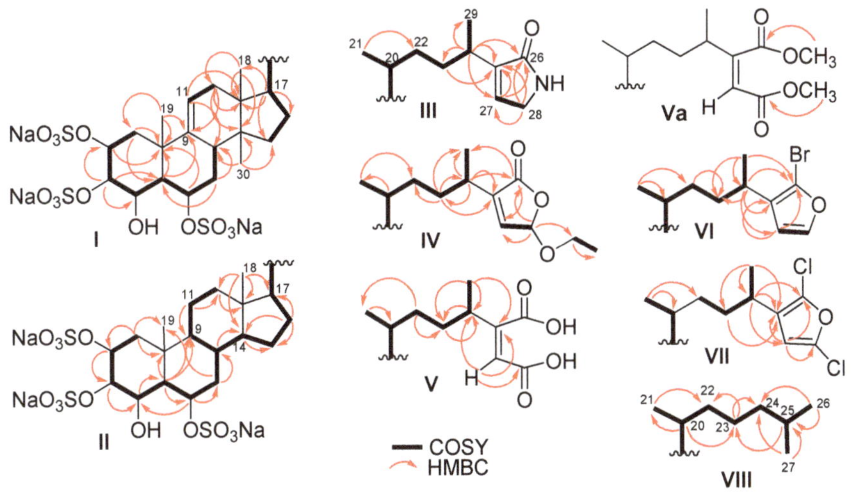

Figure 2. Substructures of **1–4** and **8–10** with the key COSY (bold line) and HMBC (arrow line) correlations.

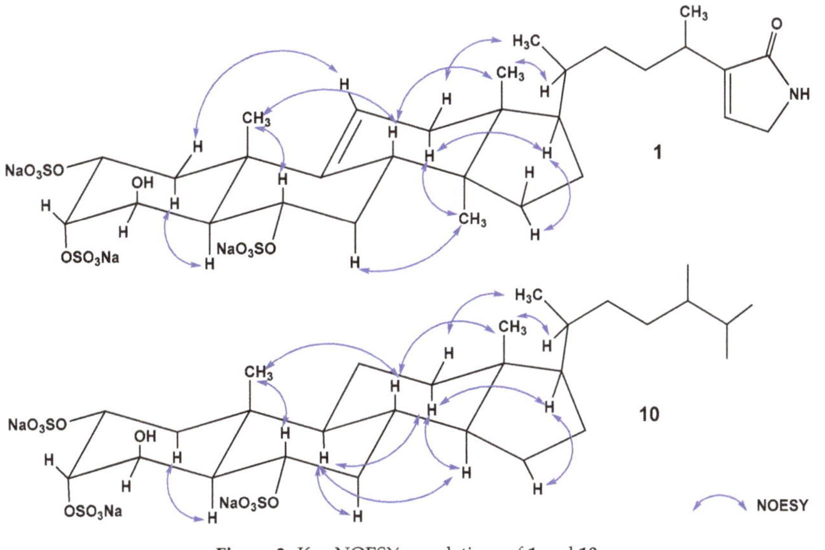

Figure 3. Key NOESY correlations of **1** and **10**.

Detailed studies of the 1D- and 2D-NMR spectra of **1–4**, **8** and **9** (including the determination of the relative configuration of stereogenic centers using NOESY data, Tables 1 and 2, Figure 3) were performed. The generated data were compared to those of the known analogs, such as topsentiasterol sulfates A–E [15], Sch 575867 [16], spheciosterol sulfates A–C [17], chlorotopsentiasterol sulfate D (**5**), and iodotopsentiasterol sulfate D (**6**) [18]. Indeed, signals of the steroid nuclei in these compounds and in the isolated polysulfated steroids were almost identical. Therefore, it was proposed that **1–4**, **8** and **9** have the same $\Delta^{9(11)}$-4β-hydroxy-14α-methyl-2β,3α,6α-trisulfated steroid nucleus, with a variation of the side chain.

The molecular formula of **2**, $C_{32}H_{47}Na_3O_{16}S_3$, was established from the $[M_{3Na} - Na]^-$ ion peak at *m*/*z* 829.1834 in the (−)-HRESIMS. In addition, the peaks at *m*/*z* 403.0980 and 261.0694 in the

(−)-HRESIMS of **2** were observed, corresponding to the doubly- and triply-charged ions ($[M_{3Na} - 2Na]^{2-}$ and $[M_{3Na} - 3Na]^{3-}$, respectively) (Figure S9).

The ^{1}H and ^{13}C NMR data (CD_3OD, Tables 1 and 2, Figures S10 and S11) of the side chain of **2** resemble those of topsentiasterol sulfate A [15], except for the presence of the methyl group at δ_H 1.24 t, J = 7.1/δ_C 16.1 (C-32) and a methylene group at δ_H 3.74, 3.85/δ_C 67.1 (C-31). Further analyses of the 2D-NMR spectral data, including COSY and HMBC spectra (Figures S12 and S14), revealed the following correlations: H-32/H-31, H-31/C-32, H-31/C-28, H-28/C-31 (Figure 2, substructure IV). In addition, HRESIMS spectrum showed that the molecular weight of **2** is 28 amu more than that of topsentiasterol sulfate A [15]. Based on these data, **2** was elucidated as the ethyl ester of topsentiasterol sulfate A [15]. Since **2** has not been previously reported, it was named topsentiasterol sulfate I.

The molecular formula of **3**, $C_{30}H_{43}Na_3O_{17}S_3$, was established from the $[M_{3Na} - H]^-$ ion peak at *m/z* 839.1253 in the (−)-HRESIMS spectrum. In addition, the peaks at *m/z* 408.0685 and 264.3826 in the HRESIMS of **3** corresponding to the doubly- and triply-charged ions ($[M_{3Na}\text{-Na-H}]^{2-}$ and $[M_{3Na}\text{-2Na-H}]^{3-}$, respectively) were observed (Figure S16).

The ^{13}C and ^{1}H NMR of **3** ($CD_3OD+CDCl_3$, ~10:1, Tables 1 and 2, Figures S17 and S18) exhibited the signals of two carboxyl carbon (δ_C 166.8 and 171.9) and a trisubstituted double bond (δ_H 5.92/δ_C 125.9, 157.9). The HMBC spectrum of **3**, recorded in DMSO-d_6 (Figure S21), displayed correlations from H-29 to C-26 and H-27 to C-28. Based on these data and mass spectrometry data, the presence of 2-substituted maleic acid in the side chain of **3** was suggested (Figure 2, substructure V). The *Z*-configuration of the double bond in this fragment was established using NOESY experiment, in which a correlation from H-29 to H-27 was observed (Figure S22).

To confirm the structure of **3**, a methylation with diazomethane was carried out. The structure of the resulting product **3a** was clarified using 2D-NMR and HRESIMS. Cross peaks from OMe-26 to C-26 and OMe-28 to C-28 were observed in the HMBC spectrum (Figure 2, substructure Va). In addition, the peaks of the $[M_{3Na} - Na]^-$and $[M_{3Na} - 2Na]^{2-}$ ions were observed in the (−)-HRESIMS at *m/z* 845.1764 and 411.0943, respectively (Figure S23). These data revealed that a dimethyl maleate was at the terminal of the side chain of the methylated derivative, as in the previously described topsensterol A, a polyhydroxylated steroid from the sponge *Topsentia sp.* [27]. Additionally, the desulfation reaction of **3** with trifluoroacetic acid was carried out. The structure of the obtained product (**11**) was established from the analysis of the HRESIMS data (Figure 4, Figure S24).

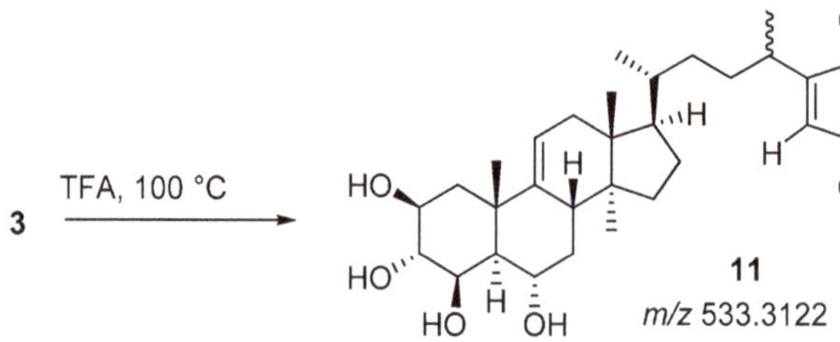

Figure 4. The scheme of the desulfation reaction of **3**.

Thus, **3** is a new analogue of polysulfated steroids from sponges, with a 2-substituted maleic acid in the terminal part of the side chain.

Compound **4** was isolated as an inseparable mixture with the previously reported chlorotopsentiasterol sulfate D (**5**) and iodotopsentiasterol sulfate D (**6**) [18] (2:7:1). Detailed analysis of the HRESIMS (Figure S25), 1D- and 2D-NMR spectra (Tables 1 and 2, Figures S26–S31) of the mixture, as well as the comparison of these data with those for the previously described compounds [15–18], led to the identification of the structure **4**. The molecular formula of **4** was determined as $C_{30}H_{42}BrNa_3O_{14}S_3$ from the (−)-HRESIMS whose peaks of singly-, doubly-, and triply-charged ions were observed (*m/z* 847.0736, $[M_{3Na} - Na]^-$, *m/z* 412.0424, $[M_{3Na} - 2Na]^{2-}$, *m/z* 267.0321, $[M_{3Na} - 3Na]^{3-}$, respectively)

(Figure S25). Measured intensities of the isotope peaks of **4** (412.0424 (100.0%), 412.5440 (36.3%), 413.0415 (122.0%), 413.5429 (41.6%), 414.0391 (61.7%) is in a good agreement with the calculation intensities of the isotope peaks for $[M_{3Na} - 2Na]^{2-}$ (412.0414 (100%), 412.5430 (35.8%), 413.0406 (119.8%), 413.5420 (41.3%), 414.0404 (24.0%)). The ^{1}H NMR spectrum (CD_3OD, Table 1, Figure S26) displayed the higher frequency-shifted three pairs of doublets corresponding to H-27 and H-28 of bromo-, chloro-, and iodo- of 3-substituted furans. Comparison of the chemical shift values of these signals to those of chloro-and iodotopsentiasterol sulfates D from the literature [18] allowed us to assign the proton signals at δ_H 6.39 (H-27) and 7.48 (H-28) to **4** (Table 1). Using the integration of the signals corresponding to H-27 and H-28 in the ^{1}H spectra of the mixture containing **4**, **5**, and **6** showed that the mixture contains about 20% bromotopsentiasterol sulfate D (**4**) and 70% and 10% of chloro- and iodo-derivatives (**5**,**6**) [18], respectively. Additional interpretation of the COSY, HSQC, and HMBC data confirmed that **4** is composed of the substructures I and VI (Figure 2, Figures S28–S30).

New trisulfated steroids, dichlorotopsentiasterol sulfate D (**8**) and bromochlorotopsentiasterol sulfate D (**9**), were isolated as an inseparable mixture. Attempts to separate **8** and **9** using repetitive HPLC failed, however, based on HRESIMS and 1D- and 2D-NMR data, it was estimated as a 9:1 mixture of **8** and **9**. The molecular formulae of the **8** and **9**, $C_{30}H_{41}Cl_2Na_3O_{14}S_3$ and $C_{30}H_{41}ClBrNa_3O_{14}S_3$, were established from the $[M_{3Na} - Na]^-$ ion peaks at *m/z* 837.0837 and 881.0340 of the (−)-HRESIMS spectrum. The predominant peaks at *m/z* 407.0480 and 429.0227 corresponded to a doubly-charged ions $[M_{3Na} - 2Na]^{2-}$, similar to that in the MS of some pentacyclic guanidine alkaloids [28–31], and two-headed sphingolipids [32]. Moreover, triply-charged ions $[M_{3Na} - 3Na]^{3-}$ in the spectra of both compounds were also observed (*m/z* 263.7026 and 278.3516, respectively) (Figure S32). Intensities of the isotope peaks calculated for **8** confirm the proposed molecular formula $C_{30}H_{41}Cl_2Na_3O_{14}S_3$ (measured: 407.0480 (100%), 407.5496 (37.2%), 408.0485 (87.6%), 408.5499 (30.8%), 409.0471 (26.6%); calculated for $[M_{3Na} - 2Na]^{2-}$: 407.0472 (100%), 407.5488 (35.8%), 408.0461 (86.5%), 408.5474 (29.36%), 409.0452 (26.7%)). Intensities of the isotope peaks calculated for **9** confirm the proposed molecular formula $C_{30}H_{41}ClBrNa_3O_{14}S_3$ (measured: 429.0227 (100.0%), 429.5244 (35.3%), 430.0219 (149.4%), 430.5233 (52.0%), 431.0213 (61.9%), 431.5225 (19.7%); calculated for $[M_{3Na} - 2Na]^{2-}$: 429.0220 (100.0%), 429.5235 (35.8%), 430.0210 (151.8%), 430.5224 (52.7%), 431.0201 (62.3%), 431.5213 (19.9%)).

The ^{1}H and ^{13}C NMR spectra of the mixture of **8** and **9** (CD_3OD, Tables 1 and 2, Figures S33 and S34) closely resembled those of chlorotopsentiasterol sulfate D (**5**) [18]. The main differences between the NMR spectra of these compounds were the singlet of H-27 at δ_H 6.31 for **8** and δ_H 6.44 for **9** (integrating these signals, a ratio of **8** to **9** was established as 9:1), instead of two characteristic doublets at δ_H 6.39 and 7.36, corresponding to H-27 and H-28 in the ^{1}H NMR spectrum of monochlorinated compound **5** [18]. Analysis of the COSY, HSQC, and HMBC spectrum confirmed the substructures I and VII (Figure 2, Figures S35–S37) in **8**.

To determine the positions of the halogen atoms in **9**, we have carried out careful analysis of the ^{1}H NMR and COSY spectra of the mixture of **4** and **5** (Table 1, Figures S28 and S37a) and detected two cross-peaks δ_H 2.45 (H-24)/δ_H 1.14 (H-29) corresponding of **4** (26-bromo) and **5** δ_H 2.56 (H-24)/δ_H 1.15 (H-29) (26-chloro) in the COSY spectrum. Therefore, in the case of a bulkier bromine substituent at C-26 the chemical shifts of H-24 and H-29 were observed in a higher field. Taking into attention, that the COSY spectra of **8** + **9** (Table 1, Figures S35 and S37a) showed only one cross-peak δ_H 2.55 (H-24)/δ_H 1.15 (H-29) similar to the cross-peak in the spectrum of **4**, the position of the chlorine atom at C-26 in **9** was established. Based on this data and the HRESIMS data (see above), structure **9** was assigned to the bromochlorotopsentiasterol sulfate D. Nevertheless, the localization of Cl- at C-26 and Br at C-28 in **9** need to be further confirmed.

Compounds **8** and **9** represent the first dihalogenated trisulfated steroids found in sponges.

The molecular formula of **10**, $C_{27}H_{45}Na_3O_{13}S_3$, was established from the $[M_{3Na} - Na]^-$ ion peak at *m/z* 719.1819 in the (−)-HRESIMS. The base peaks at *m/z* 348.0969 corresponded to the doubly-charged ion $[M_{3Na} - 2Na]^{2-}$ (Figure S38).

Detailed analysis of the ^1H and ^{13}C NMR, COSY, HSQC, HMBC, and NOESY spectra of **10** (CD_3OD, Tables 1 and 2, Figure 2, substructures II and VIII, Figures S39–S44) and a comparison of its ^1H and ^{13}C chemical shift values with those reported in the literature for the previously described trisulfated steroids [1–18], indicated that **10** is a previously unreported 4β-hydroxy derivative of halistanol sulfate C [3], which was named 4β-hydroxyhalistanol sulfate C.

Interestingly, unlike all the previously described trisulfated steroids containing 4β-hydroxy group [15–18], **10** does not contain a C-9/C-11-double bond and the α-methyl group at C-14. Thus, **10** is the first member of a new structural subgroup of trisulfated steroids from sponges.

The biosynthesis of unusual side chains of trisulfated steroids, such as **1–9**, could be hypothesized to originate from codisterol (**12**) (Figure S45) [33]. This process could proceed via the C-27 alkylation of **12**, followed by the proton loss and several reactions such as amination or hydratation of double bonds accompanied with cyclization, oxidation, hydrolysis, and halogenation, which would result in the formation of **1–6**, **8**, and **9** (Scheme 1).

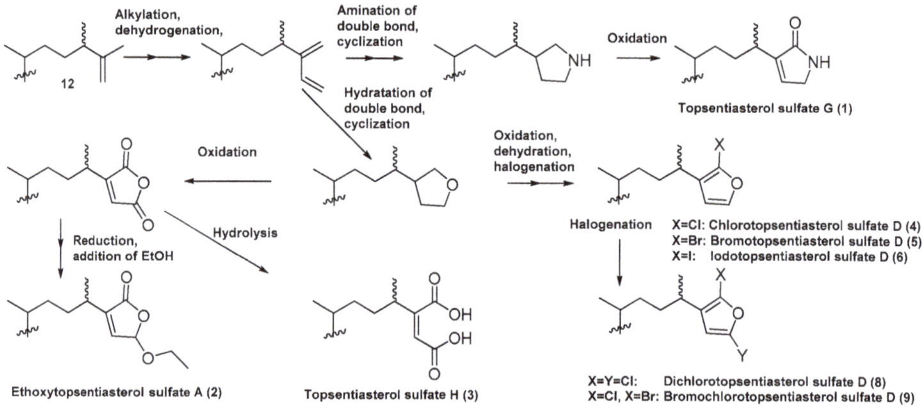

Scheme 1. Proposed biogenesis of the side chains in **1–9**.

The biological activities of **3**, **7**, and **10**, as well as of the mixtures of **4** + **5** + **6** and **8** + **9** were investigated using human prostate cancer cells PC-3 and 22Rv1. PC-3 cells are known to be androgen-independent as they do not express the androgen receptor (AR(-)). 22Rv1 expresses both the androgen receptor (AR(+)), and the androgen receptor splice variant 7 (AR-V7(+)), the expression of AR-V7 mediates the resistant of this cell line to androgen-deprivation therapy [34,35]. PSA is a downstream target gene of the androgen receptor (AR) pathway. Thus, suppression of PSA expression may indicate the inhibition of AR-signaling. AR-signaling is essential for the growth and survival of a significant number of prostate cancer cell types. In fact, downregulation of AR signaling mediated by androgen withdrawal is the standard first-line therapy for advanced human prostate cancer [36]. The isolated compounds and the mixtures were found to inhibit the expression of PSA (prostate-specific antigen) in human drug-resistant 22Rv1 cells (Figure 5A). Compound **3** and the mixture of **4** + **5** + **6**, suppressed PSA expression at a concentration as low as 10 μM (Figure 5A). Note, the IC_{50}s for all the isolated compounds determined with the MTT assay in PC-3 and 22Rv1 cells were >100 μM, which could be due to the androgen-independent nature of these particular prostate cancer cell lines.

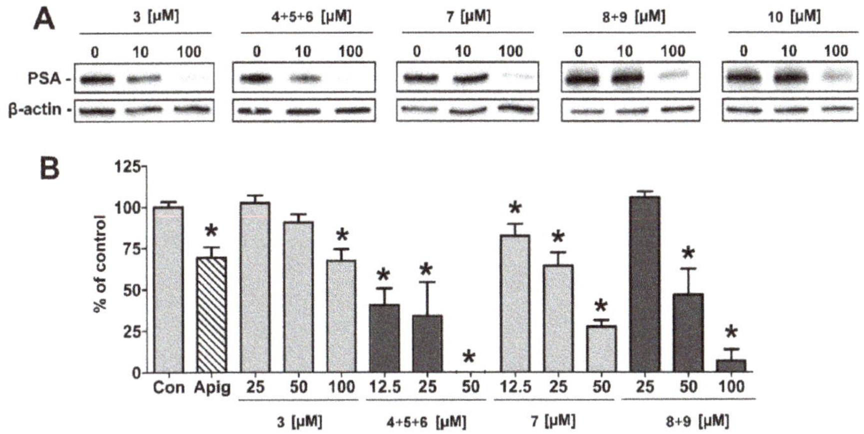

Figure 5. Effects of the compounds on prostate cancer cells. (**A**): Effect on the PSA expression. 22Rv1 cells were treated with the compounds for 24 h, then the proteins were extracted and examined with Western blotting. β-Actin was used as a loading control. (**B**): Effect on glucose uptake. PC-3 cells were seeded in the 96-well plate, treated with the test compounds for 24 h in FBS- and glucose-free media, incubated with 2-NBDG, and then the fluorescence was measured. Apigenin (50 µM) was used as a positive control (Apig). Cells treated with vehicle (DMSO) were used as a control (Con). The glucose uptake was normalized to the cell viability, measured by the MTS test. Significant difference from the control is shown as follows: * $p < 0.05$ (Student's t-test).

Additionally, **3** and **7**, as well as the mixtures of **4** + **5** + **6** and **8** + **9** suppressed glucose uptake in 22Rv1 cells (Figure 5B), whereas **10** did not exhibit this effect (data not shown). Cancer cells are characterized by increased glucose consumption, which is related to their rapid growth and metabolism [37]. Inhibition of glucose uptake either by nutrient deprivation or inhibitors, may suppress cancer cells proliferation and/or sensitize cancer cells to standard therapies. Moreover, recent studies suggested a possible crosstalk between glycolysis and AR-signaling [38]. However, cytotoxic effects and proliferation inhibition were observed only at high concentrations of the isolated compounds (data not shown). Nevertheless, due to the promising activity on AR-receptor signaling and glucose uptake, **3** and **7**, as well as the mixtures of **4** + **5** + **6** and **8** + **9** may serve as starting compounds for a development of novel prostate cancer drugs. To the best of our knowledge, this is the very first report on the ability of marine-derived steroid compounds to suppress the PSA expression/androgen receptor signaling, as well as glucose uptake in cancer cells.

3. Materials and Methods

3.1. General Procedures

Optical rotations were measured using a Perkin-Elmer 343 polarimeter. The ^{1}H- and ^{13}C NMR spectra were recorded on an Avance III-700 spectrometer at 700 and 175 MHz, respectively. Chemical shifts were referenced to the corresponding residual solvent signal (δ_H 3.30/δ_C 49.60 in CD_3OD). The HRESIMS spectra were recorded on a Bruker maXis Impact II mass spectrometer (Bruker, Germany). Low-pressure column liquid chromatography was performed using YMC-GEL ODS-A. HPLC was performed using an Agilent Series 1100 Instrument equipped with a differential refractometer RIDDE14901810 and an YMC-ODS-A (250 × 10 mm) column. Sorbfil Si gel plates (4.5 × 6.0 cm, 5–17 µm, Sorbpolimer, Krasnodar, Russia) were used for thin-layer chromatography. MTT reduction was measured using the F200PRO reader (TECAN, Männedorf, Switzerland).

3.2. *Animal Material*

The sponge *Halichondria vansoesti* (order Suberitida, family Halichondriidae; Figure S46) was collected at a depth of 5–12 m by hand via scuba diving during the 49th scientific cruise on board R/V "Academik Oparin", in the period from 10 November, 2016 to 3 January, 2017, in the South China Sea (the territorial waters of Vietnam, 12°34′02 N; 109°24′26 E). The sponge material was identified by Grebnev B.B. A voucher specimen is kept under the registration number N 049-232 in the marine invertebrate collection of the G. B. Elyakov Pacific Institute of Bioorganic Chemistry (Vladivostok, Russia).

3.3. *Extraction and Isolation*

The sample of the sponge *Halichondria vansoesti* was immediately frozen after collection and kept at −20 °C. The biological materials (dry weight 13.7 g) were chopped into small pieces and extracted with EtOH (200 mL × 3). The combined EtOH solution was concentrated to obtain the crude ethanol extract (7.9 g), which was partitioned between *n*-hexane and aqueous EtOH (9:4). The aqueous ethanol-soluble materials (6.4 g) was concentrated and further fractionated by CC on YMC-GEL (2.5 × 15 cm) and eluted successively with H_2O→EtOH:H_2O (3:7)→EtOH:H_2O (2:3)→EtOH:H_2O (1:1)→EtOH:H_2O (3:2). Each of the subfractions obtained by elution with EtOH:H_2O (3:7) to EtOH:H_2O (3:2) were then concentrated (243 mg, 213 mg, 120 mg, 153 mg, respectively) and subjected to repeated preparative HPLC (YMC-ODS-A, 65:35:1 EtOH/H_2O/1M CH_3COONH_4 to give 1 (3.3 mg), 2 (2.3 mg), 7 (15.0 mg), 10 (13.5 mg) and mixtures of 4 + 5 + 6 (12.8 mg) and of 8 + 9 (11.0 mg). The subfraction eluted with H_2O was further extracted with BuOH, after which the butanol extract was concentrated (691 mg) and subjected to preparative HPLC (YMC-ODS-A, 30:70:1 EtOH/H_2O/1M CH_3COONH_4 to give **3** (4.7 mg).

3.4. *Compound Characterization Data*

Topsentiasterol sulfate G (**1**). Yield 0.024% of the dry weight of the sponge; amorphous powder; $[\alpha]_D^{20}$: + 48 (*c* 0.23, MeOH); ^{1}H- and ^{13}C NMR data, see Tables 1 and 2; HRESIMS *m/z* 784.1724 $[M_{3Na} - Na]^-$, 380.5927 $[M_{3Na} - 2Na]^{2-}$, 246.0657 $[M_{3Na} - 3Na]^{3-}$ (calc. for $C_{30}H_{44}NNa_3O_{14}S_3$ 784.1725, 380.5916, 246.0647, respectively).

Topsentiasterol sulfate I (**2**). Yield 0.017% of the dry weight of the sponge; amorphous powder; $[\alpha]_D^{20}$: + 69 (*c* 0.15, MeOH); ^{1}H- and ^{13}C NMR data, see Tables 1 and 2; HRESIMS *m/z* 829.1834 $[M_{3Na} - Na]^-$, 403.0980 $[M_{3Na} - 2Na]^{2-}$, 261.0694 $[M_{3Na} - 3Na]^{3-}$ (calc. for $C_{32}H_{47}Na_3O_{16}S_3$, 829.1827, 403.0967, 261.0681, respectively).

Topsentiasterol sulfate H (**3**). Yield 0.034% of the dry weight of the sponge; amorphous powder; $[\alpha]_D^{20}$: + 39 (*c* 0.19, EtOH); ^{1}H- and ^{13}C NMR data, see Tables 1 and 2; HRESIMS *m/z* 839.1253 $[M_{3Na} - H]^-$, 408.0685 $[M_{3Na} - Na - H]^{2-}$, 264.3826 $[M_{3Na} - 2Na - H]^{3-}$ (calc. for $C_{30}H_{43}Na_3O_{17}S_3$ 839.1283, 408.0695, 264.3833, respectively).

Bromotopsentiasterol sulfate D, (**4**, in mixture with **5** and **6**). Amorphous powder; ^{1}H- and ^{13}C-NMR data (of **4**), see Tables 1 and 2; HRESIMS *m/z* 847.0736 $[M_{3Na} - Na]^-$, 412.0424 $[M_{3Na} - 2Na]^{2-}$, 267.0321 $[M_{3Na} - 3Na]^{3-}$ (calc. for $C_{30}H_{42}BrNa_3O_{14}S_3$, 847.0721, 412.0414, 267.0312, respectively).

Mixture of the dichlorotopsentiasterol sulfate D and bromochlorotophentiasterol sulfate D (**8** + **9**, 9:1). Amorphous powder; ^{1}H- and ^{13}C-NMR data (for **8**), see Tables 1 and 2; HRESIMS (for **8** and **9**) *m/z* 837.0837 and 881.0340 $[M_{3Na} - Na]^-$, 407.0480 and 429.0227 $[M_{3Na} - 2Na]^{2-}$, 263.7026 and 278.3516 $[M_{3Na} - 3Na]^{3-}$ (calc. for $C_{30}H_{41}Cl_2Na_3O_{14}S_3$ and $C_{30}H_{41}ClBrNa_3O_{14}S_3$, 837.0836 and 881.0331, 407.0472, and 429.0220, 263.7017 and 278.3513, respectively).

4β-hydroxyhalistanol sulfate C (**10**). Yield 0.099% of the dry weight of the sponge; amorphous powder; $[\alpha]_D^{20}$: + 40 (*c* 0.28, MeOH); ^{1}H- and ^{13}C-NMR data, see Tables 1 and 2; HRESIMS *m/z* 719.1819 $[M_{3Na} - Na]^-$, 348.0969 $[M_{3Na} - 2Na]^{2-}$, (calc. for $C_{27}H_{45}Na_3O_{13}S_3$ 719.1823, 348.0965, respectively).

3.5. Methylation of 3

Compound **3** (0.5 mg) was converted to methyl ester **3a** by treatment with an excess (1.5 mL) of a saturated solution of diazomethane in diethyl ether. The obtained derivative **3a** was analyzed using 2D-NMR and HRESIMS (Figure 2, substructure Va, Figure S23).

3.6. Desulfation of 3

Compound **3** (<0.1 mg) was dissolved in 500 μL H_2O and 16 μL of concentrated TFA was added and kept at 100 °C for 4 h. The reaction mixture was concentrated and purified by CC on YMC-GEL (1.5 × 2 cm) and eluted successively with $H_2O \rightarrow EtOH$. The subfraction eluted with EtOH was concentrated to give **11**. The obtained derivative was analyzed using HRESIMS (Figure 4, Figure S24).

3.7. Bioactivity Assay

3.7.1. Reagents

The MTT reagent (Thiazolyl blue tetrazolium bromide) was purchased from Sigma (Taufkirchen, Germany). The MTS reagent (Cell Titer 96 Aqueous One Solution Reagent) was purchased from Promega (Madison, WI, USA).

3.7.2. Cell Lines and Culture Conditions

22Rv1 and PC-3 cell lines (human prostate cancer cell lines) were purchased from ATCC. Cells were cultured in monolayer in 10% FBS/RPMI media according to the manufacture's protocols and were regularly checked for mycoplasma contamination.

3.7.3. In Vitro MTT- and MTS-Based Drug Sensitivity Assay

The in vitro cytotoxic activity of the isolated compounds was evaluated by the MTT assay (performed as described previously [39]). For glucose uptake assay (3.7.5. Glucose uptake assay, see below) the viability was determined using the MTS assay (performed as described previously [40]). Treatment time was 48 h.

3.7.4. Western Blotting

Preparation of the samples and Western blotting were performed as described previously [41]. For the detection of PSA and β-actin expression, the anti-PSA/KLK3 (Cell Signaling, #5365, 1:1000) and anti-β-actin-HRP (Santa Cruz, sc-1616, 1:10,000) antibodies were used. Treatment time was 24 h.

3.7.5. Glucose Uptake Assay

The examination of the effect of the compounds on glucose uptake was carried out using PC-3 cells and the Glucose Uptake Cell-Based Assay Kit (Cayman Chemicals, Ann Arbor, MI, USA) and normalized to the cell viability measured using the MTS test [40]. 12,000 cells per well were seeded in two 96-well plates in 100 μL of media per well, incubated overnight, and treated with the drugs in 100 μL of FBS-free and glucose-free RPMI media per well for 24 h. For glucose uptake measurements, 10 μL of the 2-NBDG solution in FBS-free and glucose-free RPMI media (glucose uptake measurements, final 2-NBDG concentration in the wells was 50 μg/mL) of the vehicle (for cell viability measurements) was added to each well. After 6 h of incubation, the cells were washed twice with PBS (200 μL/well). Next, for the evaluation of glucose uptake, 100 μL of PBS was added to each well. The fluorescence was measured using Infinite F200PRO reader (TECAN, Männedorf, Switzerland). For cell viability measurements, the 100 μL of culture media containing MTS reagent was added to each well, and cell viability was measured using an Infinite F200PRO reader according to the manufacture's protocol.

3.7.6. Statistical Analysis

All assays were repeated at least three times. Results are expressed as the mean ± standard deviation (SD). Student's t-test was used to estimate the significance: * $p < 0.05$.

4. Conclusions

Ten polysulfated steroids **1–10** were isolated from the Vietnamese marine sponge *Halichondria vansoesti*. The structures of seven previously unreported compounds (**1–4** and **8–10**) were established by 1D- and 2D-NMR spectroscopy, HRESIMS, and chemical transformations. Compounds **1–4**, **8**, and **9** are new analogues of topsentiasterol sulfates. The characteristic $\Delta^{9(11)}$-4β-hydroxy-14α-methyl-2β, 3α, 6α-trisulfated steroid nucleus and unusual side chains, not previously described in trisulfated steroids from sponges, were found in the structures of these compounds. Compound **10** is a new analogue of halistanol sulfate, containing a 4β-hydroxy-2β, 3α, 6α-trisulfated steroid nucleus and this is the first report of this structure in sponge polar steroids. We proposed hypothetical pathways for the biosynthesis of the side chains in new topsentiasterol sulfates. Some of the isolated trisulfated steroids were able to suppress PSA expression and glucose uptake in human prostate cancer cells and thus may serve as starting compounds for the development of novel prostate cancer drugs.

Supplementary Materials: The following are available online at http://www.mdpi.com/1660-3397/17/8/445/s1, Figure S1: List of the previously described polysulfated steroids, combined into subgroups in accordance with the structural features of the steroid nucleus, Figures S2–S44: Copies of HRESIMS, 1D- and 2D-NMR spectra of **1–10**, Figure S45: Structure of codisterol (**12**), Figure S46: Photo of the studied sample of sponge *Halichondria vansoesti* (registration number N 049-232).

Author Contributions: K.M.T. isolated the metabolites; T.N.M. and K.M.T. elucidated the structures; S.A.D. performed the PSA expression and glucose uptake assays; V.A.D. performed the NMR spectra; R.S.P. and P.S.D. performed the mass spectra; B.B.G. performed species identification of the sponge; C.B., G.v.A., and N.X.C. assisted the results discussion; K.M.T., T.N.M., and S.A.D. wrote the paper, which was revised and approved by all the authors.

Funding: The isolation: the establishment of chemical structures, and the determination of cytotoxic activity were partially supported by Grant No. 18-53-54002 Viet-a from the RFBR and QTRU01.04/18-19 from VAST. The study of the effects of isolated metabolites on the expression of PSA and glucose uptake in human prostate cancer cells was supported by grant No. 18-74-10028 from RSF (Russian Science Foundation).

Acknowledgments: We thank Academician Valentin A. Stonik, for reading the manuscript and helpful advices.

Conflicts of Interest: The authors declare no conflict of interest.

References

1. Fusetani, N.; Matsunaga, S.; Konosu, S. Bioactive marine metabolites II. Halistanol sulfate, an antimicrobial novel steroid sulfate from the marine sponge *Halichondria* cf. moorei Bergquist. *Tetrahedron Lett.* **1981**, *22*, 1985–1988. [CrossRef]
2. Makarieva, T.N.; Shubina, L.K.; Kalinovsky, A.I.; Stonik, V.A.; Elyakov, G.B. Steroids in porifera. II. Steroid derivatives from two sponges of the family *Halichondriidae*. Sokotrasterol sulfate, a marine steroid with a new pattern of side chain alkylation. *Steroids* **1983**, *42*, 267–281. [CrossRef]
3. Kanazawa, S.; Fusetani, N.; Matsunaga, S. Halistanol sulfates A-E, new steroid sulfates, from a marine sponge, *Epipolasis* sp. *Tetrahedron* **1992**, *48*, 5467–5472. [CrossRef]
4. Umeyama, A.; Adachi, K.; Ito, S.; Arihara, S. New 24-Isopropylcholesterol and 24-Isopropenylcholesterol sulfate from the marine sponge *Epipolasis* Species. *J. Nat. Prod.* **2000**, *63*, 1175–1177. [CrossRef] [PubMed]
5. Bifulco, G.; Bruno, I.; Minale, L.; Riccio, R. Novel HIV-inhibitory halistanol sulfates F-H from a marine sponge, *Pseudoaxinissa digitata*. *J. Nat. Prod.* **1994**, *57*, 164–167. [CrossRef] [PubMed]
6. Nakamura, F.; Kudo, N.; Tomachi, Y.; Nakata, A.; Takemoto, M.; Ito, A.; Tabei, H.; Arai, D.; de Voogd, N.; Yoshida, M.; et al. Halistanol sulfates I and J, new SIRT1–3 inhibitory steroid sulfates from a marine sponge of the genus *Halichondria*. *J. Antibiot.* **2018**, *71*, 273–278. [CrossRef]

7. Gunasekera, S.P.; Sennett, S.H.; Kelly-Borges, M.; Bryant, R.W. Ophirapstanol trisulfate, a new biologically active steroid sulfate from the deep water marine sponge *Topsentia ophiraphidites*. *J. Nat. Prod.* **1994**, *57*, 1751–1754. [CrossRef]
8. Makarieva, T.N.; Stonik, V.A.; Dmitrenok, A.S.; Krasokhin, V.B.; Svetashev, V.I.; Vysotskii, M.V. New polar steroids from the sponges *Trachyopsis halichondroides* and *Cymbastela coralliophila*. *Steroids* **1995**, *60*, 316–320. [CrossRef]
9. Morinaka, B.I.; Masuno, M.N.; Pawlik, J.R.; Molinski, T.F. Amaranzole A, a new *N*-imidazolyl steroid from *Phorbasam aranthus*. *Org. Lett.* **2007**, *9*, 5219–5222. [CrossRef]
10. Morinaka, B.I.; Pawlik, J.R.; Molinski, T.F. Amaranzoles B-F, imidazole-2-carboxy steroids from the marine sponge *Phorbasam aranthus*. C24-N- and C24-O-analogues from a divergent oxidative biosynthesis. *J. Org. Chem.* **2010**, *75*, 2453–2460. [CrossRef]
11. Dai, J.; Sorribas, A.; Yoshida, W.Y.; Kelly, M.; Williams, P.G. Topsentinols, 24-isopropyl steroids from the marine sponge *Topsentia* sp. *J. Nat. Prod.* **2010**, *73*, 1597–1600. [CrossRef] [PubMed]
12. McKee, T.C.; Cardellinaii, J.H.; Tischler, M.; Snader, K.M.; Boyd, M.R. Ibisterol sulfate, a novel HIV-inhibitory sulfated sterol from the deep water sponge *Topsentia* sp. *Tetrahedron Lett.* **1993**, *34*, 389–392. [CrossRef]
13. Lerch, M.L.; Faulkner, D.J. Unusual polyoxygenated sterols from a Philippines sponge *Xestospongia* sp. *Tetrahedron* **2001**, *57*, 4091–4094. [CrossRef]
14. Aoki, S.; Naka, Y.; Itoh, T.; Furukawa, T.; Rachmat, R.; Akiyama, S.; Kobayashi, M. Lembehsterols A and B, novel sulfated sterols inhibiting thymidine phosphorylase, from the marine sponge *Petrosia strongylata*. *Chem. Pharm. Bull.* **2002**, *50*, 827–830. [CrossRef] [PubMed]
15. Fusetani, N.; Takahashi, M.; Matsunaga, S. Topsentiasterol sulfates, antimicrobial sterol sulfates possessing novel side chains, from a marine sponge, *Topsentia* sp. *Tetrahedron* **1994**, *50*, 7765–7770. [CrossRef]
16. Yang, S.W.; Chan, T.M.; Pomponi, S.A.; Chen, G.; Loebenberg, D.; Wright, A.; Patel, M.; Gullo, V.; Pramanik, B.; Chu, M. Structure elucidation of a new antifungal sterol sulfate, Sch 575867, from a deep-water marine sponge (Family: *Astroscleridae*). *J. Antibiot.* **2003**, *56*, 186–189. [CrossRef] [PubMed]
17. Whitson, E.L.; Bugni, T.S.; Chockalingam, P.S.; Concepcion, G.P.; Harper, M.K.; He, M.; Hooper, J.N.A.; Mangalindan, G.C.; Ritacco, F.; Ireland, C.M. Spheciosterol sulfates, PKCζ inhibitors from a Philippine sponge *Spheciospongia* sp. *J. Nat. Prod.* **2008**, *71*, 1213–1217. [CrossRef] [PubMed]
18. Guzii, A.G.; Makarieva, T.N.; Denisenko, V.A.; Dmitrenok, P.S.; Burtseva, Y.V.; Krasokhin, V.B.; Stonik, V.A. Topsentiasterol sulfates with novel iodinated and chlorinated side chains from the marine sponge *Topsentia* sp. *Tetrahedron Lett.* **2008**, *49*, 7191–7193. [CrossRef]
19. Carvalhal, F.; Correia-da-Silva, M.; Sousa, E.; Pinto, M.; Kijjoa, A. Sources and biological activities of marine sulfated steroids. *J. Mol. Endocrinol.* **2018**, *61*, 211–231. [CrossRef]
20. Marinho, P.R.; Simas, N.K.; Kuster, R.M.; Duarte, R.S.; Fracalanzza, S.E.L.; Ferreira, D.F.; Romanos, M.T.V.; Muricy, G.; Giambiagi-DeMarval, M.; Laport, M.S. Antibacterial activity and cytotoxicity analysis of halistanol trisulphate from marine sponge *Petromica citrina*. *J. Antimicrob. Chemother.* **2012**, *67*, 2396–2400. [CrossRef]
21. Kossuga, M.H.; de Lira, S.P.; Nascimento, A.M.; Gambardella, M.T.P.; Berlinck, R.G.S.; Torres, Y.R.; Nascimento, G.G.F.; Pimenta, E.F.; Silva, M.; Thiemann, O.H.; et al. Isolation and biological activities of secondary metabolites from the sponges *Monanchora* aff. *arbuscula*, *Aplysina* sp. *Petromica ciocalyptoides* and *Topsentia ophiraphidies*, from the ascidian *Didemnum ligulum* and from the octocoral *Carijoa riisei*. *Quim. Nova* **2007**, *30*, 1194–1202. [CrossRef]
22. Guimaraes, T.; Quiroz, C.G.; Borges, C.R.; Oliveira, S.Q.; Almeida, M.T.; Bianco, E.M.; Moritz, M.I.; Carraro, J.L.; Palermo, J.A.; Cabrera, G.; et al. Anti HSV-1 activity of halistanol sulfate and halistanol sulfate C isolated from Brazilian marine sponge *Petromica citrina* (Demospongiae). *Mar. Drugs* **2013**, *11*, 4176–4192. [CrossRef]
23. McKee, T.C.; Cardellina, J.H.; Riccio, R.; D'Auria, M.V.; Iorizzi, M.; Minale, L.; Moran, R.A.; Gulakowski, R.J.; McMahon, J.B. HIV-inhibitory natural products. 11. Comparative studies of sulfated sterols from marine invertebrates. *J. Med. Chem.* **1994**, *37*, 793–797. [CrossRef] [PubMed]
24. Yang, S.W.; Buivich, A.; Chan, T.M.; Smith, M.; Lachowicz, J.; Pomponi, S.A.; Wright, A.E.; Mierzwa, R.; Pate, M.; Gullo, V.; et al. A new sterol sulfate, Sch 572423, from a marine sponge, *Topsentia* sp. *Bioorg. Med. Chem. Lett.* **2003**, *13*, 1791–1794. [CrossRef]
25. Murphy, S.; Larrivee, B.; Pollet, I.; Craig, K.S.; Williams, D.E.; Huang, X.H.; Abbott, M.; Wong, F.; Curtis, C.; Conrads, T.P.; et al. Identification of sokotrasterol sulfate as a novel proangiogenic steroid. *Circ. Res.* **2006**, *99*, 257–265. [CrossRef] [PubMed]

26. Slate, D.L.; Lee, R.H.; Rodriguez, J.; Crews, P. The marine natural product, halistanol trisulfate, inhibits pp60v-src protein tyrosine kinase activity. *Biochem. Biophys. Res. Commun.* **1994**, *203*, 260–264. [CrossRef] [PubMed]
27. Chen, M.; Wu, X.D.; Zhao, Q.; Wang, C.Y. Topsensterols A–C, cytotoxic polyhydroxylated sterol derivatives from a marine sponge *Topsentia* sp. *Mar. Drugs* **2016**, *14*, 146. [CrossRef]
28. Makarieva, T.N.; Tabakmaher, K.M.; Guzii, A.G.; Denisenko, V.A.; Dmitrenok, P.S.; Kuzmich, A.S.; Lee, H.S.; Stonik, V.A. Monanchomycalins A and B, unusual guanidine alkaloids from the sponge *Monanchora pulchra*. *Tetrahedron Lett.* **2012**, *53*, 4228–4231. [CrossRef]
29. Tabakmakher, K.M.; Guzii, A.G.; Denisenko, V.A.; Dmitrenok, P.S.; Lee, H.S.; Makarieva, T.N. Monanchomycalin C, a new pentacyclic guanidine alkaloid from the Far-Eastern marine sponge *Monanchora pulchra*. *Nat. Prod. Commun.* **2013**, *8*, 1399–1402. [CrossRef]
30. Tabakmakher, K.M.; Makarieva, T.N.; Denisenko, V.A.; Guzii, A.G.; Dmitrenok, P.S.; Kuzmich, A.S.; Stonik, V.A. Normonanchocidins A, B and D, new pentacyclic guanidine alkaloids from the Far-Eastern marine sponge *Monanchora pulchra*. *Nat. Prod. Commun.* **2015**, *10*, 913–916. [CrossRef]
31. Tabakmakher, K.M.; Makarieva, T.N.; Denisenko, V.A.; Popov, R.S.; Kuzmich, A.S.; Shubina, L.K.; Lee, H.S.; Lee, Y.J.; Fedorov, S.N. Normonanchocidins G and H, new pentacyclic guanidine alkaloids from the Far-Eastern marine sponge *Monanchora pulchra*. *Nat. Prod. Commun.* **2017**, *12*, 1029–1032. [CrossRef]
32. Makarieva, T.N.; Dmitrenok, P.S.; Zakharenko, A.M.; Denisenko, V.A.; Guzii, A.G.; Li, R.; Skepper, C.K.; Molinski, T.F.; Stonik, V.A. Rhizochalins C and D from the sponge *Rhizochalina incrustata*. A rare threo–sphingolipid and a facile method for determination of the carbonyl position in α, ω–bifunctionalized ketosphingolipids. *J. Nat. Prod.* **2007**, *70*, 1991–1998. [CrossRef] [PubMed]
33. Djerassi, C.; Theobald, N.; Kokke, W.C.M.C.; Pak, C.S.; Carlson, R.M.K. Recent progress in the marine sterol field. *Pure Appl. Chem.* **1979**, *51*, 1815–1828. [CrossRef]
34. Dyshlovoy, S.A.; Otte, K.; Tabakmakher, K.M.; Hauschild, J.; Makarieva, T.N.; Shubina, L.K.; Fedorov, S.N.; Bokemeyer, C.; Stonik, V.A.; von Amsberg, G. Synthesis and anticancer activity of the derivatives of marine compound rhizochalin in castration resistant prostate cancer. *Oncotarget* **2018**, *9*, 16962–16973. [CrossRef] [PubMed]
35. Antonarakis, E.S.; Lu, C.; Wang, H.; Luber, B.; Nakazawa, M.; Roeser, J.C.; Chen, Y.; Mohammad, T.A.; Chen, Y.; Fedor, H.L.; et al. AR-V7 and resistance to enzalutamide and abiraterone in prostate cancer. *N. Engl. J. Med.* **2014**, *371*, 1028–1038. [CrossRef] [PubMed]
36. Nelson, P.S. Targeting the androgen receptor in prostate cancer—A resilient foe. *N. Engl. J. Med.* **2014**, *371*, 1067–1069. [CrossRef] [PubMed]
37. Calvaresi, E.S.; Hergenrother, P.J. Glucose conjugation for the specific targeting and treatment of cancer. *Chem. Sci.* **2013**, *4*, 2319–2333. [CrossRef] [PubMed]
38. Mitsuhashi, K.; Senmaru, T.; Fukuda, T.; Yamazaki, M.; Shinomiya, K.; Ueno, M.; Kinoshita, S.; Kitawaki, J.; Katsuyama, M.; Tsujikawa, M.; et al. Testosterone stimulates glucose uptake and GLUT4 translocation through LKB1/AMPK signaling in 3T3-L1 adipocytes. *Endocrine* **2016**, *51*, 174–184. [CrossRef] [PubMed]
39. Dyshlovoy, S.A.; Venz, S.; Hauschild, J.; Tabakmakher, K.M.; Otte, K.; Madanchi, R.; Walther, R.; Guzii, A.G.; Makarieva, T.N.; Shubina, L.K.; et al. Anti-migratory activity of marine alkaloid monanchocidin A-proteomics-based discovery and confirmation. *Proteomics* **2016**, *16*, 1590–1603. [CrossRef]
40. Pelageev, D.N.; Dyshlovoy, S.A.; Pokhilo, N.D.; Denisenko, V.A.; Borisova, K.L.; von Amsberg, G.; Bokemeyer, C.; Fedorov, S.N.; Honecker, F.; Anufriev, V.P. Quinone-carbohydrate nonglucoside conjugates as a new type of cytotoxic agents: Synthesis and determination of in vitro activity. *Eur. J. Med. Chem.* **2014**, *77*, 139–144. [CrossRef]
41. Dyshlovoy, S.A.; Tabakmakher, K.M.; Hauschild, J.; Makarieva, T.N.; Guzii, A.G.; Ogurtsova, E.S.; Otte, K.; Shubina, L.K.; Fedorov, S.N.; Madanchi, R.; et al. Anticancer activity of eight rare guanidine alkaloids isolated from marine sponge *Monanchora pulchra*. *Mar. Drugs* **2016**, *14*, 133. [CrossRef] [PubMed]

marine drugs

MDPI

Article

Oxysterols from a Marine Sponge *Inflatella* sp. and Their Action in 6-Hydroxydopamine-Induced Cell Model of Parkinson's Disease

Sophia A. Kolesnikova [1,*,†], Ekaterina G. Lyakhova [1,†], Anatoly I. Kalinovsky [1], Roman S. Popov [1], Ekaterina A. Yurchenko [1] and Valentin A. Stonik [1,2]

1 G.B. Elyakov Pacific Institute of Bioorganic Chemistry (PIBOC), Prospect 100-let Vladivostoku 159, Vladivostok 690022, Russia; elyakhova@inbox.ru (E.G.L.); kaaniv@piboc.dvo.ru (A.I.K.); prs_90@mail.ru (R.S.P.); dminae@mail.ru (E.A.Y.); office@piboc.dvo.ru or schoolNS@dvfu.ru or stonik@piboc.dvo.ru (V.A.S.)

2 School of Natural Science, Far Eastern Federal University, Sukhanova St., 8, Vladivostok 690000, Russia

* Correspondence: sovin81@inbox.ru; Tel.: +7-423-231-1168

† These authors contributed equally to the work.

Received: 25 October 2018; Accepted: 19 November 2018; Published: 21 November 2018

Abstract: Four new oxysterols **1–4** along with previously known oxygenated sterols **5–14** were isolated from the sponge *Inflatella* sp., collected from the Sea of Okhotsk. Structures of **1–4** were elucidated by the detailed NMR spectroscopic and mass-spectrometric analyses as well as by comparison of the corresponding experimental data with those reported in literature. The influence of compounds **1–14** on the viability of neuronal Neuro2a cells treated by 6-hydroxydopamine and reactive oxygen species (ROS) formation in these cells was investigated.

Keywords: secondary metabolites; oxygenated steroids; marine sponge; *Inflatella*; NMR; ROS; Parkinson's disease; structure-activity relationship

1. Introduction

Oxysterols, formed either enzymatically or by auto-oxidation, have a second oxygen function in addition to that of C-3 when compared with natural sterols. These compounds are of particular interest due to important biological functions of some of them and various bioactivities, including effects on lipid metabolism, platelet aggregation, apoptosis, different receptors and proteins [1]. Generally, oxysterols attract a great attention by the contribution to many physiological processes, including those connected with pathophysiology of the neurodegenerative diseases [2]. As a key trend, the roles of two brain sterols, 24*S*-hydroxycholesterol and 27-hydroxycholesterol, have been studied for years and discussed in multiple reports [3–5]. Among others, 24*S*-hydroxycholesterol has been reported to be markedly reduced in the circulation of patients with Parkinson's disease (PD) [4]. The treatment with 27-hydroxycholesterol or a combination of 24*S*-hydroxycholesterol and 27-hydroxycholesterol reduced the levels of noradrenaline, whereas the treatment with 24*S*-hydroxycholesterol alone had no effect. With these results, the authors demonstrated that oxysterols could regulate the proteins involved in the development of PD [5].

Recently, some other oxysterols were found to be exported from the brain: 7β-hydroxycholesterol, 7-ketocholesterol, 3β,5α-dihydroxycholestan-6-one, 7α-hydroxy-3-oxocholest-4-enoic acid, 7α,25-dihydroxycholest-4-en-3-one, and (25*R*)-7α,26-dihydroxycholest-4-en-3-one. It was underlined that these transfers were observed when total oxysterols were measured [6,7]. These facts give a new quest to disclose possible roles and bioactivities of non-common oxysterols, including those of marine origin, in development of PD and other neurodegenerative diseases.

Recent studies highlighted the point that even well-known oxygenated sterols might be a critical source of new medicine leads. Thus, hecogenin and cholest-4-en-3-one showed significant inhibitory activity (EC_{50} values of 116.3 and 390.6 μM, respectively) against the human β-site amyloid cleaving enzyme (BACE1), which has been considered as an effective drug target for treatment of Alzheimer's disease [8].

The search for new oxysterols in marine organisms and the studies on their action in model cell systems could be also considered as an approach to the creation of new pharmaceutical leads against neurodegenerative diseases. As a part of our chemical investigations of steroidal compounds from marine sponges [9–11], we have studied oxysterols of a cold-water marine sponge *Inflatella* sp. The sponges belonging to the genus *Inflatella* are insufficiently studied for their secondary metabolites, though some bioactivities of their extracts were noted [12]. The ethanol extract of the studied *Inflatella* sp. sample was preliminary analyzed by thin-layer chromatography during the screening of sponge samples from PIBOC collection. The results revealed that in contrast with extracts of other sponges, it contained the oxygenated steroids visually detected on chromatograms as a number of bright colored spots (Figure S1). Herein we describe the isolation and structural elucidation of fourteen individual oxysterols of *Inflatella* sp., including four new compounds as well as the results of their biotesting using a cell model of PD. Part of this work has been presented at the 3rd International Symposium on Life Sciences, Vladivostok, Russia, September 2018.

2. Results and Discussion

The ethanol extract of a sponge *Inflatella* sp., collected in the Sea of Okhotsk, was concentrated and partitioned between distilled water and $CHCl_3$. The obtained organic layer was further separated using a combination of column chromatography and normal- or reverse-phase HPLC to yield compounds **1–14** (Figure 1). To identify the structures of isolated compounds, along with the absolute stereochemistry, their NMR and HRESI MS characteristics were analyzed and compared with previously published data [13–18].

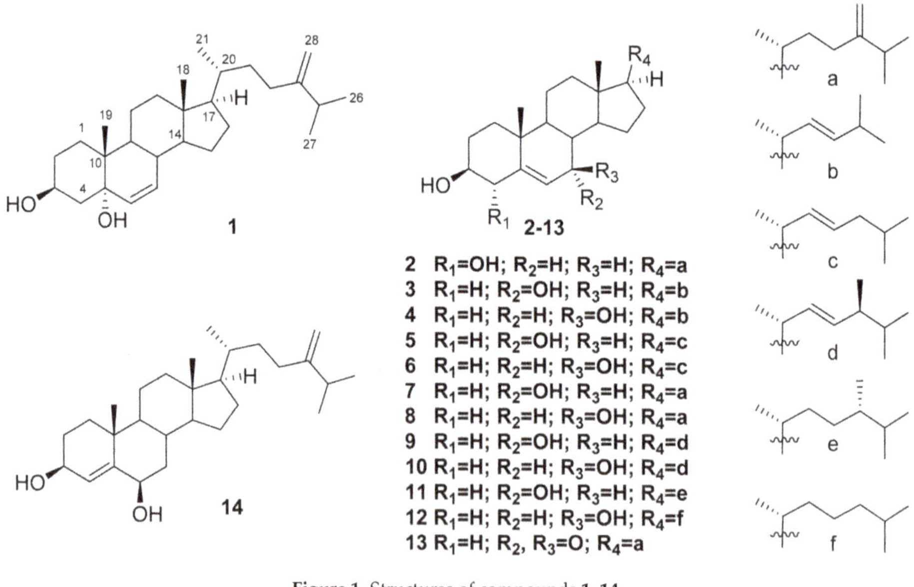

Figure 1. Structures of compounds **1–14**.

Compound **1** was isolated as white amorphous powder with molecular formula $C_{28}H_{46}O_2$, established from (+) HRESI MS (*m/z* 437.3393 $[M + Na]^+$) and ^{13}C NMR spectroscopic data (Figures S2 and S4; Table 1). The ^{1}H and ^{13}C NMR spectra (Tables 1 and 2; Figures S3 and S4) brought out signals characteristics of steroidal derivatives. Namely, the ^{1}H NMR (Table 2) and HSQC (Figure S7) spectra allowed to refer signals of five methyl groups as belonging to Me-18 (δ_H 0.71, s; δ_C 12.4), Me-19 (δ_H 0.92, s; δ_C 14.9), Me-21 (δ_H 0.96, d, *J* = 6.5 Hz; δ_C 18.9), Me-26 (δ_H 1.03, d, *J* = 6.8 Hz; δ_C 22.1), and Me-27 (δ_H 1.02, d, *J* = 6.8 Hz; δ_C 22.2). The chemical shifts at δ_H 4.12, m; δ_C 67.4, (HC-3), at δ_H 5.57, dd, *J* = 9.8, 2.7 Hz; δ_C 133.5, (HC-6) and at δ_H 5.63, dd, *J* = 9.8, 1.6 Hz; δ_C 133.4 (HC-7) along with oxygenated non-protonated carbon signal δ_C 74.2 (C-5), suggested the 3β,5α-6-ene steroidal core [13,14]. It was supported by close similarity of the corresponding ^{13}C NMR signals of **1** and known cholest-6-ene-3β,5α-diol while the epimoric compound with 3β,5β-6-ene core was quite different [13]. As the signals at δ_H 4.66 (s) and 4.72 (s) showed an exo-methylene double bond (δ_C 106.3 and 157.1), the 24(28)-ergostene side-chain was deduced for compound **1**. Therefore, the structure of new compound **1** was established as 24-methylcholesta-6,24(28)-diene-3β,5α-diol.

Table 1. ^{13}C NMR data of Compounds **1–4** (δ in ppm, $CDCl_3$).

No.	**1** [a]	**2** [a]	**3** [b]	**4** [a]
1	28.5	36.7	37.0	37.0
2	30.8	28.1	31.4	31.6
3	67.4	76.6	71.4	71.5
4	41.2	75.2	42.1	41.8
5	74.2	142.1	146.2	143.7
6	133.5	117.8	123.9	125.5
7	133.4	31.6	65.3	73.4
8	38.7	31.5	37.5	40.9
9	45.3	50.5	42.3	48.3
10	38.3	38.1	37.4	36.5
11	21.3	20.9	20.7	21.1
12	40.3	39.8	39.1	39.5
13	44.0	42.3	42.0	42.8
14	54.2	56.8	49.5	56.0
15	24.1	24.3	24.2	26.3
16	28.8	28.2	28.4	28.6
17	56.1	56.0	55.8	55.4
18	12.4	11.9	11.9	12.1
19	14.9	20.2	18.2	19.2
20	36.0	35.8	39.8	39.7
21	18.9	18.7	20.8	20.9
22	34.9	34.7	133.6	133.5
23	31.3	31.0	134.9	135.0
24	157.1	156.9		
25	34.1	33.8	30.9	30.9
26	22.1	21.9	22.7	22.7
27	22.2	22.0	22.7	22.7
28	106.3	106.0		

[a] Spectra recorded at 125.76 MHz; [b] spectra recorded at 176.04 MHz.

Compound **2** has the molecular formula $C_{28}H_{46}O_2$ that was determined by (+) HRESI MS *m/z* 437.3393 $[M + Na]^+$ and ^{13}C NMR (Figures S2 and S9; Table 1). The NMR data of **2** (Tables 1 and 2; Figures S8–S11) also confirmed its steroidal framework. At first, they showed the same type of side-chain in the structure **2** as in **1** by the presence of very close chemical shifts in the spectra of both compounds. The remaining signals were attributed to Me-18 (δ_H 0.69, s; δ_C 11.9), Me-19 (δ_H 1.03, s; δ_C 20.2), 4α-OH (δ_H 4.06, m; δ_C 75.2), and trisubstituted 5(6)-double bond (δ_H 5.74, dt, *J* = 5.5, 2.2 Hz; δ_C 117.8, HC-6 and δ_C 142.2, C-5) of the previously described 4α-hydroxylated tetracyclic system. Really, the both 4α-hydroxy- and 4β-hydroxycholesterols were obtained and well characterized during the investigation of cholesterol autoxidation [15]. As a result of the thorough comparison of 1D and 2D

NMR experimental data of **2** with published values, the structure of this new oxysterol was deduced as 24-methylcholesta-5,24(28)-diene-3β,4α-diol.

Table 2. ^{1}H NMR data of Compounds **1–4** (δ in ppm, *J* in Hz, $CDCl_3$).

No. [a]	1 [b]	2 [c]	3 [c]	4 [b]
1	α: 1.62, m β: 1.37, m	α: 1.14, m β: 1.84, m	α: 1.12, m β: 1.87, m	α: 1.06, m β: 1.85, m
2	α: 1.89, m β: 1.55, m	α: 1.89, m β: 1.60, m	α: 1.86, m β: 1.52, m	α: 1.85, m β: 1.52, m
3	4.12, m	3.27, td (10.5, 4.9)	3.39, m	3.55, m
4	α: 1.80, dd (12.4, 4.9) β: 1.64, m	4.06, m	α: 2.34, ddd (13.2, 4.9, 2.2) β: 2.29, ddt (13.2, 11.3, 1.8)	α: 2.34, ddd (13.2, 5.2, 2.3) β: 2.26, ddt (13.2, 11.3, 2.2)
5				
6	5.57, dd (9.8, 2.7)	5.74, dt (5.5, 2.2)	5.60, dd (5.3, 1.6)	5.29, br t (2.2)
7	5.63, dd (9.8, 1.6)	α: 1.58, m β: 2.10, m	3.85, br s	3.84, dt (8.3, 2.2)
8	1.93, m	1.44, m	1.47, m	1.40, m
9	1.48, dd (11.6, 3.9)	0.99, m	1.23, m	1.03, m
10				
11	α: 1.44, m β: 1.31, m	α: 1.01, m β: 1.48, m	α: 1.54, m β: 1.49, m	α: 1.53, m β: 1.47, m
12	α: 1.23, m β: 2.05, dt (12.5, 3.1)	α: 1.18, td (12.7, 5.2) β: 2.03, dt (12.7, 3.7)	α: 1.19, m β: 1.98, dt (12.6, 3.5)	α: 1.15, m β: 1.99, m
13				
14	1.23, m	1.00, m	1.44, m	1.16, m
15	α: 1.67, m β: 1.22, m	α: 1.61, m β: 1.10, m	α: 1.67, m β: 1.12, m	α: 1.77, m β: 1.40, m
16	α: 1.89, m β: 1.32, m	α: 1.87, m β: 1.29, m	α: 1.73, m β: 1.29, m	α: 1.71, m β: 1.30, m
17	1.17, m	1.14, m	1.20, m	1.12, m
18	0.71, s	0.69, s	0.70, s	0.70, s
19	0.92, s	1.03, s	1.00, s	1.35, s
20	1.43, m	1.42, m	2.01, m	2.00, m
21	0.96, d (6.5)	0.95, d (6.6)	1.01, d (6.7)	1.01, d (6.6)
22	1.16, m 1.55, m	1.16, m 1.55, m	5.18, dd (15.4, 8.4)	5.18, dd (15.4, 8.4)
23	1.88, m 2.10, ddd (15.4, 11.5, 4.8)	1.88, m 2.09, m	5.27, dd (15.3, 6.6)	5.28, dd (15.4, 6.5)
24				
25	2.23, sept (6.8)	2.23, sept (7.0)	2.19, br sept (6.7)	2.19, br sept (6.7)
26	1.03, d (6.8)	1.02, d (7.0)	0.94, d (6.7)	0.95, d (6.7)
27	1.02, d (6.8)	1.03, d (7.0)	0.94, d (6.7)	0.95, d (6.7)
28	4.66, s 4.72, s	4.66, s 4.72, s		

[a] Assignments were made with the aid of the ^{1}H-^{1}H COSY and HSQC spectra; [b] spectra recorded at 500.13 MHz; [c] spectra recorded at 700.13 MHz.

The structure of the compound **3** corresponds to the molecular formula $C_{26}H_{42}O_2$ (HRESI MS *m/z* 409.3081 $[M + Na]^+$) (Figures S2 and S14; Table 1). It has a common Δ^5-3β,7α-diol steroidal core that has been confirmed by the signals of Me-18 (δ_H 0.70, s; δ_C 11.9), Me-19 (δ_H 1.00, s; δ_C 18.2), two methines, connected with hydroxy groups (δ_H 3.59, m; δ_C 71.4, HC-3 and δ_H 3.85, br s; δ_C 65.3, HC-7), and the 5(6)-double bond (δ_H 5.60, dd, *J* = 5.3, 1.6 Hz; δ_C 123.9, HC-6 and δ_C 146.2, C-5) [16]. However, the molecular formula and characteristic signals of the 22*E*-double bond (δ_H 5.18, dd, *J* = 15.3, 6.6 Hz; δ_C 133.6, HC-22 and δ_H 5.27, dd, *J* = 15.3, 6.6 Hz; δ_C 134.9, HC-23), as well as Me-26,27 signals (δ_H 0.94, d, *J* = 6.7 Hz; 6H; δ_C 22.7) showed that this new steroid was characterized by the presence of the 22*E*-unsaturated 24-*nor*-side chain [17] (Tables 1 and 2; Figures S13–S18). Finally, the structure of new oxysterol **3** was determined as (22*E*)-24-*nor*-cholesta-5,22-diene-3β,7α-diol (**3**) that was also in good agreement with ROESY and HMBC data (Figures S16 and S18).

The $C_{26}H_{42}O_2$ molecular formula ((+) HRESI MS *m/z* 409.3081 $[M + Na]^+$) of compound **4** together with similar NMR spectral characteristics (Tables 1 and 2; Figures S2, S19–S24) suggested the presence of a side-chain the same as in compound **3**. The core parts of these compounds also demonstrated a set of close ^{1}H NMR signals except for the chemical shift values, constants, and multiplicity of H-6 (δ_H 5.29, t, J = 2.2 Hz) and H-7 (δ_H 3.85, dt, J = 8.3, 2.2 Hz). Both mentioned signals were similar to those described previously [16,18] and suggested the 7β-OH stereochemistry in **4**. All these data along with confirmation by ROESY and HMBC spectra (Figures S22 and S24) allowed to establish the (22*E*)-24-*nor*-cholesta-5,22-diene-3β,7β-diol (**4**) structure of this new oxysterol.

Additionally, the remaining ten isolated compounds **5–14** were identified as known oxygenated steroidal derivatives by spectroscopic methods and comparison with reported data including NMR spectra [16,18–20]. Most of them were described as naturally occurring metabolites possessing diverse biological activities. Thus, (22*E*)-cholesta-5,22-diene-3β,7α-diol (**5**) was originally isolated from the marine sponge *Cliona copiosa* [16], and demonstrated anti-inflammatory, analgesic and gastroprotective activities as a component of ethanolic fraction of gorgonian *Eunicella singularis* [21]. The (22*E*)-cholesta-5,22-diene-3β,7β-diol (**6**) [16] deterred starfish predators [22]. Selective activity towards DNA repair-deficient yeast mutants and cytotoxicity towards wild-type P-388 murine leukemia cells [23] were showed for 24-methylene-5-cholestene-3β,7α-diol (**7**) [18]. Moreover, the compound **7** was noted as a potential drug development candidate for Alzheimer's disease due to inhibitory potential against butyrylcholinesterase (BuChE) with IC_{50} 9.5 μM [24]. The 24-methylene-5-cholestene-3β,7β-diol (**8**) [18] was completely inactive in the screening for DNA-damaging agents in the RAD 52 yeast assay (while its epimer **7** was active with IC_{50} 7 μg/mL), and showed moderate cytotoxic activity (IC_{50} 31 μM) in the Vero cell assay, indicating that 7β-OH compound acted by a different mechanism in comparison with its α-counterpart [25]. Both compounds **7** and **8** were also noted as constituents of the royal jelly of honeybees [26].

To the best of our knowledge there are not any reported bioassay results in relation to (22*E*,24*S*)-24-methylcholesta-5,22-diene-3β,7α-diol (**9**) [16], (22*E*,24*S*)-24-methylcholesta-5,22-diene-3β,7β-diol (**10**) [16,18], and (22*E*,24*R*)-24-methylcholesta-5,22-diene-3β,7α-diol (**11**) [16,19]. 7β-Hydroxycholesterol (**12**) isolated from the Red Sea grass *Thalassodendron ciliatum* displayed an inhibitory activity against breast carcinoma cell line MCF-7 (IC_{50} 18.6 ± 0.72 μM) and liver carcinoma cell line Hep G2 (IC_{50} 25.4 ± 0.38 μM). However, it did not show the anti-inflammatory action on carrageenan-induced rat hind paw edema model [27]. When human THP-1 macrophages were exposed with an atheroma-relevant mixture of 7β-hydroxycholesterol (**12**) and 7-ketocholesterol followed by proteome analysis, the alterations in macrophage proteome were indicated with a significant differential expression of 19 proteins [28].

3β-Hydroxy-24-methylene-5-cholesten-7-one (**13**) [18] exhibited the potent inhibitory activity on the interleukin-6 production, with 54.0% inhibition at 10 μM and IC_{50} 9.4 ± 1.2 μM [29]. 24-Methylenecholest-4-ene-3β,6β-diol (**14**) [20] demonstrated the cytotoxic activity against the leukemia P-388 cell line with an IC_{50} 1 μg/mL [30].

Encouraged with the short literature review presented above, that shows different attractive bioactivities of oxysterols, we have made an attempt to evaluate the action of the isolated compounds **1–14** on viability of Neuro2a cells and reactive oxygen species (ROS) formation in these cells. In fact, neuroblastoma cells treated by 6-hydroxydopamine (6-OHDA) are used as a cell model of PD [31].

Compounds **4**, **5**, **9** and **12** did not show any notable effects on Neuro2a cell viability. Compounds **1**, **2**, **7**, **8**, **13** and **14** demonstrated slight cytotoxic activity at concentration 100 μM and decreased viability of Neuro2a cells on 25%, 17%, 44%, 27%, 38% and 33%, respectively. It is of interest that all of them have the same structural peculiarity, being the 24 (28)-unsaturated derivatives of ergostane series. No compounds decreasing cell viability more than 50% were found. At concentration of 10 μM, the oxysteroids **1–14** were non-toxic against these neuronal cells, and were used in next experiments at the non-toxic concentrations (Figure S25). Moreover, compounds **3**, **6**, **10** and **11** increased the viability of Neuro 2a cells in comparison with non-treated cells, when MTT cell viability test was used (Figure 2a and Figure S25).

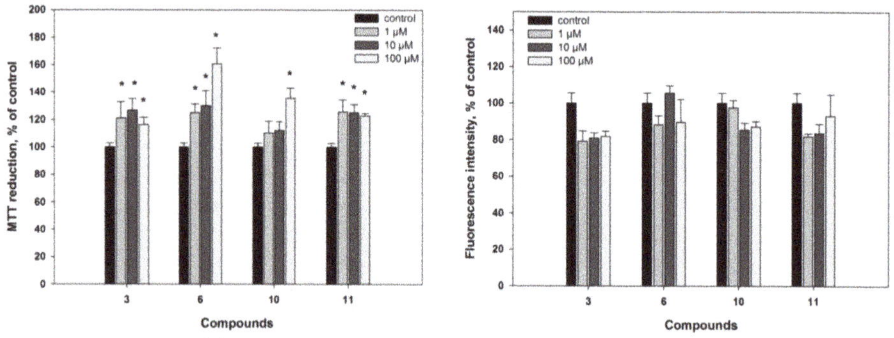

(**a**) (**b**)

Figure 2. Compounds **3**, **6**, **10** and **11**: (**a**) Caused a statistically significant overestimation of MTT reduction in MTT cell viability assay; (**b**) did not statistically significant affect activity of nonspecific esterase in fluorescein diacetate cell viability test. * Statistically significant differences ($p \leq 0.05$) between results for control cells and cells incubated with these compounds.

Applied MTT assay is one of the most widely exploited approaches in research for measuring cell proliferation, viability and drug cytotoxicity. In living cells, the water-soluble yellow dye MTT is reduced to a dark purple (blue-magenta) colored formazan precipitate, which can be analyzed colorimetrically after dissolving in an organic solvent. It was shown, that the MTT reduction site is not only mitochondria. Non-mitochondrial, cytosolic and microsomal MTT reduction makes the major contribution to an overall reduction. Changes in the activity of dozens of the mitochondrial and non-mitochondrial oxidoreductases, cellular metabolic and energy perturbations, and oxidative stress may significantly impact the MTT assay read out [32].

To study action of the tested compounds on cells in details, we additionally used fluorescein diacetate (FDA) assay based on nonspecific esterase activity measuring and thus examined the influence of compounds **3**, **6**, **10** and **11** on proliferation or/and viability of Neuro 2a cells [33]. Compounds **3**, **6**, **10** and **11** did not increase the fluorescence intensity in FDA assay in comparison with control and therefore did not influence significantly on nonspecific esterase activity in Neuro2a cells (Figure 2b). Hence, we could conclude that the observed increasing of MTT reduction was not caused by the influence of tested compounds on cell proliferation.

In fact, the overestimation in MTT assay of the compounds **3**, **6**, **10** and **11** could be caused by alternative metabolic processes. For example, the overestimation reported for rottlerin was explained by dissipation of the inner mitochondrial membrane potential, acceleration of electron transfer and increasing of dehydrogenases activity, oxygen consumption and NADH oxidation [33]. On the other hand the polyphenolic antioxidant resveratrol exhibited increasing of MTT-reducing activity without a corresponding increasing of living cells number [34]. The ability of resveratrol to down-regulate NADPH-oxidase leading to decreased ROS production and thereby provide a protective effect in cardiovascular and neurodegenerative diseases is also well known [35].

As the above reviewed reports described the influence of compounds on intracellular ROS formation, we investigated the effect of compounds **1–14** on ROS formation in Neuro 2a cells by short-time 2′,7′-dichlorodihydrofluorescein diacetate (H2DCF-DA) test. Oxysterols **1–4**, **8**, **10** and **13** at concentrations of 1 or/and 10 μM slightly decreased the ROS level in Neuro2a cells by 12–16%, while the increasing in ROS formation was not detected for all the studied compounds (Figure S26).

PD is the one of the most common age-related motoric neurodegenerative disease, regardless of countries and regions [36]. Pathogenesis of PD includes neuronal death as a result of oxidative stress involved intracellular level of ROS increasing. In this reason, compounds exhibited ROS-scavenger activities could be interesting as neuroprotective agents. All isolated compounds **1–14** were studied in

6-OHDA-induced Neuro2a cell model of PD (Figure S26). Only compounds **3**, **4** and **11** affected on viability of 6-OHDA-treated cells (Figure 3a) and ROS formation in these cells (Figure 3b).

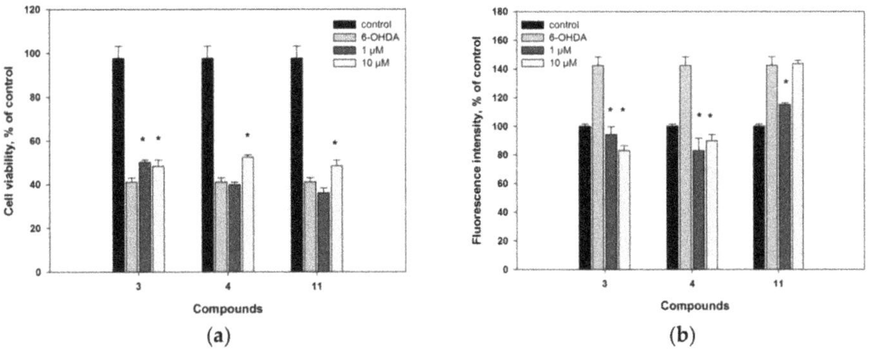

Figure 3. Influence of compounds **3**, **4** and **11** in 6-OHDA-treated Neuro2a cells: (**a**) on cell viability; (**b**) on ROS formation. * Statistically significant differences ($p \leq 0.05$) between results for 6-OHDA-treated cells and cells incubated with compounds.

As a result, compound **3** increased the viability of 6-OHDA-treated cells by 18% (at the dose of 10 μM) and 22% (1 μM), while compounds **4** and **11** increased cell viability by 28% (10 μM) and 18% (10 μM), correspondingly. All these compounds decreased ROS formation in 6-OHDA-treated cells to normal value in similar manner. Thus, compound **4** exhibits the essential neuroprotective activity in 6-OHDA-induced model of Parkinson's disease, probably due to ROS scavenging effect. Oxysterols **3**, **6**, **10** and **11** may positively influence on metabolic processes in the Neuro2a cells because they show the overestimation of survival in MTT assay.

3. Materials and Methods

3.1. General Methods

Optical rotations were measured on a Perkin-Elmer 343 digital polarimeter (Perkin Elmer, Waltham, MA, USA). The ^{1}H and ^{13}C NMR spectra were recorded in $CDCl_3$ using Bruker Avance III 500 (Bruker BioSpin GmbH, Rheinstetten, Germany) (500.13/125.77 MHz) or Avance III 700 Bruker FT-NMR (Bruker BioSpin GmbH, Rheinstetten, Germany) (700.13/176.04 MHz) spectrometers. HRESI and ESI mass spectra were recorded on an Agilent 6510 Q-TOF LC/MS mass spectrometer (Agilent Technologies, Santa Clara, CA, USA), and samples were dissolved in methanol (*c* 0.01 mg/mL). TLC was carried out on silica gel plates (CTX-1A, 5-17 μm, Sorbfil, Russia) and spots were visualized by spraying with aqueous 10% H_2SO_4 followed by heating. Column chromatography (CC) was performed on silica gel (KSK, 50−160 mesh, Sorbfil, Russia) and YMC ODS-A (12 nm, S-75 um, YMC Co., Ishikawa, Japan). HPLC was performed using an Agilent 1100 Series chromatograph with a differential refractometer (Agilent Technologies, Santa Clara, CA, USA). The reversed-phase columns (YMC-Pack ODS-A, YMC Co., Ishikawa, Japan, 10 mm × 250 mm, 5 μm and 4.6 mm × 250 mm, 5 μm) and normal-phase column (Ultrashere-Si, Beckman Instruments, Inc., Berkeley, CA, USA, 10 mm × 250 mm, 5 μm) were used for HPLC. Yields are based on dry weight of the sponge.

3.2. Animal Material

The samples of an *Inflatella* sp. sponge were collected by dredging near Kashevarov Bank, the Sea of Okhotsk (55°30′ N; 146°05′ E, Russia) at a depth of 214–197 m and were freeze dried after collection. The species was identified by Dr. Krasokhin V. B. from G.B. Elyakov Pacific Institute of Bioorganic

Chemistry, FEB RAS. A voucher specimen (PIBOC O07-33(11)) is deposited at the G.B. Elyakov Pacific Institute of Bioorganic Chemistry, FEB RAS (Vladivostok, Russia).

3.3. Extraction and Isolation

The sponge material (dry weight 216 g) was chopped into pieces and extracted with EtOH at room temperature. The ethanol soluble materials (21.0 g) were obtained after concentration of the extract was dissolved in distilled water (300 mL) and partitioned in turn with $CHCl_3$ (200 mL × 3). Evaporation of the chloroform extracts gave dark green gum (12.7 g) that was further separated on a silica gel column (7 cm × 10 cm) using the mixtures of $CHCl_3$/EtOH as stepwise eluent systems to yield the fractions A–F (Figure S1).

Fraction D (301.4 mg), eluted with $CHCl_3$/EtOH (15:1), was separated by column chromatography (CC) (YMC ODS-A, 15 mm × 100 mm, MeOH/H_2O, 90–100%) to yield three subfractions (D1–D3). The subfraction D1 (128.5 mg) was further subjected to silica gel CC (hexane/EtOAc stepwise systems) to obtain three subfractions. The subfraction D1.2 (17.0 mg) was purified by normal-phase HPLC (Ultrasphere-Si, hexane/EtOAc, 1:1, 2 mL/min) to yield compound **13** (6.3 mg, 0.003%). Subfraction D1.3 (6.6 mg) was separated by reverse-phase HPLC (YMC-Pack ODS-A, 10 mm × 250 mm, 95% MeOH, 2 mL/min) to obtain compounds **1** (0.8 mg, 0.0004%), **3** (0.4 mg, 0.003%) and **7** (1.8 mg, 0.012%).

Fraction E (904.4 mg), eluted with $CHCl_3$/EtOH (10:1), was fractionated by silica gel CC (25 mm × 60 mm, hexane/EtOAc, 1:1) to yield four smaller fractions. Fraction E2 (227.4 mg) was subjected to normal-phase HPLC (Ultrasphere-Si, hexane/EtOAc, 1:1, 2 mL/min) resulting in three subfractions. The first subfraction E2.1 (4.0 mg) was purified using reverse-phase HPLC (YMC-Pack ODS-A, 4.6 mm × 250 mm, 90% EtOH, 0.6 mL/min) to afford compound **2** (0.8 mg, 0.0004%) and to re-isolate metabolite **13** (1.1 mg). As a result of the process of E2.2 (22.9 mg) reverse-phase separation (YMC-Pack ODS-A, 10 mm × 250 mm, 2 mL/min) in 95% MeOH, the compounds **4** (1.0 mg, 0.0005%), **6** (2.4 mg, 0.001%), **8** (6.3 mg, 0.003%), **10** (2.0 mg, 0.0009%) and **12** (1.7 mg, 0.0008%) were obtained. The last mentioned HPLC procedures and 94% MeOH as eluent were used for the subfraction E2.3 that allowed us to isolate the individual steroids **5** (6.8 mg, 0.003%), **9** (3.3 mg, 0.002%), **11** (8.0 mg, 0.004%), **14** (1.3 mg, 0.0006%) and to gain new portions of the metabolites **3** (5.8 mg) and **7** (24.3 mg).

3.3.1. 24-Methylcholesta-6,24(28)-diene-3β,5α-diol (**1**)

White amorphous powder; $[\alpha]_D^{22}$ +45.0 (*c* 0.02, $CHCl_3$); ^1H and ^{13}C NMR data ($CDCl_3$), see Tables 1 and 2; EIMS *m/z*: 414 $[M]^+$ (10), 396 $[M - H_2O]^+$(100), 378 (15), 363 (20), 312 (8), 276 (8), 141 (12), 109 (14); (+) HRESI MS *m/z* 437.3393 $[M + Na]^+$ (calcd. for $C_{28}H_{46}O_2Na$, 437.3390).

3.3.2. 24-Methylcholesta-5,24(28)-diene-3β,4α-diol (**2**)

White amorphous powder; $[\alpha]_D^{22}$ +50.0 (*c* 0.08, $CHCl_3$); ^1H and ^{13}C NMR data ($CDCl_3$), see Tables 1 and 2; (+) HRESI MS *m/z* 437.3393 $[M + Na]^+$ (calcd. for $C_{28}H_{46}O_2Na$, 437.3390).

3.3.3. (22*E*)-24-Nor-cholesta-5,22-diene-3β,7α-diol (**3**)

White amorphous powder; $[\alpha]_D^{22}$ −47.5 (*c* 0.04, $CHCl_3$); ^1H and ^{13}C NMR data ($CDCl_3$), see Tables 1 and 2; (+) HRESI MS *m/z* 409.3081 $[M+Na]^+$ (calcd. for $C_{26}H_{42}O_2Na$, 409.3077).

3.3.4. (22*E*)-24-Nor-cholesta-5,22-diene-3β,7β-diol (**4**)

White amorphous powder; $[\alpha]_D^{22}$ −9.0 (*c* 0.10, $CHCl_3$); ^1H and ^{13}C NMR data ($CDCl_3$), see Tables 1 and 2; (+) HRESI MS *m/z* 409.3081 $[M + Na]^+$ (calcd. for $C_{26}H_{42}O_2Na$, 409.3077).

3.4. Biological Activities

3.4.1. Cell Line and Culture Condition

The neuroblastoma cell line Neuro2a was purchased from ATCC. Cells were cultured according to the manufacturer instructions in DMEM medium containing 10% fetal bovine serum (Biolot, Russia) and 1% penicillin/streptomycin (Invitrogen). Cells were incubated at 37 °C in a humidified atmosphere containing 5% (*v*/*v*) CO_2.

3.4.2. MTT Assay

Cell suspension (1×10^3 cells/well) was incubated with different concentration of compounds during 24 h. After that, cell viability was determined by MTT (3-(4,5-dimethylthiazol-2-yl)-2,5-diphenyltetrazolium bromide) method as manufacturer described (Sigma-Aldrich, St. Louis, MO, USA).

3.4.3. Nonspecific Esterase Activity Assay

Cell suspension (1×10^3 cells/well) was incubated with different concentrations of the studied compounds during 24 h. A stock solution of the fluorescein diacetate (FDA) (Sigma-Aldrich, USA) in DMSO (1 mg/mL) was prepared. After incubation of the cells with compounds, FDA solution (50 μg/mL) was added to each well and the plate was incubated at 37 °C for 15 min. Cells were washed with phosphate buffer saline and fluorescence was measured with a Fluoroskan Ascent plate reader (ThermoLabsystems, Finland) at λ_{ex} = 485 nm and λ_{em} = 518 nm. Cell viability was expressed as the percent of control.

3.4.4. 6-OHDA-Induced In Vitro Model of Parkinson's Disease

The neuroprotective activity of the studied compounds in 6-hydroxydopamine-induced cell model of Parkinson's disease was investigated as described previously [37]. Neuroblastoma Neuro2a line cells (1×10^3 cells/well) were treated with compounds at concentrations of 1 and 10 μM during 1 h, after that 6-OHDA (Sigma-Aldrich, USA) at concentration of 50 μM was added in each well and neuroblastoma cells were cultivated during 24 h. After that, viability of cells was measured by MTT assay. The results were presented as percent of control data.

3.4.5. Reactive Oxygen Species (ROS) Level Analysis

Cell suspensions (1×10^3 cells/well) were incubated during 1 h with 1 and 10 μM solutions of the tested compounds. Non-treated and treated with 6-OHDA at concentration of 50 μM (Sigma-Aldrich, USA) cells were used as negative and positive controls, respectively. The portion (20 μL) of 2′,7′-dichlorodihydrofluorescein diacetate (H2DCF-DA) stock solution (Molecular Probes, Eugene, OR, USA) with concentration of 100 mM was added in each well and the microplate was incubated for an additional 10 min at 37 °C. The intensity of dichlorofluorescin fluorescence was measured at λ_{ex} = 485 nm, and λ_{em} = 518 nm with plate reader PHERAstar FS (BMG Labtech, Ortenberg, Germany). The data were processed by MARS Data Analysis v. 3.01R2 (BMG Labtech, Ortenberg, Germany). In other experiments, cells were incubated with compounds during 1 h. Then, 6-OHDA (50 μM) was added in each well for 30 min and ROS levels were measured. All obtained results were presented as percent of negative control data.

4. Conclusions

A sponge *Inflatella* sp. contains a variety of oxysterols differing from each other in positions of additional hydroxy or oxo groups of their tetracyclic core and in structures of side chains. Fourteen oxidized sterols, including four previously unknown compounds, were isolated. Structures of new oxysterols have been established. Previously known compounds were structurally identified by comparison of their NMR and MS spectra with those reported in literature. All of the obtained compounds were studied in the 6-hydroxydopamine-induced cell model of Parkinson's disease. At least, one new oxysterol, (22*E*)-24-*nor*-cholesta-5,22-diene-3β,7β-diol (**4**), showed a substantial activity in this test and might be used for the further studies as a drug candidate.

Supplementary Materials: ^{1}H and ^{13}C spectra of new compounds **1–4** are available online at http://www.mdpi.com/1660-3397/16/11/458/s1, Figure S1: Experimental Section, Figure S2: HRESI MS Spectra (Positive Ion Mode) of compounds **1–4** in $CDCl_3$, Figure S3: ^{1}H NMR (500.13 MHz) spectrum of **1** in $CDCl_3$, Figure S4: ^{13}C NMR (125.76 MHz) spectrum of **1** in $CDCl_3$, Figure S5: COSY NMR (700.13 MHz) spectrum of **1** in $CDCl_3$, Figure S6: ROESY NMR (500.13 MHz) spectrum of **1** in $CDCl_3$, Figure S7: HSQC NMR (700.13 MHz) spectrum of **1** in $CDCl_3$, Figure S8: ^{1}H NMR (700.13 MHz) spectrum of **2** in $CDCl_3$, Figure S9: ^{13}C NMR (125.76 MHz) spectrum of **2** in $CDCl_3$, Figure S10: COSY NMR (700.13 MHz) spectrum of **2** in $CDCl_3$, Figure S11: ROESY NMR (700.13 MHz) spectrum of **2** in $CDCl_3$, Figure S12: HSQC NMR (700.13 MHz) spectrum of **2** in $CDCl_3$, Figure S13: ^{1}H NMR (700.13 MHz) spectrum of **3** in $CDCl_3$, Figure S14: ^{13}C NMR (176.04 MHz) spectrum of **3** in $CDCl_3$, Figure S15: COSY NMR (700.13 MHz) spectrum of **3** in $CDCl_3$, Figure S16: ROESY NMR (700.13 MHz) spectrum of **3** in $CDCl_3$, Figure S17: HSQC NMR (700.13 MHz) spectrum of **3** in $CDCl_3$, Figure S18: HMBC NMR (700.13 MHz) spectrum of **3** in $CDCl_3$, Figure S19: ^{1}H NMR (500.13 MHz) spectrum of **4** in $CDCl_3$, Figure S20: ^{13}C NMR (125.76 MHz) spectrum of **4** in $CDCl_3$, Figure S21: COSY NMR (500.13 MHz) spectrum of **4** in $CDCl_3$, Figure S22: ROESY NMR (500.13 MHz) spectrum of **4** in $CDCl_3$, Figure S23: HSQC NMR (500.13 MHz) spectrum of **4** in $CDCl_3$, S24: HSQC NMR (500.13 MHz) spectrum of **4** in $CDCl_3$, Figure S25: Viability of Neuro2a cells, Figure S26 ROS formation in Neuro2a cells, Figure S27: Viability of Neuro2a cells treated with 6-OHDA.

Author Contributions: Conceptualization, S.A.K., E.G.L.; methodology, S.A.K., E.G.L.; formal analysis, S.A.K., E.G.L.; investigation, S.A.K., E.G.L. and E.A.Y.; data curation S.A.K., E.G.L.; writing—original draft preparation, S.A.K., E.G.L.; writing—review and editing, S.A.K., E.G.L. and V.A.S; visualization, S.A.K., E.G.L.; bioassay, E.A.Y; NMR data providing, A.I.K.; HRESI MS and EIMS spectra providing, R.S.P.; supervision, V.A.S.; project administration, V.A.S.; funding acquisition, V.A.S.

Funding: This work was supported by the Grant No. 17-14-01065 from the RSF (Russian Science Foundation).

Acknowledgments: The study was carried out on the equipment of the Collective Facilities Center, The Far Eastern Center for Structural Molecular Research (NMR/MS) of PIBOC FEB RAS.

Conflicts of Interest: The authors declare no conflict of interest.

References

1. Schroepfer, G.J., Jr. Oxysterols: Modulators of cholesterol metabolism and other processes. *Physiol. Revs.* **2000**, *80*, 361–554. [CrossRef] [PubMed]
2. Doria, M.; Maugest, L.; Moreau, T.; Lizard, G.; Vejux, A. Contribution of cholesterol and oxysterols to the pathophysiology of Parkinson's disease. *Free Radic. Biol. Med.* **2016**, *101*, 393–400. [CrossRef] [PubMed]
3. Griffiths, W.J.; Abdel-Khalik, J.T.; Yutuc, H.E.; Morgan, A.H.; Wang, Y. Current trends in oxysterol research. *Biochem. Soc. Trans.* **2016**, *44*, 652–658. [CrossRef] [PubMed]
4. Lee, C.Y.J.; Seet, R.C.S.; Huang, S.H.; Long, L.H.; Halliwell, B. Different patterns of oxidized lipid products in plasma and urine of dengue fever, stroke, and Parkinson's disease patients: Cautions in the use of biomarkers of oxidative stress. *Antioxyd. Redox Signal.* **2009**, *11*, 407–420. [CrossRef] [PubMed]
5. Marwarha, G.; Rhen, T.; Schommer, T.; Ghribi, O. The oxysterol 27-hydroxycholesterol regulates α-synuclein and tyrosine hydroxylase expression levels in human neuroblastoma cells through modulation of liver X receptors and estrogen receptors–relevance to Parkinson's disease. *J. Neurochem.* **2011**, *119*, 1119–1136. [CrossRef] [PubMed]
6. Iuliano, L.; Crick, P.J.; Zerbinati, C.; Tritapepe, L.; Abdel-Khalik, J.; Poirot, M.; Wang, Y.; Griffiths, W.J. Cholesterol metabolites exported from human brain. *Steroids* **2015**, *99*, 89–93. [CrossRef] [PubMed]
7. Crick, P.J.; Bentley, T.W.; Abdel-Khalik, J.; Matthews, I.; Clayton, P.T.; Morris, A.A.; Bigger, B.W.; Zerbinati, C.; Tritapepe, L.; Iuliano, L.; et al. Quantitative charge-tags for sterol and oxysterol analysis. *Clin. Chem.* **2015**, *61*, 400–411. [CrossRef] [PubMed]
8. Zhu, Y.Z.; Liu, J.W.; Wang, X.; Jeong, I.H.; Ahn, Y.J.; Zhang, C.J. Anti-BACE1 and antimicrobial activities of steroidal compounds isolated from marine *Urechis unicinctus*. *Mar. Drugs* **2018**, *16*, 94. [CrossRef] [PubMed]
9. Kolesnikova, S.A.; Lyakhova, E.G.; Kalinovsky, A.I.; Pushilin, M.A.; Afiyatullov, S.S.; Yurchenko, E.A.; Dyshlovoy, S.A.; Minh, C.V.; Stonik, V.A. Isolation, structures, and biological activities of triterpenoids from a *Penares* sp. marine sponge. *J. Nat. Prod.* **2013**, *76*, 1746–1752. [CrossRef] [PubMed]

10. Lyakhova, E.G.; Kolesnikova, S.A.; Kalinovskii, A.I.; Kim, N.Y.; Krasokhin, V.B.; Stonik, V.A. Secondary metabolites of the marine sponge *Penares cf. schulzei*, fluorescence properties of 24-methylenecholesta-4,6,8(14)-trien-3-one. *Chem. Nat. Comp.* **2015**, *51*, 334–335. [CrossRef]
11. Lyakhova, E.G.; Kolesnikova, S.A.; Kalinovsky, A.I.; Dmitrenok, P.S.; Nam, N.H.; Stonik, V.A. Further study on *Penares* sp. from Vietnamese waters: minor lanostane and *nor*-lanostane triterpenes. *Steroids* **2015**, *96*, 37–43. [CrossRef] [PubMed]
12. Berne, S.; Kalauz, M.; Lapat, M.; Savin, L.; Janussen, D.; Kersken, D.; Avguštin, J.A.; Jokhadar, Š.Z.; Jaklič, D.; Gunde-Cimerman, N.; et al. Screening of the Antarctic marine sponges (Porifera) as a source of bioactive compounds. *Polar Biol.* **2016**, *39*, 947–959. [CrossRef]
13. Holland, H.L.; Jahangir. Reactions of steroidal 4,5- and 5,6- epoxides with strong bases. *Can. J. Chem.* **1983**, *61*, 2165–2170. [CrossRef]
14. Della Greca, M.; Fiorentino, A.; Molinaro, A.; Monaco, P.; Previtera, L. Hydroperoxysterols in *Arum italicum*. *Nat. Prod. Lett.* **1994**, *5*, 7–14. [CrossRef]
15. Zielinski, Z.A.M.; Pratt, D.A. Cholesterol autoxidation revisited: debunking the dogma associated with the most vilified of lipids. *J. Am. Chem. Soc.* **2016**, *138*, 6932–6935. [CrossRef] [PubMed]
16. Notaro, G.; Piccialli, V.; Sica, D. New steroidal hydroxyketones and closely related diols from the marine sponge *Cliona copiosa*. *J. Nat. Prod.* **1992**, *55*, 1588–1594. [CrossRef]
17. Liu, T.F.; Lu, X.; Tang, H.; Zhang, M.M.; Wang, P.; Sun, P.; Liu, Z.Y.; Wang, Z.L.; Li, L.; Rui, Y.C.; et al. 3β,5α,6β-Oxygenated sterols from the South China Sea gorgonian *Muriceopsis flavida* and their tumor cell growth inhibitory activity and apoptosis-inducing function. *Steroids* **2013**, *78*, 108–114. [CrossRef] [PubMed]
18. Findlay, J.A.; Patil, A.D. Novel sterols from the finger sponge *Haliclona oculata*. *Can. J. Chem.* **1985**, *63*, 2406–2410. [CrossRef]
19. Yang, F.; Zhang, H.-J.; Liu, X.-F.; Chen, W.-S.; Tang, H.-F.; Lin, H.-W. Oxygenated steroids from marine bryozoan *Biflustra grandicella*. *Biochem. System. Ecol.* **2009**, *37*, 686–689. [CrossRef]
20. Anjaneyulu, V.; Babu, B.H.; Rao, K.M.C.A.; Rao, K.N. 24-Methylenecholest-4-ene-3β,6β-diol from a soft coral *Sinularia ovispiculata* of the Andaman and Nicobar Islands. *Ind. J. Chem. B* **1994**, *33B*, 806–808.
21. Deghrigue, M.; Festa, C.; Ghribi, L.; D'Auria, M.V.; De Marino, S.; Ben Jannet, H.; Bouraoui, A. Anti-inflammatory and analgesic activities with gastroprotective effect of semi-purified fractions and isolation of pure compounds from Mediterranean gorgonian *Eunicella singularis*. *Asian Pac. J. Trop. Med.* **2015**, *8*, 606–611. [CrossRef] [PubMed]
22. Slattery, M.; Hamann, M.T.; McClintock, J.B.; Perry, T.L.; Puglisi, M.P.; Yoshida, W.Y. Ecological role of water-borne metabolites from Antarctic soft corals. *Mar. Ecol. Prog. Ser.* **1997**, *161*, 133–144. [CrossRef]
23. Gunatilaka, A.A.L.; Samaranayake, G.; Kingston, D.G.I.; Hoffmann, G.; Johnson, R.K. Bioactive ergost-5-ene-3β,7α-diol derivatives from *Pseudobersama mossambicensis*. *J. Nat. Prod.* **1992**, *55*, 1648–1654. [CrossRef] [PubMed]
24. Lu, W.; Zhang, C.; Zheng, K.; Su, J.; Zeng, L. Spectral characteristics and cholinesterase inhibitory activities of some Δ5-3β,7β-dihydroxy sterols and their C-7 epimers. *Tianran Chanwu Yanjiu Yu Kaifa* **2006**, *18*, 893–895.
25. Heltzel, C.E.; Gunatilaka, A.A.L.; Kingston, D.G.I.; Hofmann, G.A.; Johnson, R.K. Synthesis and structure-activity relationships of cytotoxic 7-hydroxy sterols. *J. Nat. Prod.* **1994**, *57*, 620–628. [CrossRef] [PubMed]
26. Kodai, T.; Umebayashi, K.; Nakatani, T.; Ishiyama, K.; Noda, N. Compositions of royal jelly II. Organic acid glycosides and sterols of the royal jelly of honeybees (*Apis mellifera*). *Chem. Pharm. Bull.* **2007**, *55*, 1528–1531. [CrossRef] [PubMed]
27. Abdelhameed, R.F.; Ibrahim, A.K.; Yamada, K.; Ahmed, S.A. Cytotoxic and anti-inflammatory compounds from Red Sea grass *Thalassodendron ciliatum*. *Med. Chem. Res.* **2018**, *27*, 1238–1244. [CrossRef]
28. Ward, L.J.; Ljunggren, S.A.; Karlsson, H.; Li, W.; Yuan, X.M. Exposure to atheroma-relevant 7-oxysterols causes proteomic alterations in cell death, cellular longevity, and lipid metabolism in THP-1 macrophages. *PLoS ONE* **2017**, *12*, e0174475/1–e0174475/17. [CrossRef] [PubMed]
29. Thao, N.P.; Nam, N.H.; Cuong, N.X.; Tai, B.H.; Quang, T.H.; Ngan, N.T.T.; Luyen, B.T.T.; Yang, S.Y.; Choi, C.H.; Kim, S.; et al. Steroidal constituents from the soft coral *Sinularia dissecta* and their inhibitory effects on lipopolysaccharide-stimulated production of pro-inflammatory cytokines in bone marrow-derived dendritic cells. *Bull. Kor. Chem. Soc.* **2013**, *34*, 949–952.

30. Zeng, L.; Li, X.; Su, J.; Fu, X.; Schmitz, F.J. A new cytotoxic dihydroxy sterol from the soft coral *Alcyonium patagonicum*. *J. Nat.Prod.* **1995**, *58*, 296–298. [CrossRef] [PubMed]
31. Pasban-Aliabadi, H.; Esmaeili-Mahani, S.; Abbasnejad, M. Orexin-A protects human neuroblastoma SH-SY5Y cells against 6-hydroxydopamine-induced neurotoxicity: involvement of PKC and PI3K signaling pathways. *Rejuvenation Res.* **2017**, *20*, 125–133. [CrossRef] [PubMed]
32. Stockert, J.C.; Horobin, R.W.; Colombo, L.L.; Blázquez-Castro, A. Tetrazolium salts and formazan products in cell biology: Viability assessment, fluorescence imaging, and labeling perspectives. *Acta Histochem.* **2018**, *120*, 159–167. [CrossRef] [PubMed]
33. Stepanenko, A.A.; Dmitrenko, V.V. Pitfalls of the MTT assay: Direct and off-target effects of inhibitors can result in over/under estimation of cell viability. *Gene* **2015**, *574*, 193–203. [CrossRef] [PubMed]
34. Bernhard, D.; Schwaiger, W.; Crazzolara, R.; Tinhofer, I.; Kofler, R.; Csordas, A. Enhanced MTT-reducing activity under growth inhibition by resveratrol in CEM-C7H2 lymphocytic leukemia cells. *Cancer Lett.* **2003**, *195*, 193–199. [CrossRef]
35. Bitterman, J.L.; Chung, J.H. Metabolic effects of resveratrol: Addressing the controversies. *Cell. Mol. Life Sci.* **2015**, *72*, 1473–1488. [CrossRef] [PubMed]
36. Mhyre, T.R.; Boyd, J.T.; Hamill, R.W.; Maguire-Zeiss, K.A. Parkinson's Disease. *Subcell. Biochem.* **2012**, *65*, 389–455. [PubMed]
37. Pan, Z.; Niu, Y.; Liang, Y.; Zhang, X.; Dong, M. β-Ecdysterone protects SH-SY5Y cells against 6-hydroxydopamine-induced apoptosis via mitochondria-dependent mechanism: Involvement of p38(MAPK)-p53 signaling pathway. *Neurotox. Res.* **2016**, *30*, 453–466. [CrossRef] [PubMed]

marine drugs

Article

Neuroprotective Activity of Some Marine Fungal Metabolites in the 6-Hydroxydopamin- and Paraquat-Induced Parkinson's Disease Models

Ekaterina A. Yurchenko [1,*], Ekaterina S. Menchinskaya [1], Evgeny A. Pislyagin [1], Phan Thi Hoai Trinh [2,3], Elena V. Ivanets [4], Olga F. Smetanina [4] and Anton N. Yurchenko [4]

1 Laboratory of Bioassays and Mechanism of Action of Biologically Active Substances, G.B. Elyakov Pacific Institute of Bioorganic Chemistry Far Eastern Branch of Russian Academy of Sciences, Vladivostok 690022, Russia; ekaterinamenchinskaya@gmail.com (E.S.M.); pislyagin@hotmail.com (E.A.P.)
2 Department of Marine Biotechnology, Nhatrang Institute of Technology Research and Application, Vietnam Academy of Science and Technology, 02 Hung Vuong, Nha Trang 650000, Vietnam; phanhoaitrinh@nitra.vast.vn
3 Graduate University of Science and Technology, Vietnam Academy of Science and Technology, 18 Hoang Quoc Viet, Cau Giay, Ha Noi 100000, Vietnam
4 Laboratory of Chemistry of Microbial Metabolites, G.B. Elyakov Pacific Institute of Bioorganic Chemistry Far Eastern Branch of Russian Academy of Sciences, Vladivostok 690022, Russia; ev.ivanets@yandex.ru (E.V.I.); smetof@rambler.ru (O.F.S.); yurchant@ya.ru (A.N.Y.)
* Correspondence: dminae@mail.ru; Tel.: +7-4232-318832

Received: 26 October 2018; Accepted: 19 November 2018; Published: 21 November 2018

Abstract: A new melatonin analogue 6-hydroxy-*N*-acetyl-β-oxotryptamine (**1**) was isolated from the marine-derived fungus *Penicillium* sp. KMM 4672. It is the second case of melatonin-related compounds isolation from microfilamentous fungi. The neuroprotective activities of this metabolite, as well as 3-methylorsellinic acid (**2**) and 8-methoxy-3,5-dimethylisochroman-6-ol (**3**) from *Penicillium* sp. KMM 4672, candidusin A (**4**) and 4″-dehydroxycandidusin A (**5**) from *Aspergillus* sp. KMM 4676, and diketopiperazine mactanamide (**6**) from *Aspergillus flocculosus*, were investigated in the 6-hydroxydopamine (6-OHDA)- and paraquat (PQ)-induced Parkinson's disease (PD) cell models. All of them protected Neuro2a cells against the damaging influence of 6-OHDA to varying degrees. This effect may be realized via a reactive oxygen species (ROS) scavenging pathway. The new melatonin analogue more effectively protected Neuro2A cells against the 6-OHDA-induced neuronal death, in comparison with melatonin, as well as against the PQ-induced neurotoxicity. Dehydroxylation at C-3″ and C-4″ significantly increased free radical scavenging and neuroprotective activity of candidusin-related *p*-terphenyl polyketides in both the 6-OHDA- and PQ-induced PD models.

Keywords: neuroprotective activity; Parkinson's disease; ROS; DPPH-scavenging activity; 6-OHDA; paraquat; marine fungal metabolites

1. Introduction

Currently, Parkinson's disease is one of the most common age-related motoric neurodegenerative diseases, regardless of countries and regions. This disease is characterized clinically by resting tremor, bradykinesia, rigidity, and postural instability, that significantly worsen the life quality of patients [1]. Pathogenesis of PD includes neuronal death as a result of oxidative stress involving the increase in the intracellular level of reactive oxygen species (ROS) and reactive nitrogen species. The hyperproduction of ROS may cause several forms of cell damage, such as increasing DNA damage, lipid, and protein peroxidation which can promote mitochondrial injury. In addition, some of the studies show that ROS can cause mitochondrial dysfunction and activation of apoptosis-related death signaling, which lead to neuronal cell death. These findings show the requirement of using antioxidants as a therapeutic intervention in PD in addition to other protective agents [2]. To estimate the antioxidative properties of neuroprotective agents, both cell-free and cell assays may be used. One of the most popular cell-free tests in natural product antioxidant studies is the 2,2-diphenyl-1-picrylhydrazyl (DPPH) free radical scavenging assay [3]. A widely used cell test is ROS level determination using 2′,7′-dichlorofluorescin diacetate, that is deesterified intracellularly, and turns into the highly fluorescent 2′,7′-dichlorofluorescein upon oxidation [4].

PD etiology may be linked to several factors, including genetic susceptibility and environmental elements. Regarding environmental factors, several dopaminergic neurotoxins, including 6-hydroxydopamine (6-OHDA) and 1-methyl-4-phenyl-1,2,3,6-tetrahydropyridine (MPTP), have been identified. Moreover, some pesticides/herbicides, such as rotenone, paraquat (PQ), maneb (MB), and mancozeb (MZ), cause neurotoxicity, and induce a PD-like pathology. As a result, 6-OHDA and MPTP are common models used in PD research, and pesticide-based approaches have become secondary models of study [5,6].

It is known that marine fungi produce polyketides with antioxidant and neuroprotective properties [7–9]. For example, gentisyl derivatives aspergentisyls A and B, and auroglaucin-related compounds from the marine-derived *Aspergillus glaucus* exhibited a strong radical-scavenging activity in DPPH test, with an IC_{50} of 7.6–24.2 μM [7]. Terrestrol G, a dimeric derivative of gentisyl alcohol from the marine sediment-derived fungus *Penicillium terrestre*, exhibited DPPH-scavenging properties with an IC_{50} of 4.1 μM [10].

Diketopiperazines are widespread marine fungal products with different biological activities, including free radical scavenging and neuroprotection [11,12]. Gliotoxin from *Pseudallescheria* sp., neoechinulin E, and cryptoechinulin D, exhibited DPPH scavenger activity with IC_{50} values of 5.2, 46.0, and 23.6 μM, respectively [13,14]. Neoechinulin A from *Eurotium rubrum* protected PC12 cells from the cytotoxic influence of MPTP neurotoxin [15].

Some other metabolites of marine fungi also show a neuroprotective effect in the in vitro and in vivo models of Parkinson's disease [16]. Xyloketal B, from *Xylaria* sp., scavenged free radicals in DPPH assay, and protected PC12 cells against ischemia-induced cell injury and MPTP-induced neurotoxicity [17]. About 40 synthetic derivatives of xyloketal B were investigated in various in vivo Parkinson's models, and some of them showed significant activities [18]. Secalonic acid A from *Aspergillus ochraceus* and *Paecilomyces* sp. protected against MPTP-induced dopaminergic neuronal cell death in mouse PD model, in nigral neurons, and SH-SY5Y cells [19].

In this paper, we described the isolation and identification of new alkaloid and known polyketides from the marine fungus *Penicillium* sp. KMM 4672, known diketopiperazine alkaloid from *Aspergillus flocculosus*, polyketides reported earlier from *Aspergillus* sp. KMM 4676, as well as free radical scavenging and neuroprotective activities of these compounds in two cell models of Parkinson's disease induced by 6-hydroxydopamine and paraquat.

2. Results and Discussion

2.1. Isolation and Identification of Compounds

Recently, we have found new natural compounds whose structures have not been established, possibly due to their insufficient content, along with several new and known compounds from a marine algicolous fungus *Penicillium* sp. KMM 4672 [20,21]. A repeated cultivation of this fungus, in the same conditions, was carried out to obtain a sufficient amount of unidentified compounds. As a result, these compounds were identified as new melatonin derivative (**1**), known *o*-orsellinic acid (**2**) and isochromene (**3**) derivatives (Figure 1).

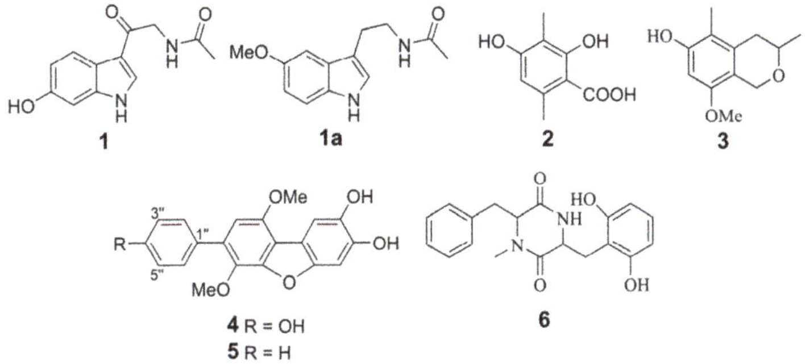

Figure 1. The structures of investigated compounds.

6-Hydroxy-*N*-acetyl-β-oxotryptamine (**1**) was isolated as a white solid. An (–)HRESIMS spectrum (Figure S8) of compound **1** contains a $[M-H]^-$ pseudomolecular peak at *m*/*z* 231.0772, which indicated a molecular formula of $C_{12}H_{12}N_2O_3$ (calcd for $C_{12}H_{11}N_2O_3$,231.0775), which corresponded to six double-bond equivalents. A careful inspection of NMR data of **1** (Table 1 and Figures S1–S7) revealed the presence of one acetyl methyl, one methylene, four sp^2-methines, four quaternary sp^2-carbons, one keto-group, and one amide carbonyl. In addition, the ^1H NMR spectrum contains the signal of three heteroatom protons. The coupling constant values of NH-1 (δ_H 11.55, d, J = 2.9 Hz), H-2 (δ_H 8.17, d, J = 2.9 Hz), H-4 (δ_H 7.89, d, J = 8.6 Hz), H-5 (δ_H 6.68, dd, J = 8.6, 1.7 Hz), and H-7 (δ_H 6.80, d, J = 1.7 Hz), together with the HMBC correlations from NH-1 to C-3a (δ_C 118.3), from H-2 to C-3a and C-7a (δ_C 137.6), from H-4 to C-3 (δ_C 114.1), C-6 (δ_C 154.0) and C-7a, from H-5 to C-3a and C-7 (δ_C 97.1), from H-7 to C-3a and C-5, and from 6-OH (δ_H 9.14) to C-5, C-6, and C-7, established the indole moiety with OH group at C-6. This suggestion was additionally proved by ROESY correlation H-1/H-7. The HMBCs from methylene H-2′ (δ_H 4.38) to C-1′ (δ_C 189.9) and C-4′ (δ_C 169.3), from H-3′ (δ_H 8.06) to C-4′, and from H-5′ (δ_H 1.90) to C-4′ showed the side chain structure. The location of the side chain at C-3 was revealed by the ROESYs of H-2′ with H-2 and H-4. Thus, the structure of **1** was elucidated to be very close to that of known *N*-acetyl-β-oxotryptamine [22]. Similar melatonin-like compounds are usually isolated from several bacterial species [23,24]. Recently, *N*-acetyl-β-oxotryptamine was reported from the medicinal basidiomycete *Inonotus vaninii* [25], and from ascomycete *Scopulariopsis* sp. [26]. To our knowledge, this study is the second case of isolation of related compounds from microfilamentous fungi.

Table 1. ^1H and ^{13}C NMR data (700/176 MHz, δ in ppm, DMSO-d_6) for 6-hydroxy-*N*-acetyl-β-oxotryptamine (**1**).

Position	δ_C, mult	δ_H (J in Hz)
1(NH)		11.55, d (2.9)
2	131.9, CH	8.17, d (2.9)
3	114.1, C	
3a	118.3, C	
4	121.5, CH	7.89, d 8.6)
5	111.9, CH	6.68, dd (8.6, 1.7)
6	154.0, C	
7	97.1, CH	6.80, d (1.7)
7a	137.6, C	
1′	189.9, C	
2′	45.4, CH_2	4.38, d (5.6)
3′(NH)		8.06, d (5.6)
4′	169.3, C	
5′	22.4, CH_3	1.90, s
6-OH		9.14, s

Together with melatonin-related **1**, the well-known fungal polyketides 3-methylorsellinic acid (**2**) and 8-methoxy-3,5-dimethylisochroman-6-ol(**3**) were isolated from this fungus. Their structures were identified by comparing the NMR and MS data (Figures S9–S13) with previously reported data [27,28].

The chemical composition of extract of an ascidian-derived fungus *Aspergillus* sp. KMM 4676 was reported earlier [29,30]. *p*-Terphenyl polyketides, candidusin A (**4**) and 4″-dehydroxycandidusin A (**5**), were major metabolites of this fungus.

The 2,5-diketopiperazine alkaloid mactanamide (**6**) was isolated from the Vietnamese sediment-derived fungus *Aspergillus flocculosus*. The NMR data (Figures S14 and S15) for this compound were identical with earlier published data [31]. It is only the third case of isolation this compound.

2.2. Biological Activities of the Studied Compounds

2.2.1. 6-Hydroxy-*N*-acetyl-β-oxotryptamine (**1**)

6-Hydroxy-*N*-acetyl-β-oxotryptamine (**1**) was not cytotoxic against neuroblastoma Neuro2a cell up to 100 μM. This compound scavenged DPPH radicals by 48% at 100 μM (Table 2).

Table 2. Radical scavenging and cytotoxicity activities of compounds **1–6**.

Compounds	DPPH Radical Scavenging		Cytotoxicity
	% at 100 μM	EC_{50}, μM	IC_{50}, μM
1	51.9 ± 1.3	-	>100
2	88.9 ± 2.9	-	>100
3	62.0 ± 4.6 [16]	-	>100
4	67.8 ± 1.1	-	75.7 ± 5.6
5	50.6 ± 1.3	101.3 ± 2.8	78.9 ± 1.9
6	83.5 ± 0.2	-	>100

Melatonin-like compound **1** showed a statistically significant reduction of reactive oxygen species (ROS) level on 18% in the neuronal 6-OHDA-treated cells in the in vitro experiment (Figure 2). Melatonin (**1a**), a well-known antioxidant and neuroprotective compound, was used to compare with **1**. It decreased ROS formation in the 6-OHDA-treated neuronal cell stronger in comparison with **1**.

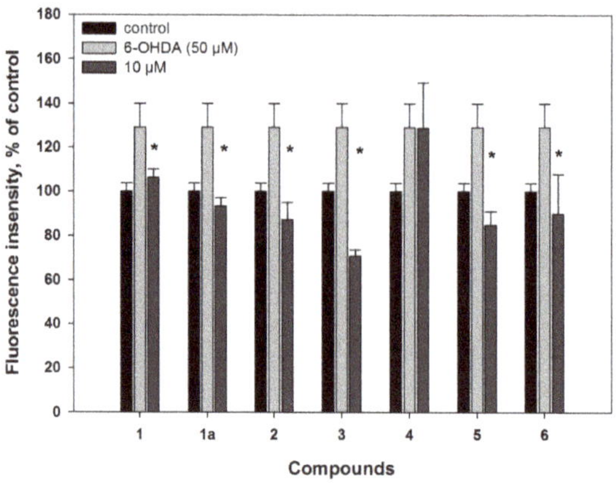

Figure 2. Influence of compounds **1–6** on reactive oxygen species (ROS) formation in Neuro2a cells treated with 6-hydroxydopamine (6-OHDA) for 30 min. * Difference between data for compounds and for 6-OHDA was statistically significant with $p \leq 0.05$.

The neuroprotective effect of **1** was shown both in the Neuro2a cells treated 1 h before, as well as 1 h after, adding of 6-OHDA by 23% and 28%, respectively, at a concentration of only 10 μM. Melatonin (**1a**) did not increase the viability of cells treated with neurotoxin in this experiment (Figure 3a). Our experiments showed that 6-hydroxy-*N*-acetyl-β-oxotryptamine (**1**) more effectively protected Neuro2a cells against 6-OHDA-induced neuronal death, in comparison with melatonin (**1a**).

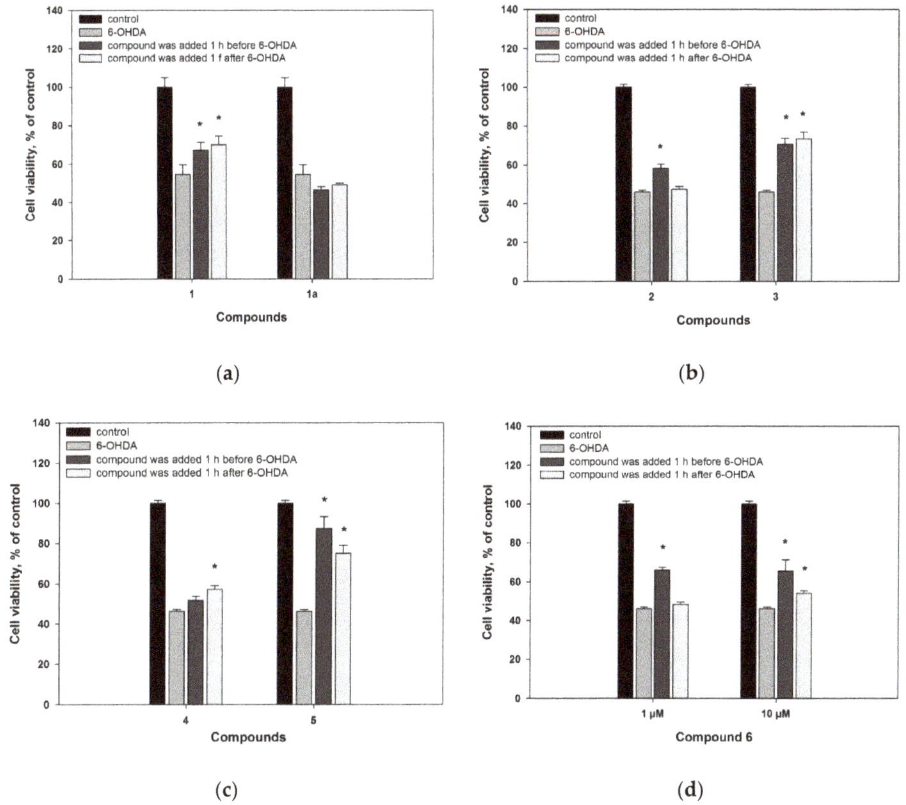

Figure 3. Neuroprotective effects of compounds **1–6** on Neuro2a cells treated with 6-OHDA (50 μM). All compounds were added to the cell suspension 1 h before treatment with 6-OHDA or 1 h after treatment with 6-OHDA. (**a**) Viability of the 6-OHDA-treated cells incubated with compounds **1** and **1a** at 10 μM; (**b**) Viability of 6-OHDA-treated cells incubated with compounds **2** and **3** at 10 μM; (**c**) Viability of 6-OHDA-treated cells incubated with compounds **4** and **5** at 10 μM; (**d**) Viability of the 6-OHDA-treated cells incubated with compound **6** (1 and 10 μM) * Difference between data for compounds and for 6-OHDA was statistically significant with $p \leq 0.05$.

In the PQ-induced PD model, compounds **1** and **1a** (at concentration of 10 μM) were more effective in comparison with their influence in the 6-OHDA-induced model, and decreased ROS formation in the PQ-treated cells by 35% and 22%, respectively (Figure 4). As a result, increase of the PQ-treated cell viability, by 40% and 24%, was observed (Figure 5).

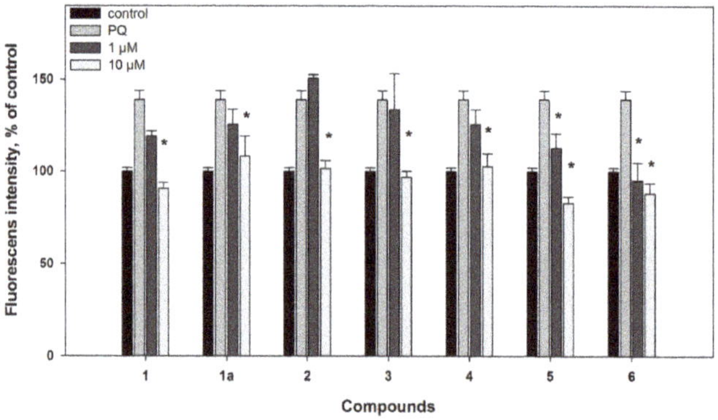

Figure 4. Effects of compounds **1–6** on ROS formation in Neuro2a cells treated with paraquat (PQ) (500 μM) for 1 h. All compounds were added to the cell suspension 1 h before treatment with PQ. * Difference between data for compounds and for PQ was statistically significant with $p \leq 0.05$.

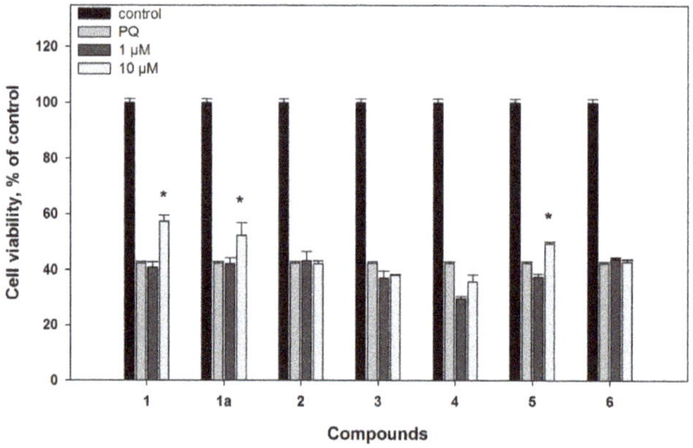

Figure 5. Neuroprotective effects of compounds **1–6** on Neuro2a cells treated with PQ (500 μM). All compounds were added to the cell suspension 1 h before treatment with PQ. * Difference between data for compounds and for PQ was statistically significant with $p \leq 0.05$.

2.2.2. 3-*O*-Methylorsellinic acid (**2**) and 8-methoxy-3,5-dimethylisochroman-6-ol (**3**)

3-*O*-Methylorsellinic acid (**2**) and 8-methoxy-3,5-dimethylisochroman-6-ol (**3**) were not cytotoxic against neuroblastoma Neuro2a cells up to 100 μM.

3-*O*-Methylorsellinic acid (**2**) at 100 μM scavenged 10% DPPH radicals in our experiments (Table 2). For orsellinic acid and its derivatives, 2,20-azinobis(3-ethylbenzothiozoline-6-sulfonate cation (ABTS·+) scavenger activities were recently reported [32]. 8-Methoxy-3,5-dimethylisochroman-6-ol (**3**) in DPPH assay was not very effective; also, at 100 μM concentration, it reduced the free radical value by 35%, as we reported earlier [33]. Nevertheless, in the 6-OHDA-treated Neuro2a cells, compounds **2** and **3** at a concentration of 10 μM significantly decreased ROS formation by 30% and 45% respectively (Figure 2).

3-*O*-Methylorsellinic acid (**2**) statistically significantly increased 6-OHDA-treated cell viability by 26%, when the compound was added to cells 1 h before adding 6-OHDA. When compound **2** was added to cells 1 h after adding 6-OHDA, it had no neuroprotective effect.

8-Methoxy-3,5-dimethylisochroman-6-ol (**3**) statistically significantly increased the neuroblastoma cell viability in the 6-OHDA-induced PD model by about 55%, regardless of when it was added to cells (Figure 3b). Compounds **2** and **3** were effective at a concentration of only 10 μM.

On the other hand, compounds **2** and **3** did not exhibit any protective effect on based on the viability of cells treated with PQ, despite the fact that they reduced ROS formation in these cells (Figures 4 and 5).

2.2.3. Candidusin A (**4**) and 4″-dehydroxycandidusin A (**5**)

Candidusin A (**4**) scavenged 32% of radicals in DPPH assay at a concentration 100 μM. 4″-Dehydroxycandidusine A (**5**) was more effective and scavenged 49% of radicals (Table 2). Candidusin B (C-3″ hydroxylated analogue of candidusin A) showed 59% DPPH radical scavenging at a concentration of 100 μg/mL [34], i.e., at a molar concentration of the compound that was more than 2.7 times higher.

Earlier, candidusin A (**4**) showed cytotoxic activities against HL-60 (IC_{50} 77.56 μM), A-549 (IC_{50} 19.34 μM), and P-388 (IC_{50} 46.83μM) tumor cells [35], while 4-dehydroxycandidusin A (**5**) exhibited cytotoxic activities against KB (IC_{50} 22.66 μM) and A 549 (IC_{50} 34.01 μM) tumor cells [36]. In our experiments, candidusin A (**4**) and 4″-dehydroxycandidusin A (**5**) had low cytotoxicity against neuroblastoma Neuro2a cells with an IC_{50} of 75.7 and 78.9 μM, respectively (Table 2). These compounds were used at a non-toxic concentration of 10 μM for the treatment of cells in PD models.

Candidusin A (**4**) did not have any effect on ROS formation in the 6-OHDA-treated cells (Figure 2). 4″-Dehydroxycandidusin A (**5**) decreased the ROS level in 6-OHDA-treated cells by 34%, being more effective as a radical scavenger. Candidusin A (**4**) had no effect on the viability of cells when it was added 1 h before treatment with 6-OHDA, and increased 6-OHDA-treated cell viability by 24% at a concentration of only 10 μM, when it was added 1 h after 6-OHDA (Figure 3c). 4″-Dehydroxycandidusin A (**5**) increased cell viability by more than 80% (when the compound was added 1 h before 6-OHDA) and 62% (when it was added 1 h after 6-OHDA). These effects were observed at a concentration of 10 μM only. When the concentration of compound **5** was reduced tenfold, its neuroprotective effect was not preserved.

In the PQ-induced model, compound **4** decreased ROS formation by 27% at a concentration of 10 μM. Compound **5** was more effective and statistically significantly decreased ROS formation by 19% and 40%, at concentrations of 1 and 10 μM, respectively (Figure 4). Nevertheless, compound **4** did not have any effect on the viability of the PQ-treated cells, but its 4″-dehydroxylated derivative (**5**) statistically significantly increased the viability of these cells by 17% at concentration of 10 μM only (Figure 5).

Thus, the presence of hydroxy groups at C-3″ and C-4″ in candidusins decreases the radical scavenging activity of these compounds in the cell-free assay. Moreover, the hydroxylation at C-4″ results in the significant decreasing their neuroprotective effect.

2.2.4. Mactanamide (**6**)

Mactanamide (**6**) was not cytotoxic against neuroblastoma Neuro2a cells up to 100 μM.

Compound **6** scavenged 15% DPPH radicals in cell-free assays at a concentration of 100 μM (Table 2). In cell experiments, this compound (**6**) demonstrated a significant antiradical effect: at 10 μM, it inhibited ROS formation in the 6-OHDA-treated neuronal cells by 30% (Figure 2).

Mactanamide (**6**) increased the 6-OHDA-treated cell viability by 42% at 10 μM in the 6-OHDA-induced PD model when the compound was added 1 h before neurotoxin. When its concentration was reduced tenfold, its neuroprotective effect was preserved (Figure 3d).

In the PQ-treated cells, mactanamide (**6**) decreased ROS formation by 32% and 37%, at concentrations of 1 and 10 μM, respectively (Figure 4). However, compound **6** did not show any neuroprotective activity on the viability of the PQ-treated cells (Figure 5).

Earlier, mactanamide showed fungistatic activity against *Candida albicans*, and an influence on osteoclast differentiation without any cytotoxicity [31,37]. Antioxidant and neuroprotective properties of mactanamide were demonstrated, for the first time, in this investigation.

Thus, compounds **1**, **2**, **3**, and **6** were non-cytotoxic for Neuro2a cells up to a concentration of 100 μM. Compounds **4** and **5** demonstrated low cytotoxicity with an IC_{50} of 75.7 and 78.9 μM, respectively. This allowed investigating the neuroprotective activity of all compounds in non-toxic concentrations of 1 and 10 μM. Neuroprotective effects of the compounds were studied in two PD in vitro models using 6-OHDA and PQ as inducers of neuronal cell damage.

Melatonin-like compound **1** demonstrated an effect in increasing cell viability in both models, but the effect on PQ-treated cells was more pronounced. In both cases, neuroprotective effects were accompanied with a decrease of ROS formation in the 6-OHDA- and PQ-treated cells. Melatonin (**1a**) decreased ROS formation in both PD models, but it increased cell viability in the PQ-induced model only.

Polyketides **2** and **3** demonstrated ROS-decreasing effects in both PD models. Nevertheless, these compounds increased cell viability in the 6-OHDA-induced model only.

Candidusin A (**4**) and 4″-dehydrocandidusin A (**5**) have minimal differences between their chemical structures but this has a significant effect on their neuroprotective activity. In the 6-OHDA and PQ models, compound **5** produced a significant increase of cell viability, whereas compound **4** did not demonstrate any effect in the PQ model, and low increased cell viability on the 6-OHDA-treated cells. A similar influence of both compounds on ROS formation in the 6-OHDA- and PQ-treated cells was observed. Compound **4** had no significant effect on ROS formation in the 6-OHDA-treated cells, and decreased ROS formation in the PQ-treated cells, at a concentration of only 10 μM. By contrast, compound **5** was very effective in the 6-OHDA-induced PD model, and decreased ROS formation in the PQ-treated cells at concentrations 1 and 10 μM.

Mactanamide (**6**) demonstrated a significant decrease of ROS formation in both the 6-OHDA- and PQ-induced PD models. However, this 2,5-diketopiperasine alkaloid increased viability of the 6-OHDA-treated cells only, and did not have any statistically significant effects on viability of the PQ-treated cells.

It should be noted that DPPH radical scavenging activity was shown for all compounds in varying degrees, and decreasing of ROS formation in 6-OHDA- and PQ-treated cells could be the result of radical scavenging by these compounds. However, differences between the effects of these compounds, on ROS formation and cell viability in different PD models, were observed.

In our investigation, two PD-like cell models, induced by neurotoxin 6-OHDA and pesticide paraquat, were used. Neurotoxins and pesticides share a common mechanism to induce damage to dopaminergic neurons that is correlated with an increased oxidative status caused by high levels of ROS, anions, and free radicals [6]. However, the effect of each of the inducers, on neurons, has the same differences.

6-OHDA has a specific neurotoxic effect on neurons containing dopamine, serotonin, and norepinephrine receptors. The structure of 6-OHDA is similar to dopamine and norepinephrine, and, therefore, this neurotoxin uses the same catecholaminergic transport system (the dopamine and norepinephrine transporters), and causes specific degeneration of dopaminergic and noradrenergic neurons [6]. Inside neurons, 6-OHDA is rapidly autooxidized to hydrogen peroxide and paraquinone, which are both highly toxic to mitochondria, by specifically affecting complex I. This process results in an increase of ROS generation and cell death [38]. Moreover, it was reported that 6-OHDA induces oxidative stress both during its autoxidation to *p*-quinone and, also, during one-electron reduction of *p*-quinone to *p*-semiquinone, catalyzed by flavoenzymes that transfer one electron [39]. In addition to these effects, 6-OHDA-induced cell death is dependent of such intracellular processes as neuroinflammation, mitochondria dysfunction, endoplasmic reticulum stress, and autophagy [40].

Paraquat causes oxidative stress in neuronal cells by another pathway. Divalent paraquat ion (PQ2+) is reduced to monovalent paraquat ion (PQ+) by NADPH-oxidase of mitochondrial complex I. Subsequently, PQ+ accumulates in dopaminergic neurons and reestablishes a new redox reaction intracellularly, leading to the generation of intracellular free radicals, such as superoxide and dopamine-reactive substances. This will eventually lead to dopaminergic neuron cell death [41].

Moreover, PQ toxicity correlates with DNA fragmentation, caspase-3 cascade modulation, and dysregulation of autophagy [5,42].

Metabolic investigations of the molecular mechanisms associated with 6-OHDA and PQ toxicity were carried out by NMR spectroscopy and mass spectrometry. It was shown that PQ selectively upregulated the pentose phosphate pathway (PPP) to increase NADPH reducing equivalents, and stimulate paraquat redox cycling, oxidative stress, and cell death. PQ also stimulated an increasing in glucose uptake, the translocation of glucose transporters to the plasma membrane, and adenosine monophosphate-activated protein kinase activation. In the contract, 6-OHDA did not demonstrate an influence on PPP. In addition, while paraquat induced a reduction in glucose-dependent glutamate-derived glutathione synthesis, 6-OHDA treatment increased this process [43,44].

In this study, we observed time differences between 6-OHDA and PQ effects on ROS formation in Neuro2a cells (Figure S16). 6-OHDA caused an increase of ROS level of 30% for 30 min after addition to the cell suspension. The effect of PQ on ROS formation was insignificant after 30 min, and an increase of ROS levels in cells, by 39%, was observed 1 h after adding of PQ to the cell suspension.

Compounds **2**, **3**, and **6** demonstrated neuroprotective effects in the 6-OHDA-induced PD model only. For this reason, they could protect Neuro2a cells against the damaging influence of products of 6-OHDA autooxidation, due to their antioxidant properties. Compound **5** increased the viability of 6-OHDA-treated cells by 80%, but it increased viability of PQ-treated cells by 17% only. This suggests the same mechanism of action.

On the other hand, compounds **1** and **1a** were more effective in the PQ-induced model, and increased cell viability by 40% and 24%, respectively, whereas in the 6-OHDA-induced model, compound **1** increased cell viability by 23% only, and melatonin (**1a**) was ineffective.

It was earlier published that melatonin and some related compounds demonstrated antioxidant activity in cell-free assays [45], and different neuroprotective effects in the in vitro experiments [46–48]. Pre-treating of PC12 cells with melatonin for 3 h increased viability of the cells, and prevented apoptosis in the 6-OHDA-induced PD model [49,50]. In addition, it was reported that melatonin diminished caspase-3 enzyme activity, cleavage of DNA fragmentation factor 45, and DNA fragmentation observed in the MPTP-treated neuroblastoma cells [46]. For this reason, melatonin-related compound **1** could influence on viability of the PQ-treated cells in a similar manner.

3. Materials and Methods

3.1. General Experimental Procedures

NMR spectra were recorded in DMSO-d_6 and acetone-d_6 on a Bruker DPX-500 and DRX-700 (Bruker BioSpin GmbH, Rheinstetten, Germany) spectrometers, using TMS as an internal standard. HRESIMS spectra were measured on a Maxis impact mass spectrometer (Bruker Daltonics GmbH, Rheinstetten, Germany).

Low-pressure liquid column chromatography was performed using silica gel (50/100 μm, Imid Ltd., Krasnodar, Russia). Plates (4.5 cm × 6.0 cm) precoated with silica gel (5–17 μm, Imid Ltd., Krasnodar, Russia) were used for thin-layer chromatography. Preparative HPLC was carried out on a Shimadzu LC-20 chromatograph (Shimadzu USA Manufacturing, Canby, OR, USA) with a Shimadzu RID-20A refractometer (Shimadzu Corporation, Kyoto, Japan) using a YMC ODS-AM (YMC Co., Ishikawa, Japan) (5 μm, 10 mm × 250 mm) and YMC SIL (YMC Co., Ishikawa, Japan) (5 μm, 10 mm × 250 mm) columns.

Melatonin (**1a**) was purchased from «JSC «PE «Obolenskoe» (Obolensk, Russia).

3.2. Fungal Strain

The strain *Penicillium* sp. KMM 4672 was isolated from brown alga *Padina* sp. (Van Phong Bay, South China Sea, Vietnam) on malt extract agar, and identified on the basis of morphological and molecular features, as described earlier [20].

The strain *Aspergillus* sp. KMM 4676 was isolated from an unidentified colonial ascidian (Shikotan Island, Pacific Ocean) on malt extract agar, and identified on the basis of morphological and molecular features as described earlier [30].

The strain *Aspergillus flocculosus* was isolated from a sediment sample (Nha Trang Bay, South China Sea, Vietnam) by inoculating on modified Sabouraud medium (peptone 10 g, glucose 20 g, agar 18 g, natural sea water 1000 mL, penicillin 1.5 g, streptomycin 1.5 g, pH 6.0–7.0). The fungus was identified according to a molecular biological protocol by DNA amplification and sequencing of the ITS region (GenBank accession number MH101466.1). BLAST search results indicated that the sequence was 100% identical (796/796 bp) with the sequence of *Aspergillus flocculosus* strain NRRL 5224 (GenBank accession number EU021616.1).

3.3. Cultivation of Fungus

All the fungal strains were cultured at room temperature for three weeks in 500 mL Erlenmeyer flasks, each containing rice (20.0 g), yeast extract (20.0 mg), KH_2PO_4 (10 mg), and natural sea water (40 mL).

3.4. Extraction and Isolation

The main part of the isolation procedures of compounds from *Penicillium* sp. KMM 4672 was described in a previous paper [20]. The *n*-hexane–EtOAc (95:5, 74.0 mg) fraction was purified by LH-20 column (80 cm × 2 cm) with $CHCl_3$ to yield **2** (12.5 mg) and **3** (14.3 mg). The *n*-hexane–EtOAc (40:60, 54.0 mg) fraction was purified by HPLC on a YMC ODS-AM column, eluting with MeOH–H_2O (65:35), and then by HPLC on a YMC SIL column, eluting with MeOH–$CHCl_3$ (5:95) to yield **1** (1.9 mg).

The main part of isolation procedures of compounds from *Aspergillus* sp. KMM 4676 were described in a previous paper [30]. The *n*-hexane–EtOAc (80:20, 59.4 mg) fraction was purified by HPLC on a YMC ODS-AM column, eluting with MeOH–H_2O (65:35) to yield **5** (3.45 mg). Another *n*-hexane–EtOAc (80:20, 157.7 mg) fraction was purified by HPLC on a YMC ODS-AM column, eluting with MeOH–H_2O (65:35), and then by HPLC on a YMC SIL column, eluting with MeOH–$CHCl_3$–NH_4Ac (10:90:1) to yield **4** (6.74 mg).

The fungal mycelia of *Aspergillus flocculosus* with the medium were extracted for 24 h with 15 L of EtOAc. Evaporation of the solvent, under reduced pressure, gave a dark brown oil (5.0 g), to which 250 mL H_2O–EtOH (4:1) was added, and the mixture was thoroughly stirred to yield a suspension. It was extracted, successively, with hexane (150 mL × 2), EtOAc (150 mL × 2), and *n*-BuOH (150 mL × 2). After evaporation of the EtOAc layer, the residual materials (3.36 g) were passed over a silica gel column (35.0 cm × 2.5 cm), which was eluted with a hexane–EtOAc gradient (1:0–0:1). The *n*-hexane–EtOAc (75:25, 41.4 mg) fraction was purified by HPLC on a YMC SIL column, eluting with MeOH–$CHCl_3$-NH_4Ac (97:3:1), and then by HPLC on a YMC ODS-AM column, eluting with MeOH–H_2O (75:25) to yield **6** (24.1 mg).

6-Hydroxy-*N*-acetyl-β-oxotryptamine (**1**): white powder; ^{1}H and ^{13}C NMR data see Table 1, Figures S1–S7; HR ESIMS m/z 231.0772 $[M-H]^-$ (calcd for $C_{12}H_{11}N_2O_3$, 231.0775, Δ + 1.4 ppm) (Figure S8).

3.5. Biological Activity of Compounds

3.5.1. Radical Scavenger Assay

DPPH radical scavenging activity of compounds was tested as described [51].

Compounds were dissolved in MeOH, and the solutions (160 μL) were dispensed into wells of a 96-well microplate. In all, 40 μL of the DPPH (Sigma-Aldrich, Steinheim, Germany) solution in MeOH (1.5×10^{-4} M) was added to each well. Concentrations of compounds in mixture were 10 and 100 μM. The mixture was shaken and left to stand for 30 min, and the absorbance of the resulting solution was measured at 520 nm with a microplate reader MultiscanFC (ThermoScientific, Waltham, MA, USA).

Radical scavenging activity of all compounds at 100 μM were presented as percent of MeOH data, and the concentration of DPPH radical scavenging at 50% (EC_{50}) was calculated for some compounds.

3.5.2. Cell Line and Culture Condition

The neuroblastoma cell line Neuro2a was purchased from ATCC. Cells were cultured in DMEM medium containing 10% fetal bovine serum (Biolot, St. Petersburg, Russia) and 1% penicillin/streptomycin (Invitrogen, Carlsbad, CA, USA). Cells were incubated at 37 °C in a humidified atmosphere containing 5% (*v*/*v*) CO_2.

3.5.3. Cell Viability Assay

Cell suspension (1×10^3 cells/well) was incubated with different concentration of compounds for 24 h. After that, cell viability was determined using the MTT (3-(4,5-dimethylthiazol-2-yl)-2,5-diphenyltetrazolium bromide) method, according to the manufacturer's instructions (Sigma-Aldrich, St. Louis, MO, USA). The results were presented as percent of control data, and concentration required for 50% inhibition of cell viability (IC_{50}) was calculated.

3.5.4. 6-Hydroxydopamine-Induced In Vitro Model of Parkinson's Disease

The neuroprotective activities of compounds in 6-hydroxydopamine-induced cell model of Parkinson's disease were examined, as described previously [52].

Neuroblastoma Neuro2a line cells (1×10^3 cells/well) were treated with 50 μM of 6-hydroxydopamine (Sigma-Aldrich, St. Louis, MO, USA) for 1 h and, after that, the investigated compounds were added to the neuroblastoma cell suspension at a concentration of 1 and 10 μM. In the other case, the substances were added to the cells 1 h before the addition of the neurotoxin. Cells incubated without 6-OHDA and compounds, and with 6-OHDA only, were used as positive and negative controls, respectively. After 24 h, viability of cells was measured using the MTT method. The results were presented as a percent of positive control data.

3.5.5. Paraquat-Induced In Vitro Model of Parkinson's Disease

Neuroblastoma Neuro2a line cells (1×10^3 cells/well) were treated with compounds at concentrations of 1 and 10 μM for 1 h, and then 500 μM of paraquat (Sigma-Aldrich, St. Louis, MO, USA) was added to the neuroblastoma cell suspension. Cells incubated without paraquat and compounds, and with paraquat only, were used as positive and negative controls, respectively. The viability of cells was measured after 24 h using the MTT method. The results were presented as percent of positive control data.

3.5.6. Reactive Oxygen Species (ROS) Level Analysis in 6-OHDA- and PQ-Treated Cells

Cell suspensions (1×10^3 cells/well) were incubated with compound solutions (10 μM) for 1 h. Then, 6-OHDA at a concentration of 50 μM was added in each well, and cells were incubated for 30 min. In other experiments, cells were incubated with PQ at a concentration of 500 μM for 30 min and 1 h. Cells incubated without 6-OHDA/PQ and compounds, and with 6-OHDA/PQ only, were used as positive and negative controls, respectively. To study ROS formation, 20 μL of 2,7-dichlorodihydrofluorescein diacetate solution (Molecular Probes, Eugene, OR, USA) was added to each well, such that the final concentration was 10 mM, and the microplate was incubated for an additional 10 min at 37 °C. The intensity of dichlorofluorescein fluorescence was measured with plate reader PHERAstar FS (BMG Labtech, Ortenberg, Germany) at λ_{ex} = 485 nm, and λ_{em} = 518 nm. The data were processed by MARS Data Analysis v. 3.01R2 (BMG Labtech, Ortenberg, Germany). The results were presented as a percentage of positive control data.

4. Conclusions

This study is the second case of isolation of melatonin-related compound from microfilamentous fungi. The neuroprotective activity in the 6-OHDA- and PQ-induced PD cell models of this and some other polyketides and alkaloids from marine-derived fungi were investigated. All of them protected Neuro2a cells against the damaging influence of 6-OHDA to varying degrees. We suppose that this effect is realized via a ROS scavenging pathway as one of the possibilities. The new melatonin analogue, 6-hydroxy-*N*-acetyl-β-oxotryptamine, protected Neuro2A cells more effectively against the 6-OHDA-induced neuronal death in comparison with melatonin. Moreover, 6-hydroxy-*N*-acetyl-β-oxotryptamine and melatonin protected Neuro2a cells against the damaging influence of PQ in a similar manner. It was shown that dehydroxylation at C-3" and C-4"significantly increases free radical scavenging and neuroprotective activity of candidusin-related *p*-terphenyl polyketides in both the 6-OHDA- and PQ-induced PD models.

Supplementary Materials: The following are available online at http://www.mdpi.com/1660-3397/16/11/457/s1, Figures S1–S15. The NMR and mass spectra of compounds **1–3** and **6**. Figure S16. ROS formation in the 6-OHDA- and PQ-treated Neuro2a cells.

Author Contributions: Conceptualization, E.A.Y. and A.N.Y.; Data curation, A.N.Y.; Formal analysis, E.A.Y. and E.A.P.; Funding acquisition, E.A.Y. and E.V.I.; Investigation, E.A.Y., E.S.M., E.A.P., P.T.H.T., E.V.I. and O.F.S.; Project administration, E.A.Y.; Resources, E.A.Y., P.T.H.T. and A.N.Y.; Supervision, E.A.Y.; Validation, E.A.Y. and O.F.S.; Visualization, E.A.Y., E.S.M. and E.A.P.; Writing—original draft, E.A.Y. and P.T.H.T.; Writing—review & editing, A.N.Y.

Funding: This research was funded by Russian Foundation for Basic Research, grant numbers 18-34-00621 (isolation and identification of compounds) and 18-34-00737 (investigation of biological activity).

Conflicts of Interest: The authors declare no conflict of interest.

References

1. Mhyre, T.R.; Boyd, J.T.; Hamill, R.W.; Maguire-Zeiss, K.A. Parkinson's Disease. *Sub-Cell. Biochem.* **2012**, *65*, 389–455.
2. Wang, Q.L.; Guo, C.; Qi, J.; Ma, J.H.; Liu, F.Y.; Lin, S.Q.; Zhang, C.Y.; Xie, W.D.; Zhuang, J.J.; Li, X. Protective effects of 3beta-angeloyloxy-8beta, 10beta-dihydroxyeremophila-7(11)-en-12, 8alpha-lactone on paraquat-induced oxidative injury in SH-SY5Y cells. *J. Asian Nat. Prod. Res.* **2018**, 1–13.
3. MacDonald-Wicks, L.K.; Wood, L.G.; Garg, M.L. Methodology for the determination of biological antioxidant capacity in vitro: A review. *J. Sci. Food Agric.* **2006**, *86*, 2046–2056. [CrossRef]
4. Cheng, G.; Zielonka, M.; Dranka, B.; Kumar, S.N.; Myers, C.R.; Bennett, B.; Garces, A.M.; Dias Duarte Machado, L.G.; Thiebaut, D.; Ouari, O.; et al. Detection of mitochondria-generated reactive oxygen species in cells using multiple probes and methods: Potentials, pitfalls, and the future. *J. Biol. Chem.* **2018**, *293*, 10363–10380. [CrossRef] [PubMed]
5. Bastias-Candia, S.; Zolezzi, J.M.; Inestrosa, N.C. Revisiting the Paraquat-Induced Sporadic Parkinson's Disease-Like Model. *Mol. Neurobiol.* **2018**. [CrossRef] [PubMed]
6. Bove, J.; Prou, D.; Perier, C.; Przedborski, S. Toxin-induced models of Parkinson's disease. *NeuroRx* **2005**, *2*, 484–494. [CrossRef] [PubMed]
7. Sun, S.W.; Ji, C.Z.; Gu, Q.Q.; Li, D.H.; Zhu, T.J. Three new polyketides from marine-derived fungus *Aspergillus glaucus* HB1-19. *J. Asian Nat. Prod. Res.* **2013**, *15*, 956–961. [CrossRef] [PubMed]
8. Li, H.L.; Li, X.M.; Liu, H.; Meng, L.H.; Wang, B.G. Two New Diphenylketones and a New Xanthone from *Talaromyces islandicus* EN-501, an Endophytic Fungus Derived from the Marine Red Alga *Laurencia okamurai*. *Mar. Drugs* **2016**, *14*, 223. [CrossRef] [PubMed]
9. Li, Y.; Li, X.; Lee, U.; Kang, J.S.; Choi, H.D.; Sona, B.W. A New Radical Scavenging Anthracene Glycoside, Asperflavin Ribofuranoside, and Polyketides from a Marine Isolate of the Fungus *Microsporum*. *Chem. Pharm. Bull.* **2006**, *54*, 882–883. [CrossRef]
10. Chen, L.; Fang, Y.; Zhu, T.; Gu, Q.; Zhu, W. Gentisyl alcohol derivatives from the marine-derived fungus *Penicillium terrestre*. *J. Nat. Prod.* **2008**, *71*, 66–70. [CrossRef] [PubMed]

11. Li, Y.; Li, X.; Kim, S.K.; Kang, J.S.; Choi, H.D.; Rho, J.R.; Son, B.W. Golmaenone, a New Diketopiperazine Alkaloid from the Marine-Derived Fungus *Aspergillus* sp. *Chem. Pharm. Bull.* **2004**, *52*, 375–376. [CrossRef] [PubMed]
12. Zhong, W.M.; Wang, J.F.; Shi, X.F.; Wei, X.Y.; Chen, Y.C.; Zeng, Q.; Xiang, Y.; Chen, X.Y.; Tian, X.P.; Xiao, Z.H.; et al. Eurotiumins A(-)E, Five New Alkaloids from the Marine-Derived Fungus *Eurotium* sp. SCSIO F452. *Mar. Drugs* **2018**, *16*. [CrossRef] [PubMed]
13. Li, D.L.; Li, X.M.; Li, T.G.; Dang, H.Y.; Wang, B.G. Dioxopiperazine alkaloids produced by the marine mangrove derived endophytic fungus *Eurotium rubrum*. *Helv. Chim. Acta* **2008**, *91*, 1888–1893. [CrossRef]
14. Li, X.; Kim, S.K.; Nam, K.W.; Kang, J.S.; Choi, H.D.; Son, B.W. A new antibacterial dioxopiperazine alkaloid related to gliotoxin from a marine isolate of the fungus *Pseudallescheria*. *J. Antibiot. (Tokyo)* **2006**, *59*, 248–250. [CrossRef] [PubMed]
15. Akashi, S.; Kimura, T.; Takeuchi, T.; Kuramochi, K.; Kobayashi, S.; Sugawara, F.; Watanabe, N.; Arai, T. Neoechinulin A Impedes the Progression of Rotenone-Induced Cytotoxicity in PC12 Cells. *Biol. Pharm. Bull.* **2011**, *34*, 243–248. [CrossRef] [PubMed]
16. Choi, D.Y.; Choi, H. Natural products from marine organisms with neuroprotective activity in the experimental models of Alzheimer's disease, Parkinson's disease and ischemic brain stroke: Their molecular targets and action mechanisms. *Arch. Pharm. Res.* **2015**, *38*, 139–170. [CrossRef] [PubMed]
17. Lu, X.l.; Yao, X.l.; Liu, Z.; Zhang, H.; Li, W.; Li, Z.; Wang, G.L.; Pang, J.; Lin, Y.; Xu, Z.; et al. Protective effects of xyloketal B against MPP+-induced neurotoxicity in Caenorhabditis elegans and PC12 cells. *Brain Res.* **2010**, *1332*, 110–119. [CrossRef] [PubMed]
18. Li, S.; Shen, C.; Guo, W.; Zhang, X.; Liu, S.; Liang, F.; Xu, Z.; Pei, Z.; Song, H.; Qiu, L.; et al. Synthesis and Neuroprotective Action of Xyloketal Derivatives in Parkinson's Disease Models. *Mar. Drugs* **2013**, *11*, 5159–5189. [CrossRef] [PubMed]
19. Zhai, A.; Zhu, X.; Wang, X.; Chen, R.; Wang, H. Secalonic acid A protects dopaminergic neurons from 1-methyl-4-phenylpyridinium (MPP(+))-induced cell death via the mitochondrial apoptotic pathway. *Eur. J. Pharmacol.* **2013**, *713*, 58–67. [CrossRef] [PubMed]
20. Yurchenko, A.; Smetanina, O.; Ivanets, E.; Kalinovsky, A.; Khudyakova, Y.; Kirichuk, N.; Popov, R.; Bokemeyer, C.; von Amsberg, G.; Chingizova, E.; et al. Pretrichodermamides D–F from a Marine Algicolous Fungus *Penicillium* sp. KMM 4672. *Mar. Drugs* **2016**, *14*, 122. [CrossRef] [PubMed]
21. Smetanina, O.F.; Yurchenko, A.N.; Ivanets, E.V.; Gerasimenko, A.V.; Trinh, P.T.H.; Ly, B.M.; Nhut, N.D.; Van, T.T.T.; Yurchenko, E.A.; Afiyatullov, S.S. Aromatic Metabolites of Marine Fungus *Penicillium* sp. KMM 4672 Associated with a Brown Alga *Padina* sp. *Chem. Nat. Compd.* **2017**, *53*, 600–602. [CrossRef]
22. Martínez-Luis, S.; Gómez, J.F.; Spadafora, C.; Guzmán, H.M.; Gutiérrez, M. Antitrypanosomal alkaloids from the marine bacterium *Bacillus pumilus*. *Molecules* **2012**, *17*, 11146–11155. [CrossRef] [PubMed]
23. Yongle, C.; Zeeck, A.; Zengxiang, C.; Zahner, H. Metabolic products of microorganisms. 222. β-Oxotryptamine derivatives isolated from *Streptomyces ramulosus*. *J. Antibiot.* **1983**, *36*, 913–915.
24. Li, D.; Wang, F.; Xiao, X.; Zeng, X.; Gu, Q.Q.; Zhu, W. A new cytotoxic phenazine derivative from a deep sea bacterium *Bacillus* sp. *Arch. Pharmacal Res.* **2007**, *30*, 552–555. [CrossRef]
25. Yang, J.; Wang, N.; Yuan, H.S.; Hu, J.C.; Dai, Y.C. A new sesquiterpene from the medicinal fungus *Inonotus vaninii*. *Chem. Nat. Compd.* **2013**, *49*, 261–263. [CrossRef]
26. Elnaggar, M.S.; Ebada, S.S.; Ashour, M.L.; Ebrahim, W.; Singab, A.; Lin, W.; Liu, Z.; Proksch, P. Two new triterpenoids and a new naphthoquinone derivative isolated from a hard coral-derived fungus Scopulariopsis sp. *Fitoterapia* **2017**, *116*, 126–130. [CrossRef] [PubMed]
27. Kawahara, N.; Nozawa, K.; Nakajima, S.; Kawai, K.I.; Udagawa, S.I. Studies on Fungal Products. XVI.: New Metabolites Related to 3-Methylorsellinate from *Aspergillus silvaticus*. *Chem. Pharm. Bull.* **1988**, *36*, 398–400. [CrossRef] [PubMed]
28. Smetanina, O.F.; Yurchenko, A.N.; Pivkin, M.V.; Yurchenko, E.A.; Afiyatullov, S.S. Isochromene Metabolite from the Facultative Marine Fungus Penicillium Citrinum. *Chem. Nat. Compd.* **2011**, *47*, 118–119. [CrossRef]
29. Yurchenko, A.N.; Ivanets, E.V.; Smetanina, O.F.; Pivkin, M.V.; Dyshlovoi, S.A.; von Amsberg, G.; Afiyatullov, S.S. Metabolites of the Marine Fungus *Aspergillus candidus* KMM 4676 Associated with a Kuril Colonial Ascidian. *Chem. Nat. Compd.* **2017**, *53*, 747–749. [CrossRef]

30. Ivanets, E.V.; Yurchenko, A.N.; Smetanina, O.F.; Rasin, A.B.; Zhuravleva, O.I.; Pivkin, M.V.; Popov, R.S.; von Amsberg, G.; Afiyatullov, S.S.; Dyshlovoy, S.A. Asperindoles A–D and a p-terphenyl derivative from the ascidian-derived fungus *Aspergillus* sp. KMM 4676. *Mar. Drugs* **2018**, *16*. [CrossRef] [PubMed]
31. Lorenz, P.; Jensen, P.R.; Fenical, W. Mactanamide, a new fungistatic diketopiperazine produced by a marine *Aspergillus* sp. *Nat. Prod. Lett.* **1998**, *12*, 55–60. [CrossRef]
32. Wu, Z.; Wang, Y.; Liu, D.; Proksch, P.; Yu, S.; Lin, W. Antioxidative phenolic compounds from a marine-derived fungus *Aspergillus versicolor*. *Tetrahedron* **2016**, *72*, 50–57. [CrossRef]
33. Smetanina, O.F.; Yurchenko, A.N.; Ivanets, E.V.; Kirichuk, N.N.; Khudyakova, Y.V.; Yurchenko, E.A.; Afiyatullov, S.S. Metabolites of the Marine Fungus *Penicillium citrinum* Associated with a Brown Alga *Padina* sp. *Chem. Nat. Compd.* **2016**, *52*, 111–112. [CrossRef]
34. Yen, G.C.; Chang, Y.C.; Sheu, F.; Chiang, H.C. Isolation and characterization of antioxidant compounds from Aspergillus candidus broth filtrate. *J. Agric. Food Chem.* **2001**, *49*, 1426–1431. [CrossRef] [PubMed]
35. Cai, S.; Sun, S.; Zhou, H.; Kong, X.; Zhu, T.; Li, D.; Gu, Q. Prenylated polyhydroxy-p-terphenyls from *Aspergillus taichungensis* ZHN-7-07. *J. Nat. Prod.* **2011**, *74*, 1106–1110. [CrossRef] [PubMed]
36. Yan, T.; Guo, Z.K.; Jiang, R.; Wei, W.; Wang, T.; Guo, Y.; Song, Y.C.; Jiao, R.H.; Tan, R.X.; Ge, H.M. New Flavonol and Diterpenoids from the Endophytic Fungus *Aspergillus* sp. YXf3. *Planta Med.* **2013**, *79*, 348–352. [CrossRef] [PubMed]
37. Shin, H.J.; Choi, B.K.; Trinh, P.T.H.; Lee, H.S.; Kang, J.S.; Van, T.T.T.; Lee, H.S.; Lee, J.S.; Lee, Y.J.; Lee, J. Suppression of RANKL-induced osteoclastogenesis by the metabolites from the marine fungus *Aspergillus flocculosus* isolated from a sponge *Stylissa* sp. *Mar. Drugs* **2018**, *16*. [CrossRef] [PubMed]
38. Rodriguez-Pallares, J.; Parga, J.A.; Munoz, A.; Rey, P.; Guerra, M.J.; Labandeira-Garcia, J.L. Mechanism of 6-hydroxydopamine neurotoxicity: The role of NADPH oxidase and microglial activation in 6-hydroxydopamine-induced degeneration of dopaminergic neurons. *J. Neurochem.* **2007**, *103*, 145–156. [CrossRef] [PubMed]
39. Villa, M.; Muñoz, P.; Ahumada-Castro, U.; Paris, I.; Jiménez, A.; Martínez, I.; Sevilla, F.; Segura-Aguilar, J. One-Electron Reduction of 6-Hydroxydopamine Quinone is Essential in 6-Hydroxydopamine Neurotoxicity. *Neurotox. Res.* **2013**, *24*, 94–101. [CrossRef] [PubMed]
40. Segura-Aguilar, J.; Kostrzewa, R.M. Neurotoxin Mechanisms and Processes Relevant to Parkinson's Disease: An Update. *Neurotox. Res.* **2015**, *27*, 328–354. [CrossRef] [PubMed]
41. Rappold, P.M.; Cui, M.; Chesser, A.S.; Tibbett, J.; Grima, J.C.; Duan, L.; Sen, N.; Javitch, J.A.; Tieu, K. Paraquat neurotoxicity is mediated by the dopamine transporter and organic cation transporter-3. *Proc. Nat. Acad. Sci. USA* **2011**, *108*, 20766–20771. [CrossRef] [PubMed]
42. Dagda, R.K.; Das Banerjee, T.; Janda, E. How Parkinsonian toxins dysregulate the autophagy machinery. *Internat. J. Mol. Sci.* **2013**, *14*, 22163–22189. [CrossRef] [PubMed]
43. Powers, R.; Lei, S.; Anandhan, A.; Marshall, D.D.; Worley, B.; Cerny, R.L.; Dodds, E.D.; Huang, Y.; Panayiotidis, M.I.; Pappa, A.; et al. Metabolic investigations of the molecular mechanisms associated with parkinson's disease. *Metabolites* **2017**, *7*. [CrossRef] [PubMed]
44. Lei, S.; Zavala-Flores, L.; Garcia-Garcia, A.; Nandakumar, R.; Huang, Y.; Madayiputhiya, N.; Stanton, R.C.; Dodds, E.D.; Powers, R.; Franco, R. Alterations in Energy/Redox Metabolism Induced by Mitochondrial and Environmental Toxins: A Specific Role for Glucose-6-Phosphate-Dehydrogenase and the Pentose Phosphate Pathway in Paraquat Toxicity. *ACS Chem. Boil.* **2014**, *9*, 2032–2048. [CrossRef] [PubMed]
45. Shirinzadeh, H.; Ince, E.; Westwell, A.D.; Gurer-Orhan, H.; Suzen, S. Novel indole-based melatonin analogues substituted with triazole, thiadiazole and carbothioamides: Studies on their antioxidant, chemopreventive and cytotoxic activities. *J. Enzyme Inhib. Med. Chem.* **2016**, *31*, 1312–1321. [CrossRef] [PubMed]
46. Chetsawang, J.; Govitrapong, P.; Chetsawang, B. Melatonin inhibits MPP+-induced caspase-mediated death pathway and DNA fragmentation factor-45 cleavage in SK-N-SH cultured cells. *J. Pineal Res.* **2007**, *43*, 115–120. [CrossRef] [PubMed]
47. Nopparat, C.; Chantadul, V.; Permpoonputtana, K.; Govitrapong, P. The anti-inflammatory effect of melatonin in SH-SY5Y neuroblastoma cells exposed to sublethal dose of hydrogen peroxide. *Mech. Ageing Dev.* **2017**, *164*, 49–60. [CrossRef] [PubMed]
48. Zhou, H.; Cheang, T.; Su, F.; Zheng, Y.; Chen, S.; Feng, J.; Pei, Z.; Chen, L. Melatonin inhibits rotenone-induced SH-SY5Y cell death via the downregulation of Dynamin-Related Protein 1 expression. *Eur. J. Pharmacol.* **2018**, *819*, 58–67. [CrossRef] [PubMed]

49. Mayo, J.C.; Sainz, R.M.; Uria, H.; Antolin, I.; Esteban, M.M.; Rodriguez, C. Melatonin prevents apoptosis induced by 6-hydroxydopamine in neuronal cells: Implications for Parkinson's disease. *J. Pineal Res.* **1998**, *24*, 179–192. [CrossRef] [PubMed]
50. Mayo, J.C.; Sainz, R.M.; Antolín, I.; Rodriguez, C. Ultrastructural confirmation of neuronal protection by melatonin against the neurotoxin 6-hydroxydopamine cell damage. *Brain Res.* **1999**, *818*, 221–227. [CrossRef]
51. Leutou, A.S.; Yun, K.; Son, B.W. Induced production of 6,9-dibromoflavasperone, a new radical scavenging naphthopyranone in the marine-mudflat-derived fungus *Aspergillus niger*. *Arch. Pharmacal Res.* **2016**, *39*, 806–810. [CrossRef] [PubMed]
52. Lyakhova, E.G.; Kolesnikova, S.A.; Kalinovsky, A.I.; Berdyshev, D.V.; Pislyagin, E.A.; Kuzmich, A.S.; Popov, R.S.; Dmitrenok, P.S.; Makarieva, T.N.; Stonik, V.A. Lissodendoric Acids A and B, Manzamine-Related Alkaloids from the Far Eastern Sponge *Lissodendoryx florida*. *Org. Lett.* **2017**, *19*, 5320–5323. [CrossRef] [PubMed]

marine drugs

MDPI

Article

Gliotoxin Enhances Autophagic Cell Death via the DAPK1-TAp63 Signaling Pathway in Paclitaxel-Resistant Ovarian Cancer Cells

Ga-Bin Park [1], Jee-Yeong Jeong [1,*] and Daejin Kim [2,*]

1 Department of Biochemistry, Kosin University College of Medicine, Busan 49267, Korea
2 Department of Anatomy, Inje University College of Medicine, Busan 47392, Korea
* Correspondence: jyjeong@kosin.ac.kr (J.-Y.J.); kimdj@inje.ac.kr (D.K.);
Tel.: +82-51-990-5425 (J.-Y.J.); +82-51-890-8651 (D.K.)

Received: 24 June 2019; Accepted: 10 July 2019; Published: 12 July 2019

Abstract: Death-associated protein kinase 1 (DAPK1) expression induced by diverse death stimuli mediates apoptotic activity in various cancers, including ovarian cancer. In addition, mutual interaction between the tumor suppressor p53 and DAPK1 influences survival and death in several cancer cell lines. However, the exact role and connection of DAPK1 and p53 family proteins (p53, p63, and p73) in drug-resistant ovarian cancer cells have not been studied previously. In this study, we investigated whether DAPK1 induction by gliotoxin derived from marine fungus regulates the level of transcriptionally active p63 (TAp63) to promote apoptosis in an autophagy-dependent manner. Pre-exposure of paclitaxel-resistant ovarian cancer cells to gliotoxin inhibited the expression of multidrug resistant-associated proteins (MDR1 and MRP1-3), disrupted the mitochondrial membrane potential, and induced caspase-dependent apoptosis through autophagy induction after subsequent treatment with paclitaxel. Gene silencing of DAPK1 prevented TAp63-mediated downregulation of MDR1 and MRP1-3 and autophagic cell death after sequential treatment with gliotoxin and then paclitaxel. However, pretreatment with 3-methyladenine (3-MA), an autophagy inhibitor, had no effect on the levels of DAPK1 and TAp63 or on the inhibition of MDR1 and MRP1-3. These results suggest that DAPK1-mediated TAp63 upregulation is one of the critical pathways that induce apoptosis in chemoresistant cancer cells.

Keywords: gliotoxin; DAPK1; TAp63; autophagy; drug resistance; ovarian cancer

1. Introduction

Death-associated protein kinase-1 (DAPK1) is a Ca^{2+}/calmodulin (CaM)-regulated serine/threonine kinase that mediates cell death [1]. Downregulation of DAPK1 by methylation in its promoter region is detected in various cancers, including pancreas, lung, and head and neck. Low DAPK1 expression in these tumors is closely related to frequent lymph node metastasis and poor clinical outcomes [2–4]. Overexpression or activation of DAPK1, as a tumor suppressor, is involved in cell death. Ectopic DAPK expression induces p53-dependent apoptosis in mouse embryo fibroblasts [5], and tumor necrosis factor-alpha (TNF-α) and interferon-gamma (IFN-γ) induce DAPK1 expression through inhibiting NF-κB activity [6]. DAPK1 activation not only requires cell cycle arrest and caspase-dependent apoptosis [7] but also contributes to autophagic cell death by reducing the interaction between Beclin-1 and Bcl-2 and Bcl-X_L [8]. Furthermore, DAPK-1 induces caspase-independent cell death through activating autophagosome formation [9]. However, DAPK1 sometimes antagonizes apoptosis in a cell-type-dependent manner. DAPK1 depletion using antisense DAPK1 cDNA promotes caspase-mediated apoptosis via TNF [10], and DAPK1 plays an essential role in the proliferation of p53-mutant estrogen receptor-negative breast cancer cells [11]. These results demonstrate that the role and molecular mechanism of DAPK1 in human cancers are not clearly understood.

Tumor suppressor p53 expression responds to various types of cellular damage and stress, including oncogenic stimuli [12,13]. Cells expressing wild-type p53 experience DAPK1 upregulation after stimulation with anticancer drugs or UV exposure [14]. In contrast, DAPK1 overexpression promotes p53 expression, resulting in the suppression of oncogenic transformation [5]. p53 mutations that reduce or abolish its function are closely associated with anticancer drug resistance in various cancers [15,16], whereas mutant p53 occurrence in ovarian cancer has no effect on apoptotic death induced by paclitaxel [17]. Ovarian cancer co-expressing p53 and Bcl-2 has been shown to have the best response to paclitaxel chemotherapy [18]. These contradictory results suggest that p53 and DAPK1 influence several different molecular pathways to induce cancer cell death, and the mutual relationship between DAPK1 and p53 is dependent on cell type and cell conditions.

The p53 family is composed of three homologous proteins, p53, p63, and p73. These proteins share essential structural domains and have similar cellular functions in proliferation, differentiation, tumorigenesis, and death [19,20]. Transcriptionally active p63 (TAp63), a p53 isoform, plays a critical role in not only intracellular fatty acid generation [21] but also tumor suppression [22] and metastasis prevention [23]. We have previously reported that TAp63 activation induces apoptosis in Epstein-Barr virus (EBV)-transformed B cells after treatment with baicalein [24], and TAp63 expression in TLR4-stimulated colon cancer cells promotes fatty acid-mediated metastasis [25]. However, the precise relationship between DAPK1 and TAp63 in modulating apoptosis in cancer is unclear, and the autophagy-related signaling pathway regulated by TAp63 in cancer needs to be investigated.

Gliotoxin, a secondary metabolite of marine fungus *Aspergillus fumigatus*, is not only a member of the epipolythiodioxopiperazine family but also characterized by a disulfide bond across a piperazine ring and an aromatic amino acid [26,27]. Treatment with gliotoxin of mouse immune cells inhibits nuclear factor kappa B (NF-κB), resulting in the downregulation of inflammatory genes activation [28]. Reactive oxygen species (ROS) induced by gliotoxin contribute to suppression of NF-κB, leading to the apoptosis of human fibrosarcoma cell line (HT1080) [29]. Gliotoxin induces apoptosis in various human cancers cells, including uterine cervix cancer cell line (Hela), chondrosarcoma cell line (SW1353), chronic lymphocytic leukemia cell, and breast cancer cell line (MCF-7) [30–32]. Recently, it has been reported that gliotoxin treatment induces apoptotic death in doxorubicin-resistant lung cancer cells through disrupting mitochondrial function and activating p53 downstream target molecules [33]. However, the expression and specific role of DAPK1 in ovarian and paclitaxel-resistant ovarian cancer cells after treatment with gliotoxin have not been studied. In this study, we investigated whether DAPK1 regulates apoptotic death in paclitaxel-resistant ovarian cancer cells and examined the relationship between DAPK1 and p53 family proteins in inducing autophagic cell death after treatment with gliotoxin.

2. Results

2.1. Treatment with Gliotoxin Suppresses Growth and Reduces Resistance in Paclitaxel-Resistant Ovarian Cancer Cells

We first determined the 50% inhibitory concentration (IC*50*) value of paclitaxel in ovarian cancer cells using Cell Counting Kit-8 (CCK-8) assays as described in the Methods section. The IC50 values of paclitaxel in CaOV3 and SKOV3 cells were 2.71 ± 0.01 nM and 5.15 ± 0.02 nM, respectively, at 48 h. Established paclitaxel-resistant ovarian cancer cells showed profound morphological differences compared to parental cell lines under microscope observation (Supplemental Figure S1A). Additionally, paclitaxel-resistant CaOV3 cells (CaOV3/PTX_R) and SKOV3 cells (SKOV3/PTX_R) sustained their proliferation rates after exposure to a high dose (100 nM) of paclitaxel (Supplemental Figure S1B). We next investigated whether treating chemoresistant ovarian cancer cells with gliotoxin prevents cell growth and induces apoptosis. Chemoresistant ovarian cancer cells not only upregulated multidrug resistant-associated proteins (MDR1 and MRP1-3) but also induced the expression of anti-apoptotic proteins, including X-linked inhibitor of apoptosis protein (XIAP), and cell survival (Figure 1A). Although exposure to gliotoxin slightly prevented the proliferation of CaOV3/PTX_R and SKOV3/PTX_R cells (Figure 1B), treating drug-resistant ovarian cancer cells with gliotoxin failed to induce cleaved caspase-9 (active p37) and caspase-3 (active p19/17) or the downstream target cleaved poly (ADP-ribose) polymerase (PARP) (Figure 1C). However, the levels of drug-resistant proteins were markedly decreased after treatment with gliotoxin (Figure 1D). These results suggest that gliotoxin renders the chemoresistant ovarian cancer cells vulnerable to cytotoxic agents, even though the drug alone could not induce the apoptotic death of cancer cells.

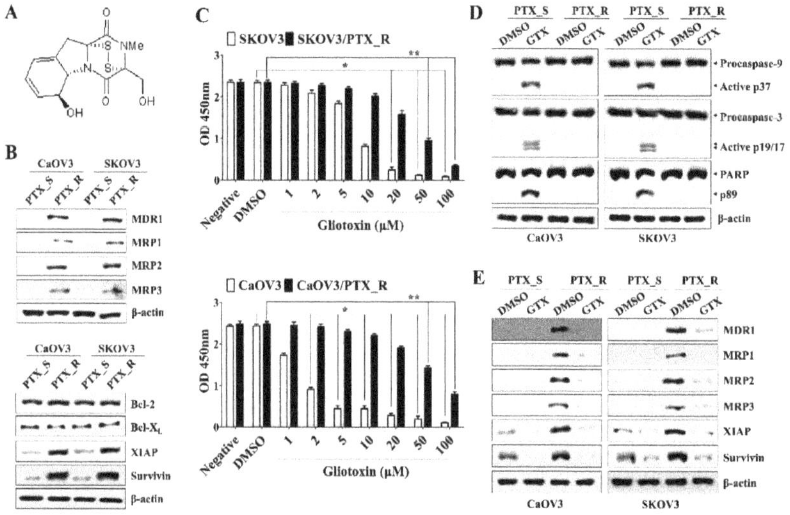

Figure 1. Treatment with gliotoxin (GTX) suppressed cell growth and reduced resistance in paclitaxel-resistant ovarian cancer cells. (**A**) The chemical structure of gliotoxin used in the whole experiment in this study. (**B**) Total protein from each group of PTX-sensitive cells (PTX_S) and PTX-resistant cells (PTX_R) was analyzed by Western blotting with the indicated antibodies. The expressions of multidrug resistant-associated proteins (MDR1-3), X-linked inhibitor of apoptosis protein (XIAP), and surviving were increased in CaOV3/PTX_R and SKOV3/PTX_R cells (**C**) Cells were treated with the indicated drug concentration for 24 h. Cell viability was measured using a Cell Counting Kit-8 assay. The absorbance at 450 nm is presented. n = 3. *$p < 0.001$ (GTX-treated PTX_S ovarian cancer cells vs. DMSO-treated PTX_S ovarian cancer cells); **$p < 0.001$ (GTX-treated PTX_R ovarian cancer cells vs. DMSO-treated PTX_R ovarian cancer cells). (**D**,**E**) Cells (1.5×10^5/well) were treated with 5 μM GTX for 24 h. Total protein was subjected to Western blot analysis with the indicated antibodies. β-actin served as an internal control. Treatment with GTX of PTX_R ovarian cancer cells reduced the expression of MDR1-3, XIAP, and surviving, but not the cleavage of caspase-9 (active p37/35) and caspase-3 (active p19/17). The results are representative of three independent experiments.

2.2. *Sequential Treatment with Gliotoxin Followed by Paclitaxel Promotes Apoptotic Death in Paclitaxel-Resistant Ovarian Cancer Cells*

As shown in Figure 1B, treatment with 5 μM GTX not only started to prevent the proliferation of PTX-sensitive SKOV3 cells but also blocked the growth of CaOV3/PTX_R and SKOV3/PTX_R cells. Furthermore, exposure to 5 μM GTX reduced in MDR1 and MRP1-3 expression in CaOV3/PTX_R and SKOV3/PTX_R cells, but not the induction of active form caspase-9 and caspase-3. We also observed that the exposure to 100 nM paclitaxel for 48 h induced nearly completely blocked the proliferation of PTX-sensitive ovarian cancer cells, whereas the growth rate of CaOV3/PTX_R and SKOV3/PTX_R cells was preserved (Figure S1). Based on these results, we next investigated whether co-treatment with gliotoxin and paclitaxel promotes apoptotic death in drug-resistant ovarian cancer cells. To verify the sensitizing effect of gliotoxin to the anti-cancer drug through reducing MDR1 and MRP1-3 in paclitaxel-resistant ovarian cancer cells, CaOV3/PTX_R and SKOV3/PTX_R cells were pre-exposed to gliotoxin (5 μM) for 8 h and then sequentially treated with paclitaxel (100 nM) for 48 h. Consecutive treatment with gliotoxin and paclitaxel significantly prevented CaOV3/PTX_R and SKOV3/PTX_R cell growth compared to co-treatment and reverse sequential treatment (Figure 2A). When CaOV3/PTX_R and SKOV3/PTX_R cells were treated with gliotoxin, and then paclitaxel, the apoptotic death of chemoresistant ovarian cancer cells was synergistically increased (Figure 2B,C). Furthermore, drug-resistant ovarian cancer cells treated with gliotoxin followed by paclitaxel exhibited activation and cleavage of caspase-9, caspase-3, and PARP (Figure 2D). These results suggest that pre-exposure to gliotoxin reverses paclitaxel resistance in chemoresistant ovarian cancer cells via the induction of apoptotic death by chemotherapeutic agents.

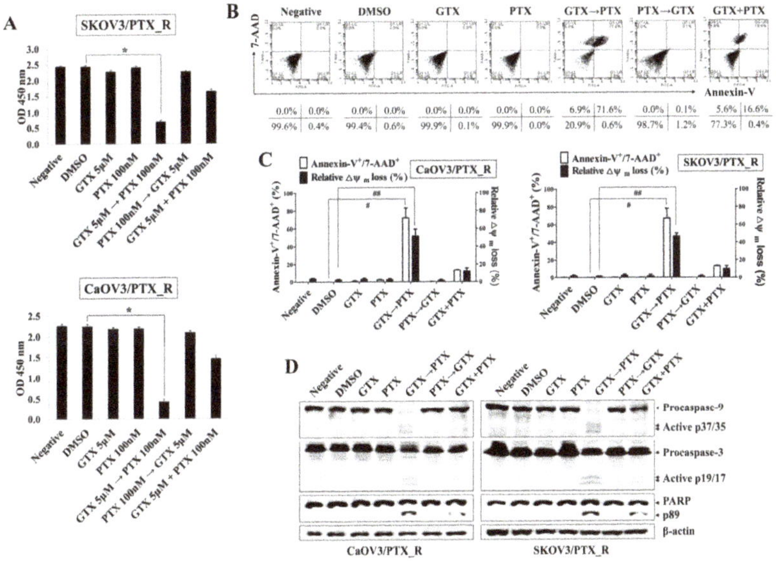

Figure 2. Sequential treatment with gliotoxin followed by paclitaxel induces apoptotic death in paclitaxel-resistant ovarian cancer cells. Cells were seeded into 96-well plates (1×10^4 cells/well) or 6-well plates (1.5×10^5 cells/well) and pre-treated with GTX (5 μM) for 8 h followed by PTX (100 nM) for 48 h. For comparison, untreated control cells were cultured with media in the presence of DMSO. (**A**) Cell viability was measured using a Cell Counting Kit-8 assay. The absorbance at 450 nm is presented. n = 3. *$p < 0.001$ (PTX_R ovarian cancer cells treated with GTX followed by PTX vs. DMSO-treated PTX_R ovarian cancer cells). (**B**,**C**) To determine the degree of apoptosis, cells were stained with annexin-V-FITC and 7-AAD and analyzed by flow cytometry. Dot-plot graphs show the percentage of viable cells (annexin-V$^-$/7-AAD$^-$), early-stage apoptotic cells (annexin-V$^+$/7-AAD$^-$), late-stage apoptotic cells (annexin-V$^+$/7-AAD$^+$), and necrotic cells (annexin-V$^-$/7-AAD$^+$). Late-stage apoptotic cells (annexin-V+/7-AAD+) were evaluated by flow cytometry. # $p < 0.005$ (PTX_R ovarian cancer cells treated with GTX, followed by PTX vs. DMSO-treated PTX_R ovarian cancer cells). To measure $\Delta\psi_m$ disruption, cells were stained with $DiOC_6$. Diminished $DiOC_6$ fluorescence (%) indicates $\Delta\psi_m$ disruption. ## $p < 0.005$ (PTX_R ovarian cancer cells treated with GTX, followed by PTX vs. DMSO-treated PTX_R ovarian cancer cells). Each value is expressed as the mean ± SD from three independent experiments (n = 3). (**D**) Whole cell lysates were subjected to Western blot analysis using the indicated antibodies. Sequential treatment with GTX followed by PTX induced the activated caspase-9 (active p37/35) and caspase-3 (active p19/17) in PTX_R ovarian cancer cells. β-actin served as an internal control. The results are representative of three independent experiments.

2.3. *Pre-Exposure to Gliotoxin Followed by Paclitaxel Upregulates the TAp63 Expression, Leading to the Caspase-Dependent Apoptosis in Drug-Resistant Ovarian Cancer Cells*

We next investigated the underlying signaling pathway to determine the role and relationship of DAPK1 and p53 family proteins. Although p53 expression was upregulated in CaOV3 and SKOV3 cells after paclitaxel stimulation (Figure 3A), exposure to gliotoxin or paclitaxel failed to induce p53 expression in CaOV3/PTX_R and SKOV3/PTX_R cells (Figure 3B). In contrast, cells treated with gliotoxin followed by paclitaxel had increased expression of DAPK1 and TAp63, a p53 family member (Figure 3B). To determine the role of TAp63 in the apoptotic death of CaOV3/PTX_R and SKOV3/PTX_R cells, we transfected TAp63-expressing plasmids into drug-resistant ovarian cancer cells. The expression of drug resistance-associated proteins was prominently lower in CaOV3/PTX_R and SKOV3/PTX_R cells with forced TAp63 expression than in cells transfected with empty vector (Figure 3C). Furthermore, TAp63 overexpression led to apoptosis in paclitaxel-resistant ovarian cancer cells after treatment with paclitaxel (Figure 3D). Sequential treatment with gliotoxin followed by paclitaxel induced the expression of autophagosome-related molecules (LC3-I/II and Beclin-1) and the apoptosis-related protein, Bax (Figure S2). Although TAp63 gene silencing had no effect on DAPK1 expression, reduced TAp63 expression prevented the induction of XIAP-associated factor 1 (XAF1), LC3-I/II, and Beclin-1, as well as the reductions in MDR1 and MRP1-3 expression, after sequential treatment with gliotoxin and paclitaxel (Figure 3E). Targeted inhibition of TAp63 also prevented the expression of cleaved and activated caspase-9, caspase-3, and PARP in CaOV3/PTX_R and SKOV3/PTX_R cells after treatment with gliotoxin followed by paclitaxel (Figure 3F). These results suggest that TAp63 expression plays an important role in enhancing apoptosis through the downregulation of multidrug resistant-associated proteins.

2.4. *DAPK1/TAp63-Mediated Autophagy Regulates Apoptotic Death in Drug-Resistant Ovarian Cancer Cells after Consecutive Treatment with Gliotoxin and Paclitaxel*

DAPK1 and p53 mutually induce apoptosis in cancer cells (6, 11). To determine the association between DAPK1 and TAp63 in inducing apoptosis in CaOV3/PTX_R and SKOV3/PTX_R cells after sequential treatment with gliotoxin and paclitaxel, we investigated the effect of DAPK1 on TAp63 expression, autophagosome-related molecule levels, and mitochondrial membrane potential changes. DAPK1-knockdown CaOV3/PTX_R and SKOV3/PTX_R cells exhibited suppressed TAp63, XAF-1, LC3-I/II, and Beclin-1 expression and downregulated MDR1 and MRP1-3 expression after sequential treatment with gliotoxin and then paclitaxel (Figure 4A). In addition, DAPK1 gene silencing using siRNA prevented the cleavage of caspase-9, caspase-3, and PARP (Figure 4B) as well as the depolarization of mitochondria membranes induced by treating paclitaxel-resistant ovarian cancer cells with gliotoxin followed by paclitaxel (Figure 4C). We finally investigated the connection between the DAPK1-TAp63 signaling pathway and autophagy-related cell death using 3-methyladenine (3-MA), an autophagy inhibitor. Pre-exposure of CaOV3/PTX_R and SKOV3/PTX_R cells to 3-MA had no effect on the expression of DAPK1, TAp63, and XAF1 after subsequent treatment with gliotoxin and paclitaxel (Figure 5A), whereas multidrug resistant-associated protein levels remained low (Figure 5A). Furthermore, 3-MA efficiently blocked the activation of the caspase-dependent apoptotic pathway and the depolarization of mitochondria membranes after sequential treatment with gliotoxin followed by paclitaxel (Figure 5B,C). These results suggest that DAPK1/TAp63-mediated autophagy is one of the key downstream target pathways that induce apoptosis in drug-resistant ovarian cancer cells and demonstrate that multidrug resistant-associated protein levels are regulated in an autophagy-independent manner after sequential treatment with gliotoxin followed by paclitaxel.

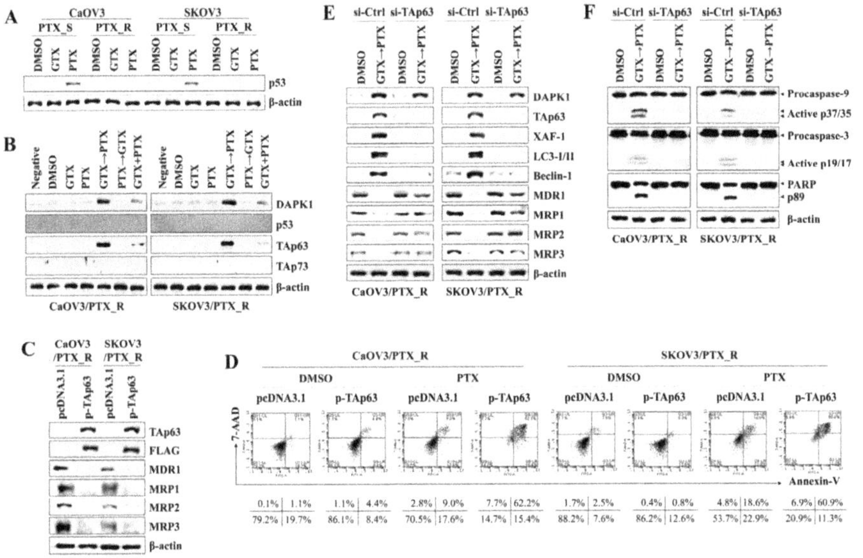

Figure 3. Pre-exposure to gliotoxin followed by paclitaxel induces caspase-dependent apoptosis in drug-resistant ovarian cancer cells by upregulating TAp63 expression. (**A**,**B**) Cells were seeded into 6-well plates (1.5×10^5 cells/well), pre-treated with GTX (5 μM) for 8 h and then treated with PTX (100 nM) for an additional 48 h. For comparison, untreated control cells were cultured with media in the presence of DMSO. Total protein was subjected to Western blot analysis with the indicated antibodies. The cells treated with GTX followed by PTX upregulated the expression of DAPK1 and TAp63. β-actin served as an internal control. (**C**,**D**) Cells were transfected with either empty vector pcDNA3.1 or TAp63 expression vector. (**C**) Transfection efficiency was determined by immunoblot using TAp63 and FLAG antibodies. Whole cell lysates were analyzed by Western blotting using the indicated antibodies. Overexpression of TAp63 downregulated the levels of MDR1 and MRP1-3. (**D**) Percentages of apoptotic cells were analyzed by annexin-V/7-AAD staining. The number of late-stage apoptotic cells (annexin-V^+/7-AAD^+) was calculated by flow cytometry. (**E**,**F**) Cells (1.5×10^5/well) were pre-treated with GTX (5 μM) for 8 h and then treated with PTX (100 nM) for an additional 24 h. Then, the cells were transfected with 200 nM siRNA against TAp63 or control. Cells were used for further experiments 40 h after transfection. The cells were analyzed by Western blotting with the indicated antibodies. Targeted inhibition of TAp63 suppressed the expression of autophagosome-related LC3-I/II and Beclin-1 (E) and prevented the upregulation of activated caspase-9 (active p37/35) and caspase-3 (active p19/17) for apoptotic death (**F**). β-actin served as an internal control. The results are representative of three independent experiments.

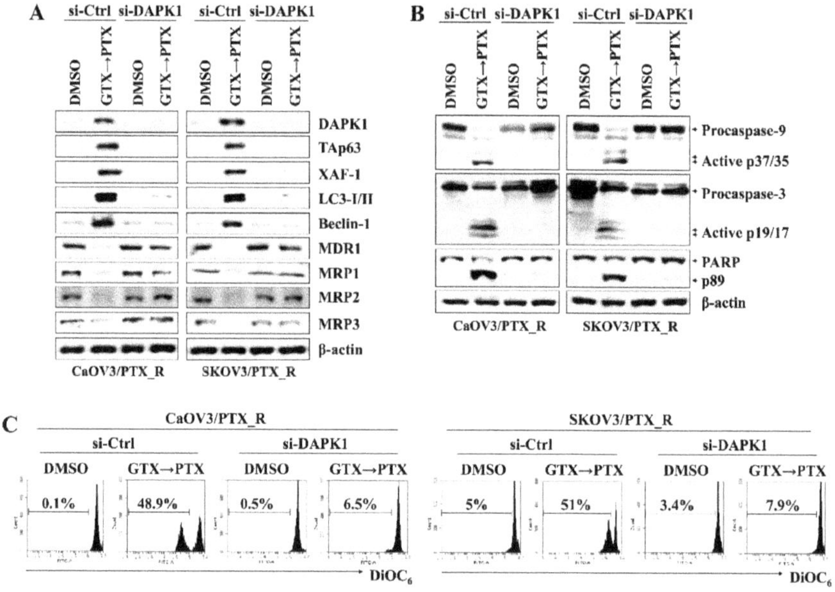

Figure 4. Increased DAPK1 induced by pre-exposure to gliotoxin and paclitaxel upregulates TAp63 expression and autophagy signaling in drug-resistant ovarian cancer cells. The cells (1.5×10^5/well) were pre-treated with GTX (5 μM) for 8 h and then treated with PTX (100 nM) for an additional 24 h. Next, cells were transfected with 200 nM siRNA against TAp63 or control. Cells were used for further experiments 40 h after transfection. (**A**,**B**) The cells were analyzed by Western blotting with the indicated antibodies. DAPK1 silencing prevented the activation of downstream target molecules, including transcriptionally active p63 (TAp63), XIAP-associated factor 1 (XAF-1), LC3-I/II, and Beclin-1 as well as the cleavage of caspase-9 (active p37/35) and caspase-3 (active p19/17) by treatment with gliotoxin followed by paclitaxel. β-actin served as an internal control. (**C**) To measure $\Delta\psi_m$ disruption, cells were stained with DiOC6 and analyzed by flow cytometry. Diminished $DiOC_6$ fluorescence (%) indicates $\Delta\psi_m$ disruption. The results are representative of three independent experiments.

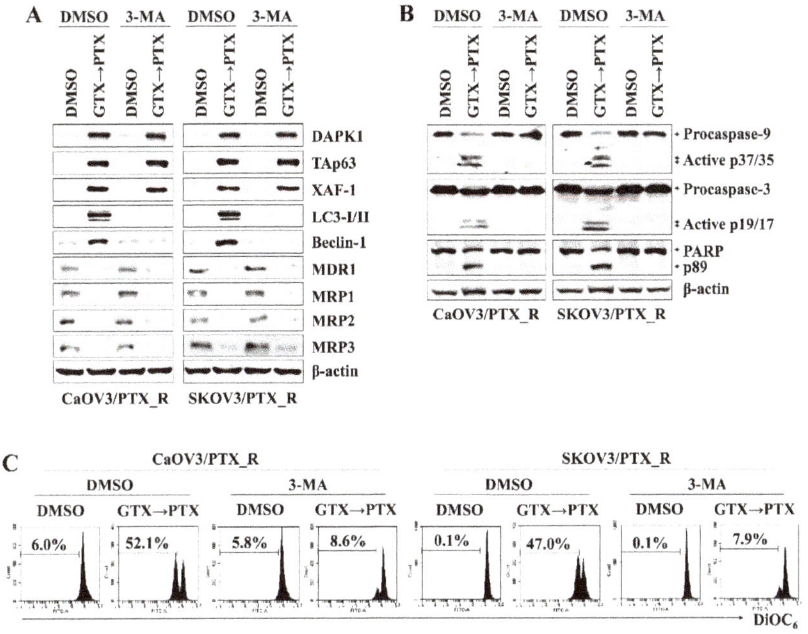

Figure 5. DAPK1/TAp63-mediated autophagy induction mediates apoptotic death in drug-resistant ovarian cancer cells after continuous treatment with gliotoxin and paclitaxel. (**A**–**C**) To inhibit autophagic signaling, cells (1.5 × 10^5/well) were pre-exposed to 3-methyladenine (3-MA) (10 mM) for 2 h. Cells were pre-treated with GTX (5 μM) for 8 h and then treated with PTX (100 nM) for an additional 48 h. For comparison, untreated control cells were cultured with media in the presence of DMSO. (**A**,**B**) Whole cell lysates were subjected to Western blot analysis using the indicated antibodies. Pretreatment with 3-MA effective prevented the expression of autophagosome-related proteins (LC3-I/II and Beclin-1) and cleaved form of caspase-9 (active p37/35) and caspase-3 (active p19/17), but had no effect on downregulation of MDR-1 and MRP1-3 after treatment with gliotoxin followed by paclitaxel. β-actin served as an internal control. (**C**) To measure $\Delta\psi_m$ disruption, cells were stained with $DiOC_6$ and analyzed by flow cytometry. Diminished $DiOC_6$ fluorescence (%) indicates $\Delta\psi_m$ disruption. The results are representative of three independent experiments.

3. Discussion

The tumor suppressor p53 promotes autophagy by inducing various autophagy-related genes, including DAPK1, a kinase acting in the early steps of autophagy [14,34]. DAPK1 overexpression also promotes the activation of cell death-associated signaling pathways, including autophagy-related apoptosis [1]. However, DAPK1 expression is frequently downregulated in B cell lymphoma and non-small cell lung cancer through multiple mechanisms, including promoter methylation [35,36]. TAp63, a p53 family member sharing a transactivation domain, has been reported to regulate the same target genes [19,20]. TAp63 not only inhibits cell growth but also prevents cell cycle progression in p53-deficient cancer cells [37]. These reports demonstrate that DAPK1 plays an important role in apoptosis induced by cytotoxic drug treatment and that the TAp63 and/or DAPK-related signaling pathways are promising candidates for controlling cancer growth in certain tumor environments. In this study, treatment with gliotoxin reversed the paclitaxel resistance of drug-resistant ovarian cancer cells through the downregulation of multidrug resistant-associated proteins. In addition, sequential treatment with gliotoxin followed by paclitaxel activated the DAPK1-mediated TAp63 signaling pathway to induce autophagic cell death in paclitaxel-resistant ovarian cancer cells (Figure 6). These results suggest that monitoring TAp63 and DAPK1 expression level is critical for detecting paclitaxel resistance and deciding whether to use paclitaxel in advanced or recurrent ovarian cancer patients.

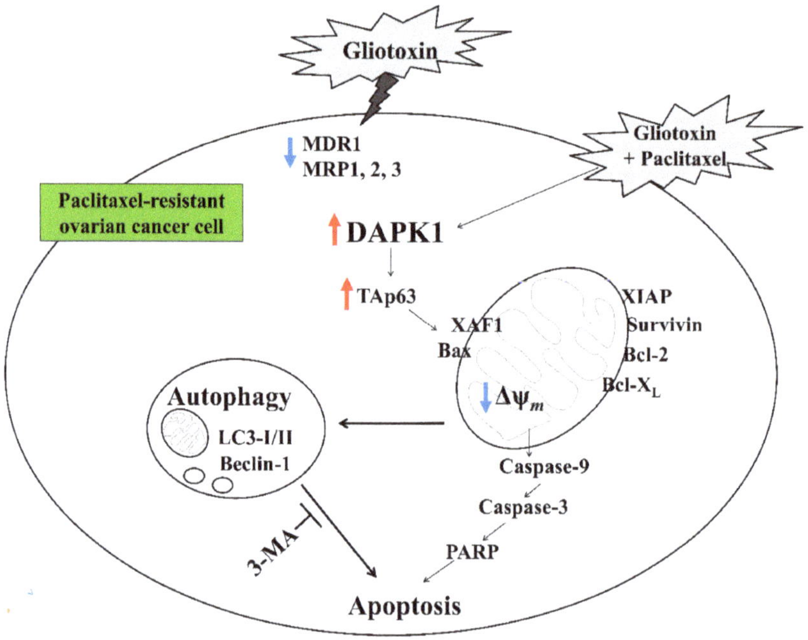

Figure 6. Schematic diagram of the intracellular signaling mechanism after sequential treatment with gliotoxin followed by paclitaxel in human ovarian cancer cells.

DAPK1 activation by cell death-inducing stimuli promotes apoptosis through the activation of p53-dependent p14/p19ARF tumor suppressor genes [5]. DAPK1 overexpression activated autophagic apoptotic death in a caspase-independent manner in breast and cervical cancer cells expressing wild-type p53 [9]. In contrast, stimulation with TGF-beta resulted in DAPK1-induced mitochondrial damage, leading to caspase-dependent apoptosis in a p53-depleted hepatoma cell line [38]. These contradictory results demonstrate that the role of DAPK1 might require further study to understand the connection with p53 or p53 family proteins in the apoptosis pathway. Although treating CaOV3 and SKOV3 cells with paclitaxel increased p53 expression, sequential exposure to gliotoxin followed by paclitaxel upregulated the levels of DAPK1 and TAp63 but not p53 and TAp73 expression in CaOV3/PTX_R and SKOV3/PTX_R cells. Furthermore, gene silencing of DAPK1 using siRNA in CaOV3/PTX_R and SKOV3/PTX_R cells prevented autophagy induction, caspase activation, and mitochondrial membrane disruption, as well as TAp63 activation. These results suggest that DAPK1 contributes to TAp63 activation to induce autophagic cell death in paclitaxel-resistant ovarian cancer cells after consecutive treatment with gliotoxin and paclitaxel. However, the precise association based on the molecular mechanism of DAPK1 and TAp63 in various cancer environments still needs to be investigated.

Cells that survive previous chemotherapy obtain resistance to several anticancer drugs through their development of various defense mechanisms, including promoting drug efflux capability, altering drug metabolism, and changing drug targets [39]. Inactivation of p53 or mutant p53 in cancer cells decreases drug accumulation through the upregulation of multidrug-resistance protein (MRP1), which mediates ATP-dependent drug efflux [40]. Although exposure to gliotoxin induces mitochondrial membrane disruption and p53-dependent apoptotic cell death in adriamycin-resistant non-small cell lung cancer cells [33], the acquired mechanism to overcome the cytotoxic effects of chemotherapeutic drugs might be very diverse in cell type- or tumor environmental-dependent manners. In addition, the contribution of other p53 family proteins in the absence of wild-type p53 to overcome anticancer drugs is still unclear. Sequential treatment with gliotoxin, followed by paclitaxel increased the level of TAp63 in paclitaxel-resistant ovarian cancer cells. Furthermore, forced expression of TAp63 by transfection with a TAp63-containing plasmid reduced the expression of multidrug resistant-associated proteins (MDR1 and MRP1-3). These results suggest that TAp63 also plays an important role in modulating drug resistance without wild-type p53.

Although pre-exposure to 3-MA before sequential treatment efficiently blocked cleaved caspase-9, caspase-3, and PARP generation and prevented mitochondrial membrane disruption, pretreatment with 3-MA still inhibited multidrug resistant-associated protein levels but failed to attenuate DAPK1-TAp63 signaling pathway activation. These results suggest that the DAPK1-TAp63 pathway controls autophagy induction and drug-resistant protein expression in an independent manner to promote the apoptotic pathway after sequential treatment with gliotoxin, followed by paclitaxel (Figure 6).

Taken together, our results suggest that gliotoxin might be a promising agent to control advanced or recurrent ovarian cancer in clinical situations by reducing paclitaxel resistance. Our data also demonstrate that DAPK1 and TAp63 levels could be used as diagnostic or determining factors of drug resistance before starting repeated chemotherapy against ovarian cancer.

4. Materials and Methods

4.1. Cell Lines and Reagents

Human ovarian cancer cell lines CaOV3 and SKOV3 (American Type Culture Collection (ATCC), Manassas, VA, USA) were used in this study. These cells were cultured in DMEM and McCoy's 5A (Corning Incorporated, Corning, NY, USA) with 10% FBS (RMBIO, Missoula, MT, USA), glutamine, and antibiotics and maintained at 37 °C under 5% CO2. Gliotoxin (GTX) and 3-methyladenine (3-MA) were obtained from TOCRIS (Bristol, UK). Paclitaxel (PTX) was purchased from Sigma-Aldrich (St. Louis, MO, USA). Paclitaxel-resistant sublines (CaOV3/PTX_R and SKOV3/PTX_R) were established in the paclitaxel-sensitive (PTX_S) parent cell lines CaOV3 and SKOV3, respectively, by sequential exposure of cells to increasing concentrations of PTX 2.5 ~ 100 nM over 6 months. Finally, the authenticity of the drug-resistant sublines was confirmed by the ATCC Standards Development Organization (SDO) through short tandem repeat profiling in accordance with the American National Standards Institute (ANSI) Standard (ASN-0002).

4.2. Proliferation Assay with Cell Counting Kit-8

Cell proliferation was measured using a Cell Counting Kit-8 (CCK-8) (Enzo Life Sciences, Farmingdale, NY, USA) as described in the supplier's protocol. Cells were seeded into 96-well plates (1×10^4 cells/well) and pre-treated with GTX (5 μM) for 8 h and then treated with PTX (100 nM) for an additional 48 h. For comparison, non-treated control cells were cultured with media in the presence of DMSO. After drug treatment, the cells were stained with 10 μL of CCK-8 dye in 90 μL of culture medium for 2 h at 37 °C. The absorbance was measured at 450 nm.

4.3. Analysis of Apoptosis by Flow Cytometry

The percentages of cells undergoing apoptosis were measured by flow cytometry with fluorescein isothiocyanate (FITC)-labeled annexin-V (BD Biosciences, San Diego, CA, USA) and 7-amino actinomycin D (7-AAD) (BD Biosciences). The cells were suspended in 100 μL of 1× annexin-V binding buffer; then, FITC-conjugated annexin-V (3 μL) and 7-AAD (3 μL) were added to the suspensions, and the cells were kept at room temperature for 15 min in the dark. The stained cells were monitored with a BD Accuri™ C6 (BD Biosciences).

4.4. Measurement of Mitochondria Membrane Potential ($\Delta\psi_m$)

Changes in mitochondrial membrane potential were determined using $DiOC_6$ (3,3′-dihexyloxacarbocyanine iodide; Molecular Probes, Eugene, OR). Cells were seeded into 96-well plates (1×10^4 cells/well), pre-treated with GTX (5 μM) for 8 h, and then treated with PTX (100 nM) for an additional 48 h. Cells were harvested, washed twice with PBS, resuspended in PBS supplemented with $DiOC_6$ (20 nM), incubated in the dark at 37 °C for 15 min, and analyzed immediately using a flow cytometer with an FL-1 filter.

4.5. Western Blot Analysis

Harvested cells were lysed with RIPA buffer (Elpis Biotech, Daejeon, Korea) supplemented with a protease inhibitor cocktail and phosphatase inhibitors (Sigma-Aldrich). Equal amounts of protein (10 μg/sample) determined with a BCA assay kit (Pierce, Rockford, IL, USA) were subsequently loaded onto SDS-PAGE gels. After electrophoresis, the proteins were transferred onto nitrocellulose membranes (Millipore Corp., Billerica, MA, USA). The membranes were blocked with 5% non-fat skim milk and probed with primary antibodies. The expression level of target proteins was determined using a chemiluminescence kit (Advansta Corp., Menlo Park, CA, USA) and an Amersham Imager 600 (GE Healthcare Life Sciences, Little Chalfont, UK). The expression levels of β-actin were used as a control.

4.6. Small Interfering RNA (siRNA) Transfection

Human TAp63-siRNA (5′-GCA CAC AGA CAA AUG AAU UUU-3′), human DAPK1-siRNA (5′-CAA CTA TGA TGT TAA CCA A-3′), and negative control-siRNA (Cat. No. SN-1001-CFG) were obtained from Bioneer (Daejeon, Korea). Cells were seeded at a density of 1.5×10^5 per well in a 6-well plate and grown overnight. The cells were then transfected with 200 nM siRNA using Lipofectamine RNAiMAX Reagent (Invitrogen, Carlsbad, CA, USA) as described in the supplier's protocol. The cells were used for further experiments at 48 h after transfection.

4.7. TAp63 Overexpression Using Transient Transfection

Transient transfection of cultured cells was performed using Lipofectamine 2000 as described in the supplier's instructions. Cells were plated on 6-well culture plates at a density of 2×10^5 cells/well and transfected the next day. Typically, 10 ng of construct DNA was transfected with 9 μL of Lipofectamine. The cultured cells were transiently transfected with either a TAp63 expression vector of TAp63 cDNA cloned into pcDNA3.1 (Addgene, Cambridge, MA, USA) or empty vector pcDNA3.1 (Invitrogen). Cells were transfected for 48 h and analyzed by Western blotting.

4.8. Statistical Analysis

Student's *t*-test and one-way analysis of variance (ANOVA) using SPSS version 24.0 statistical software (IBM Corp., Armonk, NY, USA) were used for all statistical analyses. The data are presented as the mean ± standard deviation (SD). Differences were determined to be statistically significant at $p < 0.05$ and highly significant at $p < 0.001$.

Supplementary Materials: The following are available online at http://www.mdpi.com/1660-3397/17/7/412/s1, Figure S1: Establishment of paclitaxel-resistant ovarian cancer cells, Figure S2: Effect of GTX treatment on autophagy and the Bcl-2 family in PTX-resistant ovarian cancer cells.

Author Contributions: G.-B.P. carried out all of the experiments and analyses in this study. D.K. contributed to the conception and design of the study and wrote the manuscript. G.-B.P. and D.K. elaborated study design, coordinated the research. J.-Y.J. critically reviewed and revised the manuscript.

Funding: This work was supported by the National Research Foundation of Korea (NRF) grant funded by the Korea government (Ministry of Science and ICT, MIST) (NRF-2018R1C1B6002381) and Basic Science Research Program through the National Research Foundation of Korea (NRF) funded by the Ministry of Education (NRF-2018R1D1A1B07040382).

Conflicts of Interest: The authors declare that they have no competing interest.

References

1. Bialik, S.; Kimchi, A. The death-associated protein kinases: Structure, function, and beyond. *Annu. Rev. Biochem.* **2006**, *75*, 189–210. [CrossRef] [PubMed]
2. Sanchez-Cespedes, M.; Esteller, M.; Wu, L.; Nawroz-Danish, H.; Yoo, G.H.; Koch, W.M.; Jen, J.; Herman, J.G.; Sidransky, D. Gene promoter hypermethylation in tumors and serum of head and neck cancer patients. *Cancer Res.* **2000**, *60*, 892–895. [PubMed]
3. Kim, D.H.; Nelson, H.H.; Wiencke, J.K.; Christiani, D.C.; Wain, J.C.; Mark, E.J.; Kelsey, K.T. Promoter methylation of DAP-kinase: Association with advanced stage in non-small cell lung cancer. *Oncogene* **2001**, *20*, 1765–1770. [CrossRef] [PubMed]
4. Dansranjavin, T.; Möbius, C.; Tannapfel, A.; Bartels, M.; Wittekind, C.; Hauss, J.; Witzigmann, H. E-cadherin and DAP kinase in pancreatic adenocarcinoma and corresponding lymph node metastases. *Oncol. Rep.* **2006**, *15*, 1125–1131. [CrossRef] [PubMed]
5. Raveh, T.; Droguett, G.; Horwitz, M.S.; DePinho, R.A.; Kimchi, A. DAP kinase activates a p19ARF/p53-mediated apoptotic checkpoint to suppress oncogenic transformation. *Nat. Cell Biol.* **2001**, *3*, 1–7. [CrossRef] [PubMed]
6. Yoo, H.J.; Byun, H.J.; Kim, B.R.; Lee, K.H.; Park, S.Y.; Rho, S.B. DAPk1 inhibits NF-κB activation through TNF-α and INF-γ-induced apoptosis. *Cell Signal.* **2012**, *24*, 1471–1477. [CrossRef] [PubMed]
7. Wu, B.; Yao, H.; Wang, S.; Xu, R. DAPK1 modulates a curcumin-induced G2/M arrest and apoptosis by regulating STAT3, NF-κB, and caspase-3 activation. *Biochem. Biophys. Res. Commun.* **2013**, *434*, 75–80. [CrossRef] [PubMed]
8. Zalckvar, E.; Berissi, H.; Eisenstein, M.; Kimchi, A. Phosphorylation of Beclin 1 by DAP-kinase promotes autophagy by weakening its interactions with Bcl-2 and Bcl-XL. *Autophagy* **2009**, *5*, 720–722. [CrossRef]
9. Inbal, B.; Bialik, S.; Sabanay, I.; Shani, G.; Kimchi, A. DAP kinase and DRP-1 mediate membrane blebbing and the formation of autophagic vesicles during programmed cell death. *J. Cell Biol.* **2002**, *157*, 455–468. [CrossRef]
10. Jin, Y.; Gallagher, P.J. Antisense depletion of death-associated protein kinase promotes apoptosis. *J. Biol. Chem.* **2003**, *278*, 51587–51593. [CrossRef]
11. Zhao, J.; Zhao, D.; Poage, G.M.; Mazumdar, A.; Zhang, Y.; Hill, J.L.; Hartman, Z.C.; Savage, M.I.; Mills, G.B.; Brown, P.H. Death-associated protein kinase 1 promotes growth of p53-mutant cancers. *J. Clin. Investig.* **2015**, *125*, 2707–2720. [CrossRef] [PubMed]
12. Brady, C.A.; Jiang, D.; Mello, S.S.; Johnson, T.M.; Jarvis, L.A.; Kozak, M.M.; Kenzelmann Broz, D.; Basak, S.; Park, E.J.; McLaughlin, M.E.; et al. Distinct p53 transcriptional programs dictate acute DNA-damage responses and tumor suppression. *Cell* **2011**, *145*, 571–583. [CrossRef] [PubMed]
13. Itahana, Y.; Itahana, K. Emerging Roles of p53 Family Members in Glucose Metabolism. *Int. J. Mol. Sci.* **2018**, *19*, 776. [CrossRef] [PubMed]
14. Martoriati, A.; Doumont, G.; Alcalay, M.; Bellefroid, E.; Pelicci, P.G.; Marine, J.C. dapk1, encoding an activator of a p19ARF-p53-mediated apoptotic checkpoint, is a transcription target of p53. *Oncogene* **2005**, *24*, 1461–1466. [CrossRef] [PubMed]
15. Marin, J.J.; Romero, M.R.; Martinez-Becerra, P.; Herraez, E.; Briz, O. Overview of the molecular bases of resistance to chemotherapy in liver and gastrointestinal tumours. *Curr. Mol. Med.* **2009**, *9*, 1108–1129. [CrossRef] [PubMed]
16. Hientz, K.; Mohr, A.; Bhakta-Guha, D.; Efferth, T. The role of p53 in cancer drug resistance and targeted chemotherapy. *Oncotarget* **2017**, *8*, 8921–8946. [CrossRef] [PubMed]
17. Debernardis, D.; Siré, E.G.; De Feudis, P.; Vikhanskaya, F.; Valenti, M.; Russo, P.; Parodi, S.; D'Incalci, M.; Broggini, M. p53 status does not affect sensitivity of human ovarian cancer cell lines to paclitaxel. *Cancer Res.* **1997**, *57*, 870–874. [PubMed]
18. Petty, R.; Evans, A.; Duncan, I.; Kurbacher, C.; Cree, I. Drug resistance in ovarian cancer—The role of p53. *Pathol. Oncol. Res.* **1998**, *4*, 97–102. [CrossRef] [PubMed]
19. Wei, J.; Zaika, E.; Zaika, A. p53 Family: Role of Protein Isoforms in Human Cancer. *J. Nucleic Acids* **2012**, *2012*, 687359. [CrossRef]

20. Dötsch, V.; Bernassola, F.; Coutandin, D.; Candi, E.; Melino, G. p63 and p73, the ancestors of p53. *Cold Spring Harb. Perspect. Biol.* **2010**, *2*, a004887. [CrossRef]
21. Su, X.; Gi, Y.J.; Chakravarti, D.; Chan, I.L.; Zhang, A.; Xia, X.; Tsai, K.Y.; Flores, E.R. TAp63 is a master transcriptional regulator of lipid and glucose metabolism. *Cell Metab.* **2012**, *16*, 511–525. [CrossRef] [PubMed]
22. Flores, E.R.; Sengupta, S.; Miller, J.B.; Newman, J.J.; Bronson, R.; Crowley, D.; Yang, A.; McKeon, F.; Jacks, T. Tumor predisposition in mice mutant for p63 and p73: Evidence for broader tumor suppressor functions for the p53 family. *Cancer Cell* **2005**, *7*, 363–373. [CrossRef] [PubMed]
23. Su, X.; Chakravarti, D.; Cho, M.S.; Liu, L.; Gi, Y.J.; Lin, Y.L.; Leung, M.L.; El-Naggar, A.; Creighton, C.J.; Suraokar, M.B.; et al. TAp63 suppresses metastasis through coordinate regulation of Dicer and miRNAs. *Nature* **2010**, *467*, 986–990. [CrossRef] [PubMed]
24. Park, G.B.; Kim, Y.S.; Lee, H.K.; Yang, J.W.; Kim, D.; Hur, D.Y. ASK1/JNK-mediated TAp63 activation controls the cell survival signal of baicalein-treated EBV-transformed B cells. *Mol. Cell. Biochem.* **2016**, *412*, 247–258. [CrossRef] [PubMed]
25. Park, G.B.; Chung, Y.H.; Gong, J.H.; Jin, D.H.; Kim, D. GSK-3β-mediated fatty acid synthesis enhances epithelial to mesenchymal transition of TLR4-activated colorectal cancer cells through regulation of TAp63. *Int. J. Oncol.* **2016**, *49*, 2163–2172. [CrossRef]
26. Waring, P.; Sjaarda, A.; Lin, Q.H. Gliotoxin inactivates alcohol dehydrogenase by either covalent modification or free radical damage mediated by redox cycling. *Biochem. Pharmacol.* **1995**, *49*, 1195–1201. [CrossRef]
27. Gardiner, D.M.; Waring, P.; Howlett, B.J. The epipolythiodioxopiperazine (ETP) class of fungal toxins: Distribution, mode of action, functions and biosynthesis. *Microbiology* **2005**, *151*, 1021–1032. [CrossRef]
28. López-Franco, O.; Suzuki, Y.; Sanjuán, G.; Blanco, J.; Hernández-Vargas, P.; Yo, Y.; Kopp, J.; Egido, J.; Gómez-Guerrero, C. Nuclear factor-kappa B inhibitors as potential novel anti-inflammatory agents for the treatment of immune glomerulonephritis. *Am. J. Pathol.* **2002**, *161*, 1497–1505. [CrossRef]
29. Kim, Y.S.; Park, S.J. Gliotoxin from the marine fungus Aspergillus fumigatus induces apoptosis in HT1080 fibrosarcoma cells by downregulating NF-κB. *Fish. Aquat. Sci.* **2016**, *19*, 35. [CrossRef]
30. Nguyen, V.T.; Lee, J.S.; Qian, Z.J.; Li, Y.X.; Kim, K.N.; Heo, S.J.; Jeon, Y.J.; Park, W.S.; Choi, I.W.; Je, J.Y.; et al. Gliotoxin isolated from marine fungus Aspergillus sp. Induces apoptosis of human cervical cancer and chondrosarcoma cells. *Mar. Drugs* **2013**, *12*, 69–87. [CrossRef]
31. Hubmann, R.; Hilgarth, M.; Schnabl, S.; Ponath, E.; Reiter, M.; Demirtas, D.; Sieghart, W.; Valent, P.; Zielinski, C.; Jäger, U.; et al. Gliotoxin is a potent NOTCH2 transactivation inhibitor and efficiently induces apoptosis in chronic lymphocytic leukaemia (CLL) cells. *Br. J. Haematol.* **2013**, *160*, 618–629. [CrossRef] [PubMed]
32. Pan, X.Q.; Harday, J. Electromicroscopic observations on gliotoxin-induced apoptosis of cancer cells in culture and human cancer xenografts in transplanted SCID mice. *In Vivo* **2007**, *21*, 259–265. [PubMed]
33. Manh Hung, L.V.; Song, Y.W.; Cho, S.K. Effects of the Combination of Gliotoxin and Adriamycin on the Adriamycin-Resistant Non-Small-Cell Lung Cancer A549 Cell Line. *Mar. Drugs* **2018**, *16*, 105. [CrossRef] [PubMed]
34. Harrison, B.; Kraus, M.; Burch, L.; Stevens, C.; Craig, A.; Gordon-Weeks, P.; Hupp, T.R. DAPK-1 binding to a linear peptide motif in MAP1B stimulates autophagy and membrane blebbing. *J. Biol. Chem.* **2008**, *283*, 9999–10014. [CrossRef] [PubMed]
35. Katzenellenbogen, R.A.; Baylin, S.B.; Herman, J.G. Hypermethylation of the DAP-kinase CpG island is a common alteration in B-cell malignancies. *Blood* **1999**, *93*, 4347–4353. [PubMed]
36. Esteller, M.; Sanchez-Cespedes, M.; Rosell, R.; Sidransky, D.; Baylin, S.B.; Herman, J.G. Detection of aberrant promoter hypermethylation of tumor suppressor genes in serum DNA from non-small cell lung cancer patients. *Cancer Res.* **1999**, *59*, 67–70. [PubMed]
37. Yao, J.Y.; Chen, J.K. TAp63 plays compensatory roles in p53-deficient cancer cells under genotoxic stress. *Biochem. Biophys. Res. Commun.* **2010**, *403*, 310–315. [CrossRef] [PubMed]
38. Jang, C.W.; Chen, C.H.; Chen, C.C.; Chen, J.Y.; Su, Y.H.; Chen, R.H. TGF-beta induces apoptosis through Smad-mediated expression of DAP-kinase. *Nat. Cell Biol.* **2002**, *4*, 51–58. [CrossRef]

39. Housman, G.; Byler, S.; Heerboth, S.; Lapinska, K.; Longacre, M.; Snyder, N.; Sarkar, S. Drug resistance in cancer: An overview. *Cancers* **2014**, *6*, 1769–1792. [CrossRef]
40. Sullivan, G.F.; Yang, J.M.; Vassil, A.; Yang, J.; Bash-Babula, J.; Hait, W.N. Regulation of expression of the multidrug resistance protein MRP1 by p53 in human prostate cancer cells. *J. Clin. Investig.* **2000**, *105*, 1261–1267. [CrossRef]

marine drugs

MDPI

Article

Marine Bacterium *Vibrio* sp. CB1-14 Produces Guanidine Alkaloid 6-*epi*-Monanchorin, Previously Isolated from Marine Polychaete and Sponges

Tatyana Makarieva *, Larisa Shubina, Valeria Kurilenko, Marina Isaeva, Nadezhda Chernysheva, Roman Popov, Evgeniya Bystritskaya, Pavel Dmitrenok and Valentin Stonik

G.B. Elyakov Pacific Institute of Bioorganic Chemistry (PIBOC), Russian Academy of Sciences, Prospect 100 let Vladivostoku, 159, 690022 Vladivostok, Russia; shubina@piboc.dvo.ru (L.S.); valerie@piboc.dvo.ru (V.K.); issaeva@piboc.dvo.ru (M.I.); chernysheva.nadezhda@gmail.com (N.C.); prs_90@mail.ru (R.P.); belyjane@gmail.com (E.B.); paveldmt@piboc.dvo.ru (P.D.); stonik@piboc.dvo.ru (V.S.)

* Correspondence: makarieva@piboc.dvo.ru; Tel.: +7-950-295-66-25

Received: 6 February 2019; Accepted: 2 April 2019; Published: 4 April 2019

Abstract: Twenty-three bacterial strains were isolated from the secreted mucus trapping net of the marine polychaete *Chaetopterus variopedatus* (phylum Annelida) and twenty strains were identified using 16S rRNA gene analysis. Strain CB1-14 was recognized as a new species of the genus *Vibrio* using the eight-gene multilocus sequence analysis (MLSA) and genome sequences of nineteen type *Vibrio* strains. This *Vibrio* sp. was cultured, and 6-*epi*-monanchorin (**2**), previously isolated from the polychaete and two sponge species, was found in the cells and culture broth. The presence of the 6-*epi*-monanchorin was confirmed by its isolation followed by ^{1}H NMR and HRESIMS analysis. These results showed the microbial origin of the bicyclic guanidine alkaloid **2** in *C. variopedatus*.

Keywords: guanidine alkaloids; 6-*epi*-monanchorin; HRESI MS; ^{1}H NMR spectra; marine bacteria; *Vibrio* sp.; polychaete; *Chaetopterus variopedatus*; 16S rRNA gene analysis; phylogenetic reconstruction

1. Introduction

Various guanidine-containing natural products, isolated from different marine invertebrates, demonstrate antifungal, antibacterial, antiviral, and antitumor properties [1] and are suitable compounds for drug development due to high levels of their bioactivities and water solubility. Moreover, some natural guanidine-containing compounds, such as streptomycin, have already been introduced in the clinic.

Most of the marine guanidine alkaloids found in marine sponges are polycyclic, and two bicyclic representatives of this group, namely monanchorin (**1**) and 6-*epi*-monanchorin (**2**), are known. These compounds were isolated from representatives of two phylogenetically distant taxa, namely marine sponges *Monanchora ungiculata* and *Halichondria panicea* (phylum Porifera) [2,3], and marine polychaete *Chaetopterus variopedatus* (phylum Annelida) [4]. Previously it has been reported that the compound **1** shows weak cytotoxic activity against IC2 murine mast cells [2], while compounds **1** and **2** (Figure 1) are able to inhibit the migration and colony formation of cisplatin-resistant cancer NCCIT-R cells [4].

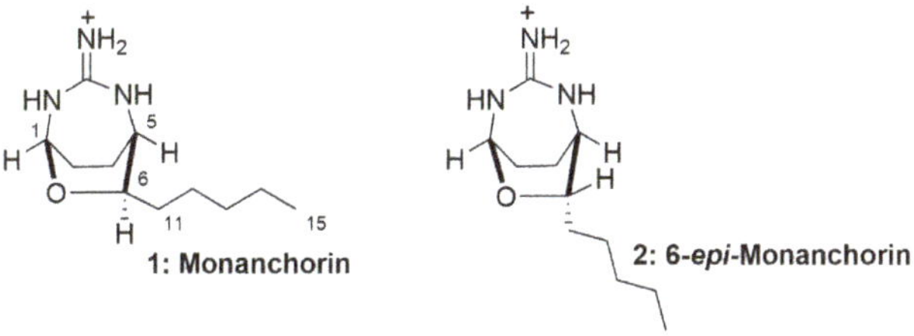

Figure 1. Structures of natural compounds **1** and **2**.

The presence of the alkaloids **1** and **2** in such different taxa could indicate that a common unidentified marine microorganism(s), accumulated in both sponges and the polychaete is a genuine producer of these secondary metabolites of unknown biogenesis. Really, the presence of the same secondary metabolites in distantly related animal taxa sometimes point to potential symbiotic or dietary sources of the corresponding substances. However, experimental evidences of their microbial origin were rarely obtained. Recently, we compared levels of these alkaloid content in different body parts of the polychaete *C. variopedatus* [5,6]. Both alkaloids were predominant into the food net parts of the animals and the content of 6-epi-monanchorin (**2**) was very high (5.0% of dry weight) [4]. These findings prompted us to undertake the present study. We have tried to identify the biogenetic origin of the above mentioned polychaete metabolites.

2. Results and Discussion

2.1. Isolation of Microorganisms

The secreted mucous net of the polychaete was pre-rinsed in sterile sea water. Pieces of tissue were aseptically removed and homogenized in sterile sea water. Bacterial strains were isolated by plating samples of tissue homogenates onto medium plates containing the modified MN medium [7]. The plates were incubated aerobically at 20 °C for 7 days. The bacterial colonies that grew on the Difco^{TM}Marine Agar 2216 Becton, Dickinson and Company (BD) with that medium were picked up and classified morphologically and biochemically. Twenty-three bacterial strains were isolated in pure cultures and then analyzed by MALDI MS.

2.2. Preliminary Identification of Potential Microorganism-Producers by Monitoring of the Compounds Giving Ion Peaks at m/z 212.17 by MALDI MS, Characteristic of 1 and 2 MS

A preliminary screening procedure was carried out using Ultrafex III MALDI TOF/TOF mass spectrometer and Biotyper Software (Bruker Daltonics) to select isolates for further analyses. Sample preparation was carried out by "direct transfer" procedure (Ver. 2.0 Biotyper). Spectra were calibrated with external calibration by *Eschercihia coli* DH5 alpha standard and protein calibration standard I (Bruker Daltonics). The majority of identified bacterial strains were represented by *Vibrio* spp. and, thus, *Vibrio* was the dominant group of bacteria cultured from the mucous net of this polychaete. The occurrence of the compounds with a peak at *m/z* 212.17 in MALDI MS, presumably corresponding to 6-*epi*-monanchorin or monanchorin (**2** or **1**), are shown in the Table 1. In total there were eleven promising strains found, seven of which were identified as *Vibrio* spp. and gave this ion peak in MS. It should be noted that the data obtained by this method should be considered as preliminary and did not allow accurate identification, neither microorganisms nor target compounds.

Table 1. Taxonomic position of microorganism-producers and occurrence of compounds with *m/z* 212.17 ion peak by MALDI MS data.

No	Strain	Taxon	*m/z* 212.17 *	No	Strain	Taxon	*m/z* 212.17
1	CB1-3	nd	nd	13	CB2-3	nd	nd
2	CB1-5	nd	nd	14	CB2-4	*Vibrio* sp.	nd
3	CB1-6	nd	nd	15	CB2-5	Vibrio sp.	nd
4	CB-1-7	*Vibrio* sp.	nd	16	CB2-6	Vibrio sp.	+
5	CB1-8	nd	nd	17	CB2-7	nd	ad
6	CB1-9	nd	ad	18	CB2-8	*Vibrio* sp.	ad
7	CB1-10	*Vibrio* sp.	ad	19	CB2-9	*Vibrio* sp.	ad
8	CB1-11	*Vibrio* sp.	ad	20	CB2-10	nd	ad
9	CB1-12	nd	nd	21	CB2-11	*Vibrio* sp.	+
10	CB1-13	nd	nd	22	CB2-12	*Vibrio* sp.	ad
11	CB1-14	nd	+	23	CB2-13	nd	nd
12	CB2-1	*Vibrio* sp.	nd				

nd, not detected; ad, ambiguous detected; +, detected.

2.3. *Identification of Compounds **1** or **2** by HRESIMS*

The authentic identification of compounds **1** and **2** into the three promising strains such as CB1-14, CB2-11, and CB2-6 (see Table 1) was carried out after isolation of these compounds by HPLC followed by analysis with HRESIMS. The strains were incubated at 200 rpm in 100 mL of modified MN liquid medium at 28 °C for 7 days. After incubation, the whole cultures were centrifuged to harvest the bacterial cells. Then cells were suspended in water (30 ml), frozen, and subjected to ultrasonic treatment. The suspension was extracted with EtOAc, and the organic phase was evaporated to dryness. The resulting mixture was dissolved in a small amount of EtOH, and extracts were subjected to HPLC on ODS-A columns. The fractions with retention times of 12 to 17 min were collected and analyzed by HRESIMS. Compounds showing ion peak with *m/z* 212.1757 $[M + H]^+$ (calcd for $C_{11}H_{22}N_3O$, 212.1757) were isolated from strains CB1-14 and CB2-11. Strain CB1-14 showed a more intense peak at *m/z* 212.1757 compared with that for CB2-11. Their mass spectra were identical to the spectra of standards. As a result, monanchorins were identified in these two strains. However, in order to determine which of two epimeric compounds was biosynthesized by these microorganisms, it was necessary to isolate the alkaloids in amounts sufficient for the obtaining of NMR data.

2.4. *Isolation and Identification of 6-epi-Monanchorin by ^1H NMR Spectroscopy*

The strain CB1-14 was chosen for preparative isolation of target compounds. After incubation of 12 L medium at 28 °C for 7 days, the culture broth of *Vibrio* sp. strain CB1-14 was separated from cells by centrifugation. The 6-*epi*-monanchorin (**2**, Figure 1) was isolated from the EtOAc extracts of both cells and lyophilized culture broth using reverse-phase HPLC. The structure was exactly identified on the basis of ^1H NMR and HRESIMS data by comparison with authentic sample [4]. As a result, it was found that the CB1-14 strain biosynthesizes 6-*epi*-monanchorin (**2**). Monanchorin itself was not found in this strain in amounts sufficient for NMR spectrum recording.

2.5. *16S rRNA Gene Sequence Analysis of Bacterial Isolates*

Twenty bacterial isolates selected for screening for compounds **1** and **2** production were identified by 16S rRNA gene analysis on the EzBiocloud server [8]. Based on the sequence comparison to reference type strains, the isolates were assigned to the two bacterial phyla (Proteobacteria and Firmicutes). Two isolates (CB1-13 and CB1-18) showed the highest similarity values with *Bacillus hwajinpoensis* SW-72^T (99.21%–99.24%) and *Bacillus hemicentroti* JSM 076093^T (98.27%). One isolate (CB1-3) shared the highest similarity value with *Pseudovibrio japonicus* WSF2^T (99.2%), *Pseudovibrio ascidiaceicola* DSM 16392^T (98.99%), and *Pseudovibrio denitrificans* DSM 17465^T (98.91%) from Alphaproteobacteria. The others were closely related to the species of the genus *Vibrio* from Gammaproteobacteria. The isolates CB1-14, CB2-10, CB2-8, and CB1-5 showed 98.96%–99.58% sequence similarity with *Vibrio hangzhouensis* CN83^{T}. The other isolates CB2-5, CB1-7, and CB2-12 had 98.79%–100% sequence similarity with *Vibrio barjaei* 3062^{T} and *Vibrio thalassae* MD16^{T}. Most of isolates (CB1-1, CB1-10, CB1-11, CB2-4, CB2-9, CB2-11, and CB2-13) shared the highest similarity values with *Vibrio mediterranei* CIP 103203^{T} (99.65%) and *Vibrio shilonii* AK1^{T} (99.59%). Three isolates (CB1-6, CB2-1 and CB2-7) showed similarity values less than 97.5% with reference type strains of the species of genus *Vibrio*.

The phylogenetic tree based on the 16S rRNA sequences (1438 bp) clearly showed that *Vibrio* isolates grouped into four clades (Figure 2), three of which included the single type strains, *V. barjaei* or *V. hangzhouensis* or *V. mediterranei*. The fourth clade was at the base of the genus *Vibrio* and did not include any type strains.

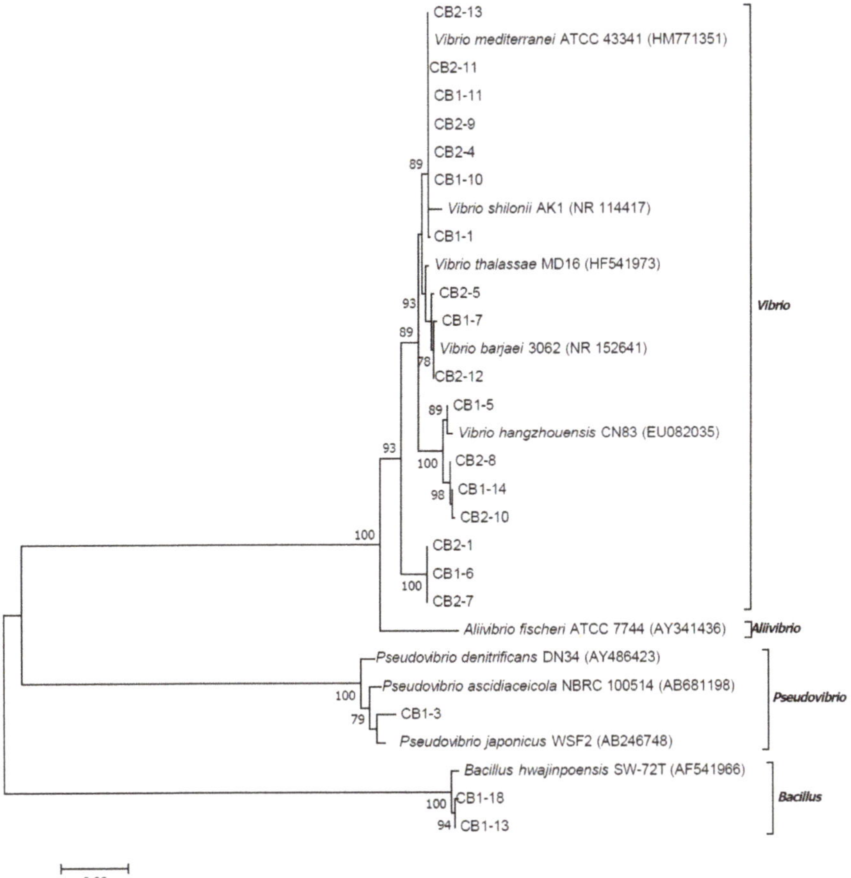

Figure 2. Bacterial phylogenetic tree on the basis of 16S rRNA gene sequences of isolates recovered from the mucus net of the *C. variopedatus* and closely related sequences of type strains. The tree topology was obtained using the maximum likelihood method based on the Tamura three-parameter model. Bootstrap values above 75% calculated from 1000 re-sampling are shown on the node. The scale bar represents the number of substitutions per site.

Guided by the cutoff value at the species level equal to 98.65% [9] and phylogenetic positions, the isolates CB1-13 and CB1-18 might be identified as *B. hwajinpoensis* and the isolate CB1-3 as *P.*

japonicus. Among *Vibrio* isolates, the isolates CB2-5, CB1-7, and CB2-12 might be identified as *V. barjaei*, the isolate CB1-5 as *V. hangzhouensis*, and the isolates CB1-1, CB1-10, CB1-11, CB2-4, CB2-9, CB2-11, and CB2-13 as *V. mediterranei*. The clades, containing CB1-14 and CB2-1, might be distinguished as candidates for new species. Thus, one of bacterial strain (CB1-14) presumably producing monanchorins was identified as *Vibrio* sp., closely related to *Vibrio hangzhouensis* CN83^{T}, but probably distinguished from this species.

Therefore, the phylogenetic analysis revealed bacterial diversity in the mucus net of the *C. variopedatus*. The dominant cultured bacteria were members of the genus *Vibrio*, belonging, at least, to three different species.

2.6. Multilocus Sequence Analysis of CB1-14

The phylogenic analysis based on 16S rRNA gene sequences showed the isolate CB1-14 was closely related to *V. hangzhouensis* CN83^{T}, sharing 98.96% identity with this strain. It means that the calculated identity value is within the boundary range proposed for delineating *Vibrio* species [10]. Since the 16S rRNA gene sequence did not help in differentiating closely related bacterial species, the eight-gene MLSA was applied as that currently used for delimitating *Vibrio* species [11,12].

To overcome difficulties in application of universal primers for the MLSA, the draft genome of CB1-14 was obtained and used to retrieve sequences of eight housekeeping genes. Following previously described MLSA scheme [11] and using available genome sequences of nineteen type strains including *V. maritimus* CAIM 1455^{T}, *V. variabilis* CAIM 1457^{T}, *V. mediterranei* NBRC 15635^{T}, and *V. hangzhouensis* CGMCC-1-7062^{T}, the MLSA study was performed. Based on phylogenies generated by ML (Maximum Likelihood), MP (Maximum Parsimony), and NJ (Neighbor Joining) methods (data are not presented) and split tree decomposition analysis (Figure 3), the MLSA placed the isolate CB1-14 into the Mediterranei clade. Within the clade, the isolate CB1-14 formed a separate branch closely related to *V. maritimus* CAIM 1455^{T} and *V. variabilis* CAIM 1457^{T}, with a high bootstrap support.

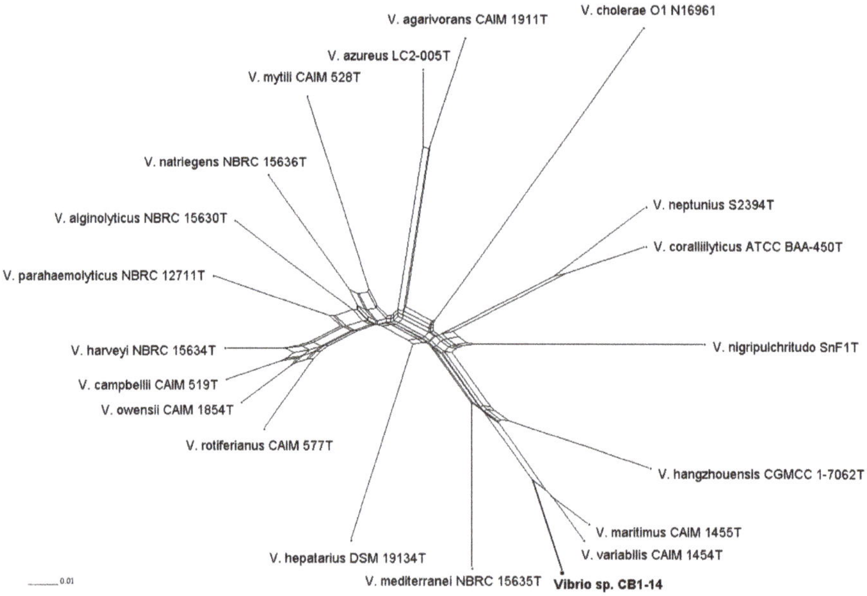

Figure 3. Concatenated split network tree based on eight gene loci. The *ftsZ*, *gapA*, *gyrB*, *mreB*, *pyrH*, *recA*, *rpoA*, and *topA* gene sequences from 20 taxa were concatenated including the isolate CB1-14 (bold font). Phylogenetic tree was generated using the SplitsTree4 program.

Thus, the phylogenetic reconstruction showed that the isolate CB1-14 should be recognized as a new species in the genus *Vibrio*. The valid description of this new species in *Vibrio* genus, isolated from an organ of the polychaete, namely from its mucous net, will be done in a special journal.

Marine invertebrates are the oldest animals on Earth, distributed over all the ocean biomes from polar to tropical waters and from shallow to very deep substrates. In the course of their evolution, marine invertebrates have acquired long-term and stable associations with a wide diversity of bacteria, cyanobacteria, archaea, and other groups of microbes, which make up to 60% of the biomass of some these animals and are essential to their survival [13]. There are a number of reports that cultures of microorganisms, isolated from marine sponge [14–19] and ascidian tissues [20], produce secondary metabolites previously isolated from these invertebrates, that indicates their microbial origin [13]. However, up to date, only biosurfactants were identified from polychaete-associated microbial isolates [21]. Production of the 6-*epi*-monanchorin by *Vibrio* sp. CB1-14 isolate is completely unprecedented. Most of the compounds so far isolated from *Vibrio* spp. were proved to be non-ribosomal peptides or their hybrids. Only a few guanidine-containing secondary metabolites were isolated from *Vibrio*, for example siderophore vanchrobactin from *Vibrio anguillarum* [22] as well as Na channel blocker tetrodotoxin and its derivatives from bacteria *V. alginolyticus*, *V. harveyi*, *V. fischeri*, and *Vibrio* sp. [23–26].

Our finding that the *Vibrio* sp. CB1-14 isolate, obtained from polychaete food net and which is able to biosynthesize compound **2**, shows that this bacterium (and probably some other close related species) has important unrecognized biosynthetic capabilities, and should be considered as a potential microbial source of monanchorins. From the biotechnological viewpoint, the cultivation of bacteria after optimization of 6-*epi*-monanchorin production could help to solve the recognized supply problem of marine-derived drugs. Identification of this producer also opens prospects of bicyclic guanidine alkaloid biosynthesis.

3. Materials and Methods

3.1. General

The ^{1}H-NMR spectra were recorded on a Bruker Avance III-700 spectrometer in $CDCl_3$. Chemical shifts were referenced to the corresponding residual solvent signal (δH 7.26/δC 77.20 for $CDCl_3$). ESI mass spectra (including HRESIMS) were obtained on a Bruker maXis Impact II LC-MS spectrometer by direct infusion in MeOH. MALDI-TOF mass spectra were obtained on a Bruker Ultraflex III TOF/TOF laser desorption spectrometer coupled with delayed extraction using a Smartbeam MALDI 200 laser with α-cyano-hydroxy cinnamic acid as the matrix. HPLC was performed on a Shimadzu instrument with a RID-10A refractive index detector using a YMC-ODS-A (250 × 10 mm) column.

3.2. Animal Material

Three specimens of the polychaete C. *variopedatus* were collected from the coastal waters by scuba at a depth of 6–10 m (salinity 33%, temperature 20) in Troitsa bay, Peter the Great Gulf, Sea of Japan, Russia, in August 2016 and identified by Dr. B. B. Grebnev (GB Elyakov Pacific Institute of Bioorganic Chemistry of Far Eastern Branch of Russian Academy of Sciences, Vladivostok, Russia).

3.3. Isolation of Microorganisms

The secreted mucous net of polychaete were pre-rinsed in sterilized sea water. Pieces of tissue (about 1 g) were aseptically removed and homogenized in 5 mL sterilized sea water. Bacterial strains were isolated by plating samples of tissue homogenate (0.1 mL) onto Petri dishes with the modified MN medium containing 75% natural sea water, 25% distilled water, 0.12 mM $CaCl_2$, 0.15 mM $MgSO_4 \times 7H_2O$, 0.09 mM $K_2HPO_4 \times 3H_2O$, 8.8 mM $NaNO_3$, 0.19 mM Na_2CO_3, 0.0013 mM disodium EDTA, 0.014 mM Citric acid × H_2O, 0.015 mM Ferric ammonium citrate, 1% Bacto agar at pH 8.5. These dishes were incubated aerobically at 20 °C for 10 days. The bacterial colonies that grew on the modified MN medium were picked up and then pure bacterial cultures were grown on Difco^{TM}Marine Agar 2216

(BD) and classified morphologically and biochemically. Bacterial strains were stored in 30% glycerol solution at −80 °C.

3.4. *Identification of Microorganisms by MALDI MS*

Bacterial isolates were stored at −80 °C on the Microbank system (VWR, Darmstadt, Germany). Selected colonies were isolated from plates using a sterile pipette tip and applied directly onto a 384-position ground steel target plate (Bruker Daltonics, Bremen, Germany). The samples were immediately mixed with 2 μL of saturated solution of α-cyano-hydroxy cinnamic acid (HCCA, Bruker Daltonics) in 50% acetonitrile (Sigma–Aldrich, Taufkirchen, Germany), supplemented with 2.5% trifluoroacetic acid (Roth, Karlsruhe, Germany). The matrix/sample spots were crystallized by air drying. Spectra of bacterial strains from the KMM collection of our Institute, as well as reference strains from different commercial collections, were used for comparison. Spectra were calibrated with external calibration by *Escherichia coli* DH5 alpha standard and protein calibration standard I (Bruker Daltonics).

3.5. *Incubation of Microorganisms for HRESI MS Analysis of Compounds*

The bacterial strains (CB1-14, CB2-11, and CB2-6) were incubated at 200 rpm, at 28 °C for 7 days, in the 100 mL liquid-modified MN medium. For preparative isolation of target compounds, the strain CB1-14 was incubated at the same conditions using 12 L of the medium.

3.6. *Isolation and Structure Identification of 6-epi-Monanchorin*

After incubation, the cells and culture broth of *Vibrio* sp. (strain CB1-14) were separated by centrifugation at 5000 rpm for 30 min. The cells were suspended in water (50 mL), frozen, and, after de-freezing, subjected to ultrasonic treatment. Then the suspension was extracted with EtOAc, and the organic phase was evaporated to dryness. Further chromatographic purification of the obtained residue with reversed-phase HPLC (YMC-ODS-A, 250 × 10 mm) using EtOH-H_2O (55:45% + 0.05% TFA) gave pure compound **2**.

6-*epi*-monanchorin (**2**, 0.2 mg), HRESI MS *m*/*z* 212.1757 $[M + H]^+$ (calcd for $C_{11}H_{22}N_3O$, 212.1757). ^1H NMR (700 MHz, $CDCl_3$): 8.74 (1H, br.s, H-2), 8.64 (1H, br.s, H-4), 7.08 (2H, br.s, H-10), 4.84 (1H, t, *J* = 3.0 Hz, H-1), 3.90 (1H, ddd, *J* = 6.0, 1.6, 7.6 Hz, H-6), 3.33 (1H, dt, *J* = 6.0, 1.6 Hz, H-5), 2.36 (1H, m, H-9a), 2.24 (2H, m, H-8), 2.13 (1H, m, H-9b), 1.74 (1H, m, H-11a), 1.52 (1H, m, H-11b), 1.40 (1H, m, H- H-12a), 1.30 (5H, m, H-12b and H_2-13 and H_2-14), 0.89 (3H, t, *J* = 6.7 Hz, H_3-15).

3.7. *DNA Isolation and Amplification and Phylogenetic Analysis of 16S rDNA Gene*

Genomic DNAs from bacterial isolates were prepared using NucleoSpin kit (Macherey-Nagel, Germany) according to the recommendation provided by the manufacturer. PCR amplification of 16S rDNA gene from all the isolates was performed according to [27], using primers BF-20 (5′-ATCACGCGTAAAAATCT-3′) and BR2-22 (5′-CCGCAATATCATTGGTGGT-3′), resulting in about a 1500 bp length PCR product. The purified PCR fragments were sequenced using the ABI PRISM 3130xl Genetic Analyzer (Applied Biosystems) and by the BigDye v.3.1 sequencing kit (Applied Biosystems) (see Table S1 in Supplementary Materials). Obtained sequences were analyzed on the highest percentage of similarities using the Ez-taxon database [8] and the MEGA program version 7 [28]. The 16S rRNA phylogenetic tree was constructed using the maximum likelihood (ML) method based on the Tamura 3-parameter model [29], with 1000 bootstrap replications in the MEGA program.

3.8. *Genome Sequencing and Multilocus Sequence Analysis of CB1-14*

A draft genome sequence of the isolate CB1-14 was obtained using 454 GS Junior (Roche Life Science, USA). A *de novo* assembly was performed using Newbler version 3.0 software Junior (Roche Life Science, USA). The genome sequence was assembled into 621 contigs with 14,322 bp of N50. The estimated genome size was 5.3 Mb. Gene prediction and automated genome annotation were carried out using RAST v. 2.0 with default parameters [30]. Sequences of eight protein-coding genes (*ftsZ*, *gapA*, *gyrB*, *mreB*, *pyrH*, *recA*, *rpoA*, and *topA*) from twenty taxa were retrieved from the CB1-14 draft genome, and from the GenBank/DDBJ/EMBL databases. The MEGA program was used to concatenate, align, and reconstruct the ML, maximum parsimony (MP), and neighbor-joining (NJ) phylogenies with 1000 bootstrap replications. The best-fit model for protein evolution determined in the MEGA program was HKY+G [31]. Split decomposition analysis was performed using SplitsTree version 4.14.3 with a neighbor net drawing and a Jukes–Cantor correction [32,33].

4. Conclusions

Our results present the first evidence of the microbial origin of 6-*epi*-monanchorin (**2**), previously isolated from the secreted mucus trapping net of the marine polychaete *C. variopedatus*. Using the 16S rRNA gene analysis, it was revealed that diverse *Vibrio* species are dominant bacteria cultured from the *C. variopedatus* mucus net. In addition, it was shown that these bacteria belong to several different species of the genus *Vibrio*. The strain CB1-14, producing alkaloid **2**, was recognized as a new species in the genus *Vibrio* by phylogenetic reconstruction using eight protein-coding genes. Our results suggest that filter-feeding polychaetes should be considered as a novel source of alkaloid-producing bacteria.

Supplementary Materials: The following are available online at http://www.mdpi.com/1660-3397/17/4/213/s1. HRESIMS spectra of 6-*epi*-monanchorin (**2**) isolated from polychaete *Chaetopterus variopedatus* and marine bacterium Vibrio sp. CB1-14; ^{1}H NMR spectra for 6-*epi*-monanchorin (**2**) isolated from polychaete *Chaetopterus variopedatus* and marine bacterium *Vibrio* sp. CB1-14; HPLC chromatograms of culture medium extract and cells extracts of CB1-14 and Table S1. Accession numbers and Chimera identification of 16S rRNA of bacterial isolates. The GenBank accession numbers for all 16S rRNA nucleotide sequences will be available on online on the NCBI server after 20 July 2019.

Author Contributions: T.M., V.S., M.I., L.S., and V.K. wrote the paper; L.S. isolated and purified 6-*epi*-monanchorin; E.B. performed 16S rDNA study; N.C. and M.I. performed genome sequencing of CB1-14 and MLSA study; R.P. and P.D. performed MS study.

Funding: This work was supported by the Grant No. 17-14-01065 from the RSF (Russian Science Foundation).

Acknowledgments: The authors are grateful to Guzev K.V. for nucleotide sequencing of 16S rDNA sequences and Dr. Grebnev B.B. for the animal identification. The spectral data were obtained on the equipment of the Collective Facilities Center (The Far Eastern Center for Structural Molecular Research (NMR/MS) PIBOC FEB RAS).

Conflicts of Interest: The authors declare no conflict of interest. The founding sponsors had no role in the design of the study; in the collection, analyses, or interpretation of data; in the writing of the manuscript, and in the decision to publish the results.

References

1. Berlinck, R.G.S.; Bertonha, A.F.; Takaki, M.; Rodriguez, J.P.G. The chemistry and biology of guanidine natural products. *Nat. Prod. Rep.* **2017**, *34*, 1264–1301. [CrossRef]
2. Meragelman, K.M.; McKee, T.C.; McMahon, J.B. Monanchorin, a bicyclic alkaloid from the sponge *Monanchora ungiculata*. *J. Nat. Prod.* **2004**, *67*, 1165–1167. [CrossRef]
3. Abdjul, D.B.; Yamazaki, H.; Kanno, S.; Takahashi, O.; Kirikoshi, R.; Ukai, K.; Namikoshi, M. Haliclonadiamine derivatives and 6-*epi*-monanchorin from the marine sponge *Halichondria panicea* collected at Iriomote Island. *J. Nat. Prod.* **2016**, *79*, 1149–1154. [CrossRef] [PubMed]
4. Shubina, L.K.; Makarieva, T.N.; Denisenko, V.A.; Dmitrenok, P.S.; Dyshlovoy, S.A.; von Amsberg, G.; Glazunov, V.P.; Silchenko, A.S.; Stonik, I.V.; Lee, H.S.; et al. Absolute configuration and body part distribution of alkaloid 6-*epi*-monanchorin from the marine polychaete *Chaetopterus variopedatus*. *Nat. Prod. Commun.* **2016**, *11*, 1253–1257. [CrossRef] [PubMed]
5. Enders, H.E. A study of the life history and habits of *Chaetopterus variopedatus*. *J. Morphol.* **1909**, *20*, 479–531. [CrossRef]
6. MacGinitie, G.E. The method of feeding in Chaetopterus. *Biol. Bull.* **1939**, *77*, 115–118. [CrossRef]
7. Waterbury, J.B.; Stanier, R.Y. Isolation and Growth of Cyanobacteria from Marine and Hypersaline Environments. In *The Prokaryotes*; Starr, M.P., Stolp, H., Trüper, H.G., Balows, A., Schlegel, H.G., Eds.; Springer: Berlin, Germany, 1981; pp. 221–223.

8. Kim, O.S.; Cho, Y.J.; Lee, K.; Yoon, S.H.; Kim, M.; Na, H.; Park, S.C.; Jeon, Y.S.; Lee, J.H.; Yi, H.; et al. Introducing EzTaxon-e: A prokaryotic 16S rRNA gene sequence database with phylotypes that represent uncultured species. *Int. J. Syst. Evol. Microbiol.* **2012**, *62*, 716–721. [CrossRef]
9. Kim, M.; Oh, H.S.; Park, S.C.; Chun, J. Towards a taxonomic coherence between average nucleotide identity and 16S rRNA gene sequence similarity for species demarcation of prokaryotes. *Int. J. Syst. Evol. Microbiol.* **2014**, *64*, 346–351. [CrossRef]
10. Kita-Tsukamoto, K.; Oyaizu, H.; Nanba, K.; Simidu, U. Phylogenetic relationships of marine bacteria, mainly members of the family *Vibrionaceae*, determined on the basis of 16S rRNA sequences. *Int. J. Syst. Bacteriol.* **1993**, *43*, 8–19. [CrossRef] [PubMed]
11. Sawabe, T.; Kita-Tsukamoto, K.; Thompson, F.L. Inferring the evolutionary history of *Vibrios* by means of multilocus sequence analysis. *J. Bacteriol.* **2007**, *189*, 7932–7936. [CrossRef] [PubMed]
12. Sawabe, T.; Ogura, Y.; Matsumura, Y.; Gao, F.; Amin, A.K.M.; Mino, S.; Nakagawa, S.; Sawabe, T.; Kumar, R.; Fukui, Y.; Satomi, M. Updating the *Vibrio* clades defined by multilocus sequence phylogeny: Proposal of eight new clades, and the description of *Vibrio tritonius* sp. nov. *Front. Microbiol.* **2013**, *4*, 414. [CrossRef]
13. Rizzo, C.; Lo Giudice, A. Marine Invertebrates: Underexplored Sources of Bacteria Producing Biologically Active Molecules. *Diversity (Basel)* **2018**, *10*, 52. [CrossRef]
14. Schmitz, F.J.; Vanderah, D.J.; Hollenbeak, K.H.; Enwall, C.E.L.; Gopichand, Y.; Sengupta, P.K.; Hossain, M.B.; van der Helm, D. Metabolites from the marine sponge Tedania ignes—A new atisanediol and several known diketopiperazines. *J. Org. Chem.* **1983**, *48*, 3941–3945. [CrossRef]
15. Nicacio, K.J.; Ioca, L.P.; Froes, A.M.; Leomil, L.; Appolinario, L.R.; Thompson, C.C.; Thompson, F.L.; Ferreira, A.G.; Williams, D.E.; Andersen, R.J.; et al. Cultures of the Marine Bacterium *Pseudovibrio denitrificans* Ab134 Produce Bromotyrosine-Derived Alkaloids Previously Only Isolated from Marine Sponges. *J. Nat. Prod.* **2018**, *80*, 235–240. [CrossRef]
16. Stierle, A.C.; Cardellina, J.H., II; Singleton, F.L. A marine micrococus produces metabolites ascribed to the sponge *Tedania ignis*. *Experientia* **1988**, *44*, 1021. [CrossRef]
17. Elyakov, G.B.; Kuznetsova, T.A.; Mikhailov, V.V.; Maltsev, I.I.; Voinov, V.G.; Fedoreyev, S.A. Brominated diphenyl ethers from a marine bacterium associated with the sponge *Dysidea* sp. *Experientia* **1991**, *47*, 632–633. [CrossRef]
18. Agarwal, V.; El Gamal, A.A.; Yamanaka, K.; Poth, D.; Kersten, R.D.; Schorn, M.; Allen, E.E.; Moore, B.S. Biosynthesis of polybrominated aromatic organic compounds by marine bacteria. *Nat. Chem. Biol.* **2014**, *10*, 640–647. [CrossRef]
19. Unson, M.D.; Faulkner, D.J. Cyanobacterial symbiont biosynthesis of chlorinated metabolites from *Dysidea herbacea* (Porifera). *Experientia* **1993**, *49*, 349–353. [CrossRef]
20. Oclarit, J.M.; Okada, H.; Ohta, S.; Kaminura, K.; Yamaoka, Y.; Iizuka, T.; Miyashiro, S.; Ikegami, S. Anti-bacillus substance in the marine sponge *Hyatella* species, prodiced by an associated *Vibrio* species bacterium. *Microbios* **1994**, *78*, 7–16.
21. Schmidt, E.W.; Donia, M.S.; McIntosh, J.A.; Fricke, W.F.; Ravel, J. Origin and Variation of Tunicate Secondary Metabolites. *J. Nat. Prod.* **2012**, *75*, 95–304. [CrossRef]
22. Rizzo, C.; Michaud, L.; Hormann, B.; Gerce, B.; Syldatk, C.; Hausmann, R.; De Domenico, E.; Lo Giudice, A. Bacteria associated with sabellids (Polychaeta: Annelida) as a novel source of surface active compounds. *Mar. Pollut. Bull.* **2013**, *70*, 125–133. [CrossRef]
23. Lemos, M.L.; Balado, M.; Osorio, C.R. Anguibactin- *versus* vanchrobactin-mediated iron uptake in *Vibrio anguillarum*: Evolution and ecology of a fish pathogen. *Environ. Microbiol. Rep.* **2010**, *2*, 19–26. [CrossRef]
24. Noguchi, T.; Hwang, D.F.; Arakawa, O.; Sugita, H.; Deguchi, Y.; Shida, Y.; Hashimoto, K. *Vibrio alginolyticus*, a tetrodotoxin-producing bacterium, in the intestines of the fish Fugu-*Vermicularis vermicularis*. *Mar. Biol.* **1987**, *94*, 625–630. [CrossRef]
25. Lee, M.J.; Jeong, D.Y.; Kim, W.S.; Kim, H.D.; Kim, C.H.; Park, W.W.; Park, Y.H.; Kim, K.S.; Kim, H.M.; Kim, D.S. A tetrodotoxin-producing *Vibrio* strain, LM-1, from the puffer fish Fugu *Vermicularis radiatus*. *Appl. Environ. Microbiol.* **2000**, *66*, 1698–1701. [CrossRef]
26. Noguchi, T.; Ali, A.E.; Arakawa, O.; Miyazawa, K.; Kanoh, S.; Shida, Y.; Nishio, S.; Hashimoto, K. Tetrodonic acid-like substance—A possible precursor of tetrodotoxin. *Toxicon* **1991**, *29*, 845–855. [CrossRef]

27. Noguchi, T.; Jeon, J.K.; Arakawa, O.; Sugita, H.; Deguchi, Y.; Shida, Y.; Hashimoto, K. Occurrence of tetrodotoxin and anhydrotetrodotoxin in *Vibrio* sp. isolated from the intestines of a xanthid crab, *Atergatis floridus*. *J. Biochem.* **1986**, *99*, 311–314. [CrossRef]
28. Stenkova, A.M.; Isaeva, M.P.; Shubin, F.N.; Rasskazov, V.A.; Rakin, A.V. Trends of the Major Porin Gene (ompF) Evolution: Insight from the Genus Yersinia. *PLoS ONE* **2011**, *6*, e20546. [CrossRef]
29. Kumar, S.; Stecher, G.; Tamura, K. MEGA7: Molecular evolutionary genetics analysis version 7.0 for bigger datasets. *Mol. Biol. Evol.* **2016**, *33*, 1870–1874. [CrossRef]
30. Tamura, K. Estimation of the number of nucleotide substitutions when there are strong transition-transversion and G+C-content biases. *Mol. Biol. Evol.* **1992**, *9*, 678–687. [CrossRef]
31. Aziz, R.K.; Bartels, D.; Best, A.A.; DeJongh, M.; Disz, T.; Edwards, R.A.; Zagnitko, O. The RAST Server: Rapid annotations using subsystems technology. *BMC Genomics* **2008**, *9*, 75. [CrossRef]
32. Hasegawa, M.; Kishino, H.; Yano, T. Dating of the human-ape splitting by a molecular clock of mitochondrial DNA. *J. Mol. Evol.* **1985**, *22*, 160–174. [CrossRef]
33. Bandelt, H.J.; Dress, A.W.M. Split decomposition: A new and useful approach to phylogenetic analysis of distance data. *Mol. Phylogenet. Evol.* **1992**, *1*, 242–252. [CrossRef]

marine drugs

Article

Magnificamide, a β-Defensin-Like Peptide from the Mucus of the Sea Anemone *Heteractis magnifica*, Is a Strong Inhibitor of Mammalian α-Amylases

Oksana Sintsova [1,*], Irina Gladkikh [1], Aleksandr Kalinovskii [1,2], Elena Zelepuga [1], Margarita Monastyrnaya [1], Natalia Kim [1], Lyudmila Shevchenko [1], Steve Peigneur [3], Jan Tytgat [3], Emma Kozlovskaya [1] and Elena Leychenko [1,*]

1 G.B. Elyakov Pacific Institute of Bioorganic Chemistry, Far Eastern Branch, Russian Academy of Sciences, 159, Pr. 100 let Vladivostoku, Vladivostok 690022, Russia; irinagladkikh@gmail.com (I.G.); alekck96@mail.ru (A.K.); zel@piboc.dvo.ru (E.Z.); rita1950@mail.ru (M.M.); natalya_kim@mail.ru (N.K.); lshev@piboc.dvo.ru (L.S.); kozempa@mail.ru (E.K.)

2 School of Natural Sciences, Far Eastern Federal University, 8, Sukhanova St, Vladivostok 690090, Russia

3 Toxicology and Pharmacology, University of Leuven (KU Leuven), Campus Gasthuisberg, O&N2, Herestraat 49, P.O. Box 922, Leuven B-3000, Belgium; steve.peigneur@kuleuven.be (S.P.); jan.tytgat@kuleuven.be (J.T.)

* Correspondence: sintsova0@gmail.com (O.S.); leychenko@gmail.com (E.L.); Tel.: +79-147185918 (O.S.); +79-084406268 (E.L.)

Received: 19 August 2019; Accepted: 17 September 2019; Published: 21 September 2019

Abstract: Sea anemones' venom is rich in peptides acting on different biological targets, mainly on cytoplasmic membranes and ion channels. These animals are also a source of pancreatic α-amylase inhibitors, which have the ability to control the glucose level in the blood and can be used for the treatment of prediabetes and type 2 diabetes mellitus. Recently we have isolated and characterized magnificamide (44 aa, 4770 Da), the major α-amylase inhibitor of the sea anemone *Heteractis magnifica* mucus, which shares 84% sequence identity with helianthamide from *Stichodactyla helianthus*. Herein, we report some features in the action of a recombinant analog of magnificamide. The recombinant peptide inhibits porcine pancreatic and human saliva α-amylases with Ki's equal to 0.17 ± 0.06 nM and 7.7 ± 1.5 nM, respectively, and does not show antimicrobial or channel modulating activities. We have concluded that the main function of magnificamide is the inhibition of α-amylases; therefore, its functionally active recombinant analog is a promising agent for further studies as a potential drug candidate for the treatment of the type 2 diabetes mellitus.

Keywords: Cnidaria; sea anemones; venom; amylase inhibitors; defensin; diabetes

1. Introduction

Type 2 diabetes mellitus is a widespread disease (~8% of adults), often resulting from a metabolic disorder caused by over-feeding, an unhealthy diet, and physical inactivity [1,2]. It covers all age groups of the population, and recently it has spread epidemiologically among children and adolescents [3,4]. The blood glucose levels of diabetic patients reaches abnormally high values, which leads to serious damage to many body systems, especially nerves and blood vessels, causing heart and kidney diseases, blindness, and even the amputation of limbs [5]. The preferred way to maintain good health for people with type 2 diabetes or prediabetes is a control of the input of glucose from the digestive tract into the blood stream [6–8]. For this purpose, the medicines based on inhibitors of pancreatic α-amylase are used. Glucobay^{TM}, the active ingredient of which, acarbose, inhibits porcine pancreatic α-amylase (PPA) and human saliva α-amylases (HSA) with Ki's of 0.797 and 1.265 μM, respectively, is one of the most common of that type of drug [9]. In some countries, medicinal plants are traditionally used to treat diabetes; the study of their composition revealed the presence of low molecular weight substances inhibiting mammalian α-amylases [10,11]. Since the effectiveness of currently existing drugs is limited and they have some side effects, the search for new highly effective inhibitors of pancreatic α-amylase is an attractive goal in the field of drug discovery.

The medicines based on proteins and peptides are poorly represented in the pharmacological market, but attract the interest of specialists due to their high selectivity and effectiveness, combined with relative safety and good tolerability. A large number of proteinaceous α-amylase inhibitors have been isolated from plants, but they are highly specific and interacted with plant α-amylases to control the breakdown of stored starch or with insect α-amylases for defense [12]. Several very effective proteinaceous inhibitors of mammalian, but not plant or microbial α-amylases were found in bacteria belonging to the genus *Streptomyces* [13–16]. However, it was shown that α-amylase inhibitors isolated from bacteria, for example, tendamistat (Ki 9–200 pM), have a high immunogenicity due to their β-sandwich fold and cannot be used in clinical practice [17].

Among animals, amylase inhibitors were found only in sea anemones, ancient sessile predators inhabiting marine environment. Helianthamide (PPA, Ki = 100 pM; human pancreatic α-amylase (HPA), Ki = 10 pM), the first representative of a new group of α-amylase inhibitors belonging to the β-defensins family, was isolated from *Stichodactyla helianthus* in 2016 [18]. This inhibitor is very active, and in contrast to tendamistat, has a more compact structure, which significantly decreases the likelihood of an immune response. Recently, as a result of the proteomic analysis of the sea anemone *H. magnifica* mucus, we have revealed that α-amylase inhibitors are major components, numbering dozens isoforms [19]. Major α-amylase inhibitor, magnificamide, was identified and sequenced (44 aa, 4770 Da) [19]. It shares 84% of sequence identity to helianthamide (44 aa, 4716 Da). The biological relevance of the presence of inhibitors of α-amylases in the mucus of Cnidaria, such as the sea anemone *H. magnifica*, remains largely unexplained. It is hypothesized that inhibition of α-amylase activity intervenes with the metabolism of starch, which forms a major source of nutrition for many organisms. Organisms exposed to α-amylase inhibitors, therefore, suffer from a reduced availability of carbohydrates that serve as an energy resource.

The results presented here are a continuation of an in depth study of magnificamide, more precisely, of a recombinant analog of the peptide with a detailed investigation of its biological activity.

2. Results

2.1. Peptide Expression and Purification

To study the properties of peptides and then to develop peptide-based drugs, it is necessary to obtain their recombinant analogues at sufficient qualities and quantities. The plasmid vector pET32b(+) containing the gene of thioredoxin ensures high yields of cysteine-containing polypeptides with native conformations, and was, therefore, chosen to create an expression construct. The synthetic gene encoding magnificamide was cloned into pET32b(+) using restriction sites KpnI and XhoI (Figure 1a). The resulting plasmid was transferred into *Escherichia coli* BL21(DE3) cells by electroporation and expressed as a fusion protein Trx-magnificamide (Figure 1b).

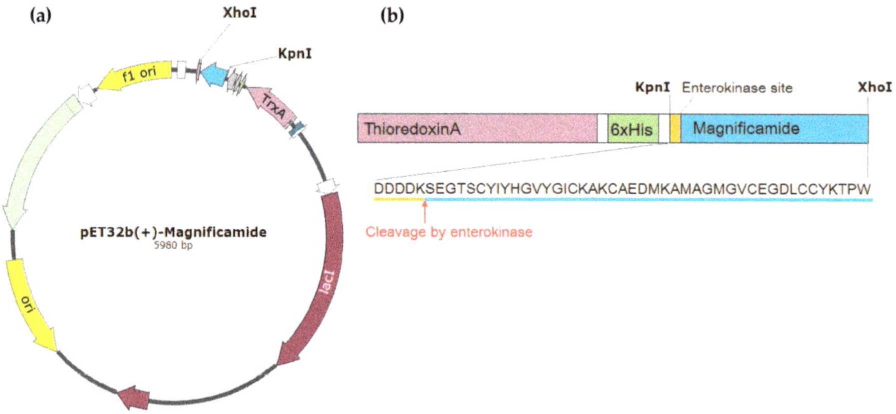

Figure 1. (**a**) Map of the pET32b(+)-magnificamide expression plasmid. A synthetic gene encoding the magnificamide and enterokinase sites was cloned using the restriction sites for KpnI and XhoI. (**b**) The scheme of fusion protein Trx-magnificamide and sequence of magnificamide (UniProtKB—C0HK71).

The fusion protein was isolated from the cell lysate by metal affinity chromatography, desalted, hydrolyzed by enterokinase, and then the recombinant magnificamide (r-magnificamide) was purified by RP-HPLC (Figure 2). After HPLC two fractions which inhibited PPA were obtained, one of them contained the mature r-magnificamide (Figure 3a); the other one contained peptide with incorrect folding (Figure 3b). The average yield of target peptide was equal to 4 mg per 1 L of cell culture (OD A_{600} = 0.6–0.8).

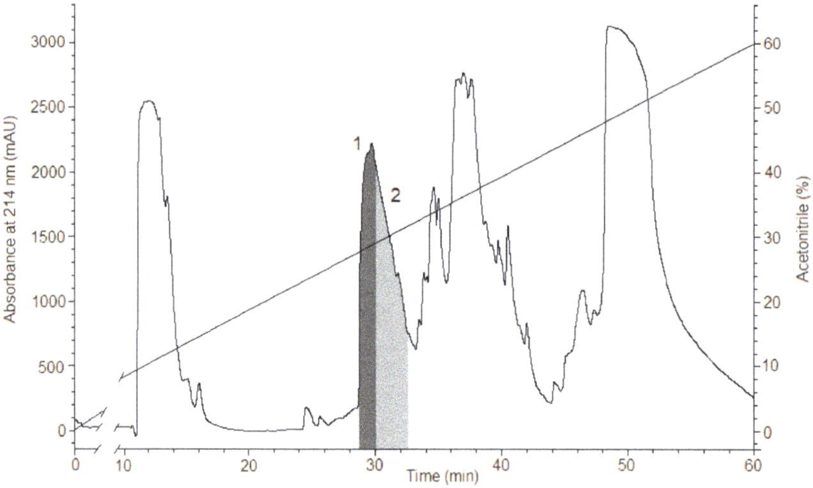

Figure 2. The RP-HPLC elution profile of r-magnificamide, obtained as the result of hydrolysis of the fusion protein Trx-magnificamide by enterokinase, on a Jupiter C4 column (Phenomenex, Torrance, CA, USA) equilibrated by 0.1% TFA, pH 2.2, in a gradient of acetonitrile concentration (0%–70%) for 70 min at 2 mL/min. Fraction 1 containing the mature peptide r-magnificamide (4770 Da) (Figure 3a) is filled by dark grey color; fraction 2 containing peptide with incorrect folding (4777 Da) (Figure 3b) is filled by light grey color.

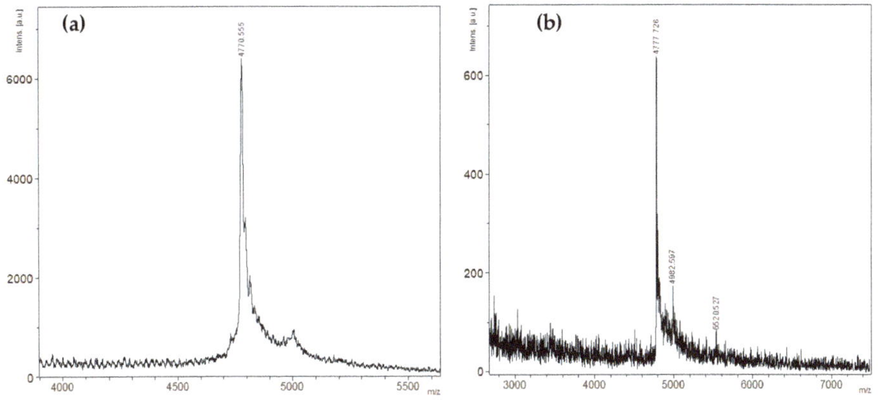

Figure 3. Mass spectra, m/z, of the peptides isolated by RP-HPLC (Figure 2): (**a**) mature r-magnificamide from fraction 1 and (**b**) incorrectly folded r-magnificamide from fraction 2. m/z—mass-to-charge ratio; a. u.—arbitrary units.

2.2. Secondary Structure of Peptides

To calculate the secondary structural elements of recombinant and native magnificamide, the circular dichroism spectroscopy method was used. The spectra in the far UV region (190–240 nm) were characterized by a minimum at 212 nm and a maximum at 203 nm. In the 225–235 nm range, distinct shoulders were observed on the spectra's curves due to the contribution of the disulfide groups' absorption (Figure 4). The similarity between the circular dichroism (CD) spectra of magnificamide and its recombinant analogue suggested that the recombinant peptide should be functional and can be used successfully to study its biological activity. Moreover, the calculation of secondary structure elements using Provenzer–Glockner method [20] revealed the complete identities of the peptides at the secondary structure level (Table 1). It should be noted that content of α-helices of the magnificamide was significantly lower than that of helianthamide, which might be reflected in the difference in their spatial structures and biological activity.

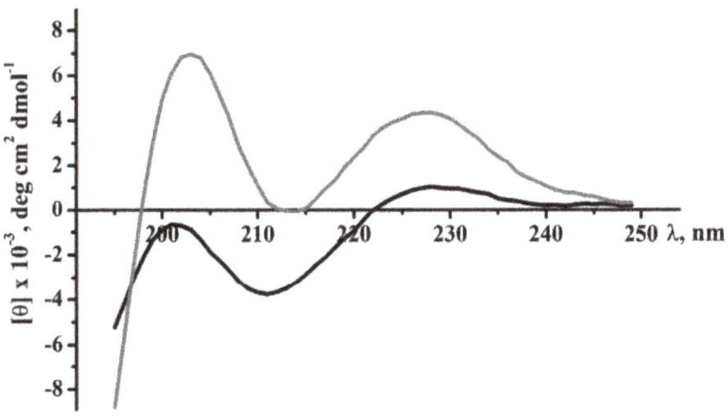

Figure 4. Circular dichroism (CD) spectra of native magnificamide (black line) and recombinant magnificamide (grey line) in 0.01M phosphate buffer, pH 7.0, far or peptide bond UV region.

Table 1. Secondary structural elements of the natural and recombinant magnificamide and helianthamide (percentages).

Sample	α-Helix			β-Structure			β-Turn	Unordered Structure
	I	II	III	I	II	III		
Magnificamide	0.0	1.7	1.7	21.4	13.7	35.1	24.3	38.9
r-Magnificamide	0.1	1.1	1.2	18.2	14.7	32.9	22.2	43.7
Helianthamide			19			32	18	31
r-Helianthamide			11			33	23	33

2.3. Molecular Modeling

The spatial structure models of magnificamide were generated using the homology modeling approach with MOE 2016.08 software (Montreal, QC, Canada) [21]. The atom coordinates of the helianthamide from *S. helianthus*, extracted from the complex with porcine pancreatic α-amylase (PDB ID 4XON) were used as a template. Then the solvated models were optimized using the 400 ns MD simulations in Amber10: EHT force field and the most energetically favorable state of magnificamide was selected (Figure 5b). The molecule has a characteristic fold stabilized by 3 disulfide bridges, including a β-sheet, formed by four strands, an α-helix, and several loops, as well as sufficiently mobile C and N-terminal regions. The content of secondary structure elements agrees well with the data of CD spectroscopy of the native peptide. Despite the relatively high RMSD value for 44 Cα atoms of magnificamide model relative to the prototype—2.46 Å, the model quality assessment showed no conformational constraints (ψ and φ-angles) of amino acid residues, which indicates the good quality of the generated model. It turned out that the largest deviation (from 2 Å to 5.6 Å) involved the flexible parts of the structure in the sequence regions 1–4, 10–12, 18–20, and 32–33. It should be noted that these areas either included variable amino acid residues or were localized in close proximity to those (Figure 5a). The mapping of magnificamide variable residues revealed an interesting feature. In fact, the variability affected only one part of the molecule, while another one remained conservative.

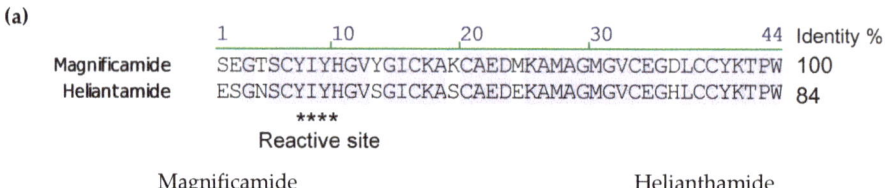

(a)

	1 10 20 30 44	Identity %
Magnificamide	SEGTSCYIYHGVYGICKAKCAEDMKAMAGMGVCEGDLCCYKTPW	100
Heliantamide	ESGNSCYIYHGVSGICKASCAEDEKAMAGMGVCEGHLCCYKTPW	84
	**** Reactive site	

Magnificamide Helianthamide

(b)

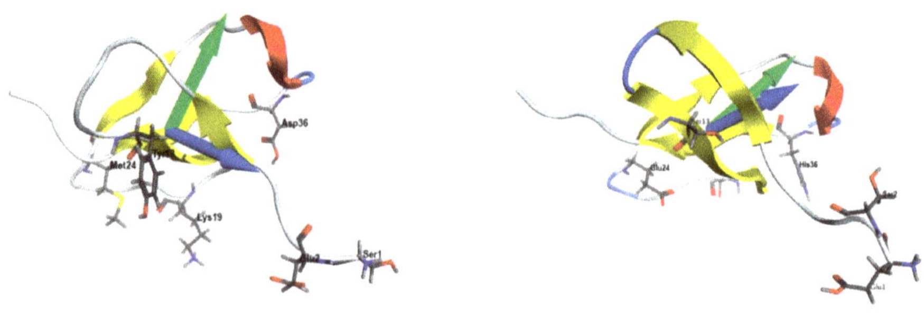

Figure 5. *Cont.*

(c)

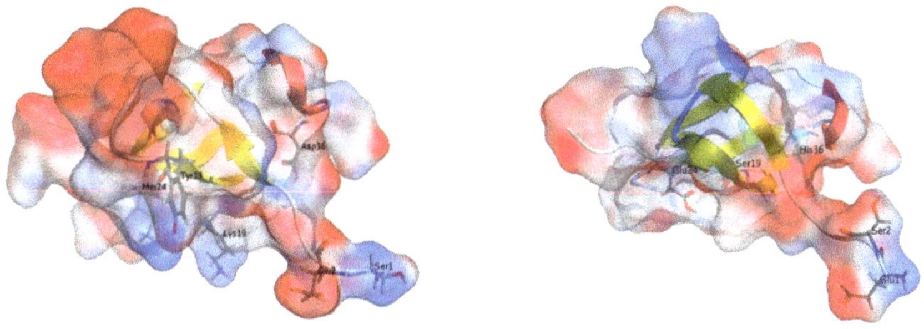

Figure 5. (**a**) Alignment of sea anemone α-amylase inhibitors: magnificamide *H. magnifica* [18] and helianthamide from *S. helianthus* [17] amino acid sequences and their spatial structures. (**b**) The ribbon diagrams of magnificamide and helianthamide spatial structures are colored according to the structure elements; the side chains of the variable residues magnificamide are shown as sticks and labeled. Molecular dipole and hydrophobic moments are indicated by blue and green arrows, respectively. (**c**) Magnificamide and helianthamide molecular surfaces are colored according to surface charge distribution.

Using the MOE 2016.08 program, the physicochemical characteristics of the inhibitor were evaluated and the surface properties of magnificamide were analyzed to compare them with helianthamide (Table 2). It was shown that, despite its greater compactness, this molecule was characterized by a larger hydrophobic surface area, as well as a redistribution of the localization of charged regions (Figure 5c). This is manifested in a change in both the magnitude and direction of the dipole, and in the hydrophobic moments of the molecules (Figure 5b; Table 2).

Table 2. Physico-chemical characteristics of the α-amylase inhibitors.

Physico-Chemical Characteristics	Magnificamide	Helianthamide (PDB ID 4XON)
Radius of hydration (Å)	10.25	10.21
Hydrophilic surface area ($Å^2$)	2009.0	1976.3
Hydrophobic surface area ($Å^2$)	1553.0	1275.4
WDW volume ($Å^3$)	3727.1	4157.9
Isoelectric point	5.81	5.33
Charge	−1.21	−1.82
Dipole moment (D)	161.86	96.07
Hydrophobic moment	145.7	165.9

2.4. *Study of Antimicrobial Activity*

Since the main function of defensins in most organisms-producers is the protection against microorganisms [22–28], we performed a screening of potential antimicrobial activity displayed by r-magnificamide. It did not reveal activity against fungi, Gram-positive or Gram-negative bacteria (Table 3).

Table 3. Antimicrobial activity of r-magnificamide.

	Organisms	r-Magnificamide (1, 5, 10, 20 μM)
Gram-positive	*Staphylococcus aureus* ATCC 21027 *Bacillus subtilis* ATCC6633	Not active Not active
Gram-negative	*Escherichia coli* VKPM B-7935 *Pseudomonas aeruginosa* ATCC 27853	Not active Not active
Fungi	*Candida albicans KMM* 455	Not active

2.5. Study of Channel Modulating Activity

Since defensins are widely present in animal venoms, also known as toxins with modulating effects on the activity of ion channels [23,29–33], we performed an extensive electrophysiological screening of r-magnificamide against 18 subtypes of voltage-gated potassium and voltage gated sodium channels (mammalian channels: $K_V1.1$, $K_V1.2$, $K_V1.3$, $K_V1.4$, $K_V1.5$, $K_V1.6$, $K_V2.1$, $K_V3.1$, $K_V4.2$, $K_V10.1$, hERG, $Na_V1.2$, $Na_V1.4$, $Na_V1.5$, $Na_V1.6$ and $Na_V1.8$; insect channels: Shaker and $BgNa_V1$) (Table 4). r-Magnificamide did not reveal ion channel modulating activity, from which it can be surmised, to conclude, that the main biological function of magnificamide is the inhibition of α-amylases.

Table 4. Electrophysiological study of r-magnificamide.

	Channels	r-Magnificamide (10 μM)
Voltage-gated potassium channels	$K_V1.1$, $K_V1.2$, $K_V1.3$, $K_V1.4$, $K_V1.5$, $K_V1.6$, $K_V2.1$, $K_V3.1$, $K_V4.2$, $K_V10.1$, hERG, Shaker *	Not active
Voltage-gated sodium channels	$Na_V1.2$, $Na_V1.4$, $Na_V1.5$, $Na_V1.6$, $Na_V1.8$, $BgNa_V1$ *	Not active

* insect channels.

2.6. Study of Mammalian α-Amylase Inhibition

Since magnificamide shared a high sequential and structural similarity with the competitive tight-binding inhibitor helianthamide, it was predicted to possess analogous kinetic features. For a quantitative assessment of tight-binding inhibitor potency, Morrison's method was applied [34,35]. This method uses the Morrison quadratic equation (Equation (1)) for fitting inhibitor-response data and determining Ki *app* as a nonlinear regression parameter.

$$\frac{v}{v_0} = 1 - \frac{\left([E] + [I] + K_i^{app}\right) - \sqrt{\left([E] + [I] + K_i^{app}\right)^2 - 4[E][I]}}{2[E]_0} \quad (1)$$

True Ki values are calculated from the Equation (2), suggesting a competitive mode of inhibition.

$$K_i^{app} = K_i\left(1 + \frac{[S]}{K_M}\right) \quad (2)$$

Recombinant magnificamide inhibition constants against porcine pancreatic α-amylase (PPA) and human salivary α-amylase (HSA) were determined. Kinetic assays revealed that recombinant magnificamide was indeed a potent nanomolar tight-binding inhibitor: Ki against PPA was 0.17 ± 0.06 nM; Ki against HSA was 7.7 ± 1.5 nM (Figure 6).

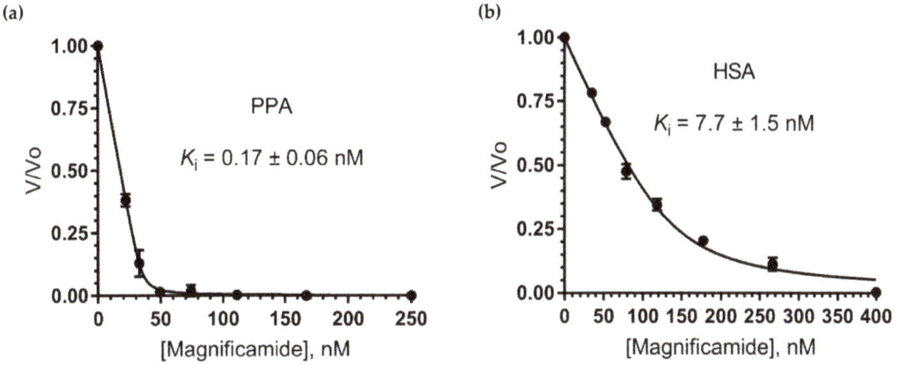

Figure 6. Amylase inhibition curves using r-magnificamide. Fixed concentrations of each enzyme (PPA on (**a**) and HSA on (**b**)) were mixed with increasing concentrations of r-magnificamide (displayed in nM). Each connecting line represents the best fits to the quadratic Morrison equation for tight binding inhibitors [35].

3. Discussion

Sea anemones are ancient sessile predators inhabiting the marine environment. They have specialized stinging cells which contain venom rich in peptides acting on different biological targets, mainly cytoplasmic membranes [36–38] and ion channels [39–44]. Venom with such a complex composition ensured the existence of sea anemones for millions of years [45]. Recently, it has been shown that sea anemones also present a source of pancreatic α-amylase inhibitors belonging to the β-defensin family [18,19]. In the venoms of sea anemones, the β-defensin fold is widely recruited to create toxins modulating ion channel activity, interestingly, often with little amino acid sequence identity, but with similar spatial structure. According to Mitchell and coauthors, cnidarian β-defensin-like toxins can be divided into four main groups: APETx-like, BDS-like, Nv1-like, and ShI-like [46]. Representatives of APETx-like and BDS-like groups interact with ASICs, hERG, voltage-gated sodium, and potassium ion channels [33,47–49]. Some of them, crassicorin I and II from *Urticina crassicornis*, reveal paralytic activity against crustaceans, as well as antimicrobial activity against Gram-positive and Gram-negative bacterial strains [33]. Nv1-like and ShI-like peptides are often a major content of sea anemones' venom and modulate voltage-gated sodium ion channels [50,51]. Helianthamide-like peptides represent a separate group [46] suggesting a different activity.

Taking into account the wide variety of sea anemone defensin-functions, we conducted a study of activity of magnificamide on various ion channels (Table 4) and found no activity. No antimicrobial activity against Gram-positive, Gram-negative bacteria, or fungi was observed either (Table 3). Thus, structural remoteness may occur due to narrow specialization of sea anemones' helianthamide-like peptides. The presence of numerous digestive enzyme (proteinases and amylases) inhibitors [19] in sea anemone venoms is per se an interesting defensive strategy, similar to plant protection from insects and herbivores.

From a practical point of view, pancreatic α-amylase inhibitors effectively control the influx of glucose into the bloodstream from the gastrointestinal tract [18,19]. Inhibitors of pancreatic α-amylase have a great pharmacological potential for the prevention and treatment of metabolic disorders and type 2 *diabetes mellitus*. In this work we have shown that magnificamide was an effective inhibitor of mammalian α-amylases. The homologue of magnificamide, helianthamide from *S. helianthus*, inhibited PPA with very close Ki (Table 5). Sea anemone inhibitors had great inhibitory activity against mammalian α-amylases (Table 5); the combination of such activity with a compact fold could be used to create new drugs.

Table 5. Mammalian α-amylase inhibitors from different sources.

Inhibitor name	Source	Mr, Da	Ki, M	Enzyme	Reference
		Peptides			
Magnificamide	*H. magnifica*	4770	1.7×10^{-10} 7.7×10^{-9}	PPA HSA	
Helianthamide	*S. helianthus*	4716	1×10^{-10} 1×10^{-11}	PPA HPA	[18]
Tendamistat (HOE-467A)	*Streptomyces tendae* 4158	7958	9×10^{-12}	PPA	[13]
Parvulustat (Z-2685)	*Streptomyces parvullus* FH-1641	8129	2.8×10^{-11} +	PPA HSA	[16]
		Low molecular compounds			
Acarbose	*Actinomycetes*	646	0.6×10^{-6} 1.3×10^{-6}	PPA HSA	[9]
Montbretin A	*Crocosmia* sp.	789	8.1×10^{-9}	HPA	[11]

Moreover, for the first time, sea anemone peptides' ability to inhibit HSA was clarified on the example of magnificamide, with Ki equal to 7.7 nM. Inhibition of salivary α-amylase allows for blocking the digestion of starch upon the first stages of entering the body. In addition, it may be useful for the treatment of diseases the of oral cavity, including caries. Caries is a multifactorial disease, a significant role in the development of which is played by oral *Streptococci*, capable of binding salivary α-amylase and using sugar that can be broken down by it for their own needs. The binding of *Streptococci* to salivary α-amylase also contributes to the formation of biofilms and the demineralization of teeth [52]. It has been shown that cherry and tea extracts exhibiting inhibitory activity for salivary α-amylase could inhibit the growth of oral *Streptococci* (in particular *Streptococcus mutans*) [53–55]. Given a stable structure and high activity of magnificamide, it may also find an application in the form of chewing gum, as was shown for cherry extract [53].

4. Materials and Methods

4.1. Obtaining the Recombinant Magnificamide

The synthetic gene encoding the target peptide was cloned into a pET32b(+) (Novagen, Germany) vector using the restriction sites for KpnI and XhoI by JSC "Eurogen" company, Moscow, Russia. The resulted construct was checked by sequencing to verify the open reading frame.

The expression construction pET32b(+)/*magnificamide* was used for the transformation of BL21(DE3) *E. coli* cells by electroporation using a Multiporator (Eppendorf, Hamburg, Germany) device. Cells were screened on LB agarose plates containing 100 μg/mL carbenicillin (Invitrogen, Carlsbad, CA, USA). Next the transformed cells were cultured in LB medium (1 L) containing 100 μg/mL carbenicillin at 37 °C to the optical density of (at A_{600}) 0.6–0.8. Isopropyl-β,D-thiogalactopyranoside (IPTG) (Invitrogen, Carlsbad, CA, USA) was added to a final concentration of 0.2 mM for induction of expression. The cells were grown for 16 h at 18 °C for the production of the fusion protein in a soluble form and then cells were precipitated from the culture medium by centrifugation at 8000 rpm for 6 min. Cells were lysed by ultra-sonication on a Sonopuls 2070 instrument (Bandeling, Berlin, Germany). The fusion protein Trx-magnificamide was isolated from the cell lysate by metal affinity chromatography on the Ni-NTA-agarose (Qiagen, Hilden, Germany) in native conditions. Then the fusion protein was desalted using Amicon Ultra-15 Centrifugal Filter Units 3000 NMWL (Millipore, Burlington, MA, USA), followed by hydrolysis by Enterokinase (NEB, Ipswich, MA, USA) according to the manufacturer's instructions. Recombinant magnificamide was purified from the reaction mixture by RP-HPLC, using a Jupiter C_4 column (Phenomenex, Torrance, CA, USA), equilibrated with 0.1% TFA at pH 2.2, in a gradient of acetonitrile (with concentrations from 0%–70%) for 70 min at 2 mL/min. The retention time of the target peptide was 30 min.

4.2. Mass Spectrometry Analysis

MALDI-TOF MS spectra of the peptide fractions obtained by RP-HPLC were recorded using an Ultra Flex III MALDI-TOF/TOF mass spectrometer (Bruker, Bremen, Germany) with a nitrogen laser (Smart Beam, 355 nm), reflector, and the potential LIFT™ tandem modes of operation. Sinapinic acid was used as a matrix. An external calibration was employed using a peptide sample [56] with *m/z* 6107 Da and its doubly-charged variant at *m/z* 3053 Da.

4.3. Assay of Porcine Pancreatic α-Amylase Inhibitory Activity

The porcine α-amylase (PPA) inhibitory activity of the peptide fractions obtained by RP-HPLC was tested by the following procedure. Experimental samples (10 μL) were added to 80 μL of 50 mM sodium phosphate, 100 mM sodium chloride buffer (pH 7.0), and PPA (A4268) (1 μg/mL) (Sigma Aldrich, St. Louis, MO, USA), and incubated for 10 min at RT. The substrate solution, 2-chloro-4-nitrophenyl α-D-maltotrioside (CNPG3) (Sigma Aldrich, St. Louis, MO, USA), was added to the reaction mixture (1 mM) and incubated for 10 min at RT. The optical absorption was measured on an xMark microplate spectrophotometer (BioRad, Hercules, CA, USA) at 405 nm. Acarbose (1mg/mL) (Sigma Aldrich, St. Louis, MO, USA) was used as a positive control.

4.4. Circular Dichroism Spectroscopy

Circular dichroism (CD) spectra were recorded on Chirascan-plus CD spectropolarimeter (Applied Photophysics, Leatherhead, UK) in quartz cells with an optical path length of 0.1 cm for the peptide region spectrum. The cuvette with the solution of the native and recombinant peptides (50 μg/mL) in a 0.01 M sodium phosphate buffer was incubated at 25 °C for 20–25 min before recording the CD spectrum. The content of secondary structure elements of peptides was calculated by the Provenzer–Glockner method [20], using advanced Provencher calculation programs from the CDPro software package (Leatherhead, UK) [57].

4.5. Homology Modeling

The generation of a theoretical model of the spatial structure of magnificamide, as well as the valuation of its physico-chemical characteristics, were performed using the specialized software MOE 2016.08 (Montreal, QC, Canada) [21]. Simulation of the molecular dynamics of magnificamide in an aqueous environment, as well as the physicochemical characteristics valuation of α-amylase inhibitors, were performed in Amber10: EHT force field.

4.6. In Vitro Antimicrobial Activity Assay

The antimicrobial activity of r-magnificamide was tested against Gram-positive (*Staphylococcus aureus* ATCC 21027 and *Bacillus subtilis* ATCC6633), Gram-negative bacteria (*Escherichia coli* VKPM B-7935 and *Pseudomonas aeruginosa* ATCC 27853), and the fungus *Candida albicans* KMM 455 by the agar dilution method. Microbial strains were taken from the American Type Culture Collection (ATCC), Russian National Collection of Industrial Microorganisms (VKPM), and Collection of Marine Microorganisms (KMM) (Pacific Institute of Bioorganic Chemistry FEB RAS). To obtain a microbial lawn, 0.1 mL of a cell suspension (0.5×10^8 cells/mL) was uniformly distributed on agar surface in Petri dishes (15 g/L tryptic soy broth, 2 g/L bacto yeast extract, 1 g/L glucose, and 20 g/L agar for bacteria; for fungi 10 g/L of glucose was added). Wells with a diameter of 6 mm were punched into the agar and filled with 100 μL of the peptide solution at concentrations 1, 5, 10, and 20 μM. The plates were then incubated for 18 h at 37 °C for bacteria, and at 30 °C for the fungus. Minimum inhibitory concentration was determined by measuring the clear zone of inhibition around each well. All assays were performed independently three times.

4.7. Electrophysiology

For the expression of Na_V channels (mammalian $rNa_V1.2$, $rNa_V1.4$, $hNa_V1.5$, $mNa_V1.6$ and $hNa_V1.8$ channels; the insect channel *Bg*Na_V1 from *Blattella germanica*; and the auxiliary subunits rβ1, hβ1, and TipE) and Kv channels (mammalian $rK_V1.1$, rKv1.2, hKv1.3, rKv1.4, $rK_V1.5$, $rK_V1.6$, $rK_V2.1$, $hK_V3.1$, $rK_V4.2$, $hK_V10.1$, and h*ERG*; and *Drosophila Shaker*'s IR) in *Xenopus laevis* oocytes; the linearized plasmids were transcribed using the T7 or SP6 mMESSAGE-mMACHINE transcription kit (Ambion, Carlsbad, CA, USA). The harvesting of stage V–VI oocytes from anesthetized female *Xenopus laevis* frog was previously described [58]. Oocytes were injected with 50 nL of cRNA at a concentration of 1 ng/nL using a microinjector (Drummond Scientific, Broomall, PA, USA). The oocytes were incubated in a solution containing 96-mM NaCl, 2-mM KCl, 1.8-mM $CaCl_2$, 2-mM $MgCl_2$, and 5-mM HEPES (pH 7.4), supplemented with 50 mg/L gentamycin sulfate.

Two-electrode voltage-clamp recordings were performed at room temperature (18–22 °C) using a Geneclamp 500 amplifier (Molecular Devices, Downingtown, PA, USA) controlled by a pClamp data acquisition system (Axon Instruments, Union City, CA, USA). Whole cell currents from oocytes were recorded 1–4 days after injection. The bath solution's composition was 96-mM NaCl, 2-mM KCl, 1.8-mM $CaCl_2$, 2-mM $MgCl_2$, and 5-mM HEPES (pH 7.4). Toxins were applied directly to the bath. Resistances of both electrodes were kept between 0.8 and 1.5 MΩ. The elicited currents were sampled at 20 kHz (Na_V) or 2 kHz (K_V), filtered at 2 kHz (Na_V) or 0.5 kHz (K_V) using a four-pole low-pass Bessel filter. Leak subtraction was performed using a -P/4 protocol. Only data obtained from cells exhibiting currents with peak amplitudes below 2 μA were considered for analysis. For the electrophysiological analysis, a number of protocols were applied from a holding potential of −90 mV with a start-to-start interval of 0.2 Hz. $K_V1.1$–$K_V1.6$ and Shaker currents were evoked by 250-ms depolarizations to 0 mV followed by a 250 ms pulse to −50 mV from a holding potential of −90 mV. Current traces of hERG channels were elicited by applying a +40 mV prepulse for 2 s followed by −120 mV for 2 s. $K_V2.1$, $K_V3.1$, and $K_V4.2$ currents were elicited by 250 ms pulses to +20 mV from a holding potential of −90 mV. $K_V10.1$ currents were evoked by 2-s depolarizing pulses to 0 mV from a holding potential of −90 mV. Sodium current traces were evoked by 100-ms depolarization to the voltage corresponding to maximal sodium current in control conditions. All data were analyzed using pClamp Clampfit 10.0 (Molecular Devices, Downingtown, PA, USA) and Origin 7.5 software (Originlab, Northampton, MA, USA).

4.8. Determination of Ki Against Porcine Pancreatic and Human Saliva α-Amylases

Kinetic assays were carried out at 37 °C in 50 mM sodium phosphate and 100 mM sodium chloride (pH 7.0). 2-Chloro-4-nitrophenyl-α-maltotrioside (CNPG3) (Sigma Aldrich, St. Louis, MO, USA) was used as the substrate and the optical absorption of the 2-chloro-4-nitrophenol was measured at 405 nm. Reactions were run with final [CNPG3] = 1 mM ($[S]/K_M = 1.41$, $K_M = 0.71$ mM), nominal $[E] = 20$ nM for PPA, [CNPG3] = 3.3 mM ($[S]/K_M = 0.97$, $K_M = 3.4$ mM), and nominal $[E] = 100$ nM for HSA to provide sufficient analytical signal. Inhibitor dilution schemes were optimized considering recommendations in [34].

The enzyme was pre-incubated with the inhibitor for 10 minutes before the addition of substrate which launched the reaction. Reactions were monitored on an xMark microplate spectrophotometer (BioRad, USA) in the kinetic mode for 30 min. The initial linear steady state region provided initial rate values for each inhibitor concentration (v), along with uninhibited rate values (v_o). Measurements were run in triplicate. Nonlinear least squares regression was carried out with GraphPad Prism 7.00 (San Diego, CA, USA). Fractional rates (v/v_o) were plotted against inhibitor concentrations and the set of data points was fitted by the Morrison Ki regression algorithm [34,35]. Ki and $[E]$ were simultaneously treated as adjustable parameters following the approach described in [59]. Derived enzyme active sites concentrations showed physically meaningful values close to nominal (34.6 and 132.5 nM for PPA and HSA respectively). Best-fit constant values were presented as mean ± SE ($n = 3$).

Author Contributions: Conceptualization, O.S., I.G., M.M., J.T., and E.L. Data curation, O.S., I.G., and E.L. Investigation, O.S., I.G., A.K., E.Z., N.K., L.S., and S.P. Methodology, O.S., S.P., and E.L. Supervision, J.T., E.K., and E.L. Validation, O.S., A.K., E.Z., N.K., L.S., S.P., and E.L. Visualization, O.S., A.K., E.Z., and N.K. Writing—original draft, O.S., I.G., A.K., E.Z., and E.L. Writing—review and editing, O.S., I.G., A.K., E.Z., M.M., S.P., J.T., E.K., and E.L. Authors guarantee the reliability of obtained data in any part of the work. All authors read and approved the final manuscript.

Funding: This research was partially (when obtaining the recombinant peptide and for determination of Ki) supported by RFBR grant number 18-38-00389. The MS and CD spectra were carried out on the equipment of the Collective Facilities Center «The Far Eastern Center for Structural Molecular Research (NMR/MS) PIBOC FEB RAS». S.P. was funded by postdoctoral grant PDM/19/164 (KU Leuven, Belgium). J.T. was funded by grants CELSA/17/047 (KU Leuven, Belgium), G0A4919N, and G0C2319N (FWO-Vlaanderen, Belgium).

Acknowledgments: We gratefully acknowledge Valery Mikhailov for conducting the antimicrobial activity research and Stanislav Anastyuk for obtaining of MS data. We would like to thank Alexandra Litavrina for the revision of the English text and Academician Valentin Stonik for editorial improvements of this manuscript.

Conflicts of Interest: The authors declare no conflict of interest. The funders had no role in the design of the study; in the collection, analyses, or interpretation of data; in the writing of the manuscript, and in the decision to publish the results.

References

1. Alam, U.; Asghar, O.; Azmi, S. General aspects of diabetes mellitus. *Handb. Clin. Neurol.* **2014**, *126*, 211–222. [CrossRef] [PubMed]
2. Pandey, A.; Chawla, S.; Guchhait, P. Type-2 diabetes: Current understanding and future perspectives. *IUBMB Life* **2015**, *67*, 506–513. [CrossRef] [PubMed]
3. Aye, T.; Levitsky, L.L. Type 2 diabetes: An epidemic disease in childhood. *Curr. Opin. Pediatr.* **2003**, *15*, 411–415. [CrossRef] [PubMed]
4. Temneanu, O.R.; Trandafir, L.M.; Purcarea, M.R. Type 2 diabetes mellitus in children and adolescents: A relatively new clinical problem within pediatric practice. *J. Med. Life* **2016**, *9*, 235–239. [PubMed]
5. Adeghate, E.; Schattner, P.; Dunn, E. An update on the etiology and epidemiology of diabetes mellitus. *Ann. N. Y. Acad. Sci.* **2006**, *1084*, 1–29. [CrossRef]
6. Scheen, A.J. Is there a role for alpha-glucosidase inhibitors in the prevention of type 2 diabetes mellitus? *Drugs* **2003**, *63*, 933–951. [CrossRef] [PubMed]
7. Chiasson, J.-L.; Josse, R.G.; Gomis, R.; Hanefeld, M.; Karasik, A.; Laakso, M.; STOP-NIDDM Trail Research Group. Acarbose for prevention of type 2 diabetes mellitus: The STOP-NIDDM randomised trial. *Lancet* **2002**, *359*, 2072–2077. [CrossRef]
8. Wu, H.; Liu, J.; Lou, Q.; Liu, J.; Shen, L.; Zhang, M.; Lv, X.; Gu, M.; Guo, X. Comparative assessment of the efficacy and safety of acarbose and metformin combined with premixed insulin in patients with type 2 diabetes mellitus. *Medicine* **2017**, *96*, e7533. [CrossRef]
9. Yoon, S.H.; Robyt, J.F. Study of the inhibition of four alpha amylases by acarbose and its 4IV-α-maltohexaosyl and 4IV-α-maltododecaosyl analogues. *Carbohydr. Res.* **2003**, *338*, 1969–1980. [CrossRef]
10. Poongunran, J.; Kumudu, H.; Perera, I.; Fernando, I.T.; Sivakanesan, R.; Fujimoto, Y. Bioassay-guided fractionation and identification of α-amylase inhibitors from *Syzygium cumini* leaves. *Pharm. Biol.* **2017**, *55*, 206–211. [CrossRef]
11. Williams, L.K.; Zhang, X.; Caner, S.; Tysoe, C.; Nguyen, N.T.; Wicki, J.; Williams, D.E.; Coleman, J.; McNeill, J.H.; Yuen, V.; et al. The amylase inhibitor montbretin A reveals a new glycosidase inhibition motif. *Nat. Chem. Biol.* **2015**, *11*, 691–696. [CrossRef]
12. Svensson, B.; Fukuda, K.; Nielsen, P.K.; Bønsager, B.C. Proteinaceous alpha-amylase inhibitors. *Biochim. Biophys. Acta* **2004**, *1696*, 145–156. [CrossRef]
13. Vértesy, L.; Oeding, V.; Bender, R.; Zepf, K.; Nesemann, G. Tendamistat (HOE 467), a tight-binding alpha-amylase inhibitor from *Streptomyces tendae* 4158. Isolation, biochemical properties. *Eur. J. Biochem.* **1984**, *141*, 505–512. [CrossRef]
14. Yokose, K.; Ogawa, K.; Sano, T.; Watanabe, K.; Maruyama, H.B.; Suhara, Y. New alpha-amylase inhibitor, trestatins. I. Isolation, characterization and biological activities of trestatins A, B and C. *J. Antibiot.* **1983**, *36*, 1157–1165. [CrossRef]

15. Wiegand, G.; Epp, O.; Huber, R. The crystal structure of porcine pancreatic alpha-amylase in complex with the microbial inhibitor Tendamistat. *J. Mol. Biol.* **1995**, *247*, 99–110. [CrossRef]
16. Sokočević, A.; Han, S.; Engels, J.W. Biophysical characterization of α-amylase inhibitor Parvulustat (Z-2685) and comparison with Tendamistat (HOE-467). *Biochim. Biophys. Acta Proteins Proteomics* **2011**, *1814*, 1383–1393. [CrossRef]
17. Gonçalves, O.; Dintinger, T.; Blanchard, D.; Tellier, C. Functional mimicry between anti-Tendamistat antibodies and alpha-amylase. *J. Immunol. Methods* **2002**, *269*, 29–37. [CrossRef]
18. Tysoe, C.; Wiliams, L.K.; Keyzers, R.; Nguyen, N.T.; Tarling, C.; Wicki, J.; Goddard-Borger, E.D.; Aguda, A.H.; Perry, S.; Foster, L.J.; et al. Potent human α-amylase inhibition by the β-defensin-like protein helianthamide. *ACS Cent. Sci.* **2016**, *2*, 154–161. [CrossRef]
19. Sintsova, O.; Gladkikh, I.; Chausova, V.; Monastyrnaya, M.; Anastyuk, S.; Chernikov, O.; Yurchenko, E.; Aminin, D.; Isaeva, M.; Leychenko, E.; et al. Peptide fingerprinting of the sea anemone *Heteractis magnifica* mucus revealed neurotoxins, Kunitz-type proteinase inhibitors and a new β-defensin α-amylase inhibitor. *J. Proteom.* **2018**, *173*, 12–21. [CrossRef]
20. Provencher, S.W.; Glöckner, J. Estimation of globular protein secondary structure from circular dichroism. *Biochemistry* **1981**, *20*, 33–37. [CrossRef]
21. Chemical Computing Group Inc. *Molecular Operating Environment (MOE) 2016.08*; Chemical Computing Group Inc.: Montreal, QC, Canada, 2016.
22. Cuesta, A.; Meseguer, J.; Esteban, M.Á. Molecular and functional characterization of the gilthead seabream β-defensin demonstrate its chemotactic and antimicrobial activity. *Mol. Immunol.* **2011**, *48*, 1432–1438. [CrossRef]
23. Shafee, T.M.A.; Lay, F.T.; Phan, T.K.; Anderson, M.A.; Hulett, M.D. Convergent evolution of defensin sequence, structure and function. *Cell. Mol. Life Sci.* **2016**, 1–20. [CrossRef]
24. Dalla Valle, L.; Benato, F.; Maistro, S.; Quinzani, S.; Alibardi, L. Bioinformatic and molecular characterization of beta-defensins-like peptides isolated from the green lizard Anolis Carolinensis. *Dev. Comp. Immunol.* **2012**, *36*, 222–229. [CrossRef]
25. Ovchinnikova, T.V.; Balandin, S.V.; Aleshina, G.M.; Tagaev, A.A.; Leonova, Y.F.; Krasnodembsky, E.D.; Men'shenin, A.V.; Kokryakov, V.N. Aurelin, a novel antimicrobial peptide from jellyfish *Aurelia aurita* with structural features of defensins and channel-blocking toxins. *Biochem. Biophys. Res. Commun.* **2006**, *348*, 514–523. [CrossRef]
26. Zhang, Z.; Zhu, S. Comparative genomics analysis of five families of antimicrobial peptide-like genes in seven ant species. *Dev. Comp. Immunol.* **2012**, *38*, 262–274. [CrossRef]
27. Tassanakajon, A.; Somboonwiwat, K.; Amparyup, P. Sequence diversity and evolution of antimicrobial peptides in invertebrates. *Dev. Comp. Immunol.* **2014**, *48*, 324–341. [CrossRef]
28. Ganz, T. Defensins: Antimicrobial peptides of innate immunity. *Nat. Rev. Immunol.* **2003**, *3*, 710–720. [CrossRef]
29. Torres, A.M.; Kuchel, P.W. The β-defensin-fold family of polypeptides. *Toxicon* **2004**, *44*, 581–588. [CrossRef]
30. Rodríguez, A.A.; Garateix, A.; Salceda, E.; Peigneur, S.; Zaharenko, A.J.; Pons, T.; Santos, Y.; Arreguín, R.; Ständker, L.; Forssmann, W.G.; et al. PhcrTx2, a new crab-paralyzing peptide toxin from the sea anemone Phymanthus crucifer. *Toxins* **2018**, *10*, 72. [CrossRef]
31. Zhu, S.; Gao, B.; Deng, M.; Yuan, Y.; Luo, L.; Peigneur, S.; Xiao, Y.; Liang, S.; Tytgat, J. Drosotoxin, a selective inhibitor of tetrodotoxin-resistant sodium channels. *Biochem. Pharmacol.* **2010**, *80*, 1296–1302. [CrossRef]
32. Zhu, S.; Peigneur, S.; Gao, B.; Umetsu, Y.; Ohki, S.; Tytgat, J. Experimental conversion of a defensin into a neurotoxin: Implications for origin of toxic function. *Mol. Biol. Evol.* **2014**, *31*, 546–559. [CrossRef]
33. Kim, C.-H.; Lee, Y.J.; Go, H.-J.; Oh, H.Y.; Lee, T.K.; Park, J.B.; Park, N.G. Defensin-neurotoxin dyad in a basally branching metazoan sea anemone. *FEBS J.* **2017**, *284*, 3320–3338. [CrossRef]
34. Copeland, R.A. *Evaluation of Enzyme Inhibitors in Drug Discovery: A Guide for Medicinal Chemists and Pharmacologists*, 2nd ed.; John Wiley and Sons: Hoboken, NJ, USA, 2013.
35. Morrison, J.F. Kinetics of the reversible inhibition of enzyme-catalysed reactions by tight-binding inhibitors. *Biochim. Biophys. Acta Enzymol.* **1969**, *185*, 269–286. [CrossRef]

36. Monastyrnaya, M.; Leychenko, E.; Isaeva, M.; Likhatskaya, G.; Zelepuga, E.; Kostina, E.; Trifonov, E.; Nurminski, E.; Kozlovskaya, E. Actinoporins from the sea anemones, tropical *Radianthus macrodactylus* and northern *Oulactis orientalis*: Comparative analysis of structure–function relationships. *Toxicon* **2010**, *56*, 1299–1314. [CrossRef]
37. Leychenko, E.; Isaeva, M.; Tkacheva, E.; Zelepuga, E. Multigene Family of Pore-forming Toxins from Sea Anemone *Heteractis Crispa*. *Mar. Drugs* **2018**, *16*, 183. [CrossRef]
38. Valle, A.; Alvarado-Mesén, J.; Lanio, M.E.; Álvarez, C.; Barbosa, J.A.R.G.; Pazos, I.F. The multigene families of actinoporins (part I): Isoforms and genetic structure. *Toxicon* **2015**, *103*, 176–187. [CrossRef]
39. Kalina, R.; Gladkikh, I.; Dmitrenok, P.; Chernikov, O.; Koshelev, S.; Kvetkina, A.; Kozlov, S.; Kozlovskaya, E.; Monastyrnaya, M. New APETx-like peptides from sea anemone *Heteractis crispa* modulate ASIC1a channels. *Peptides* **2018**, *104*, 41–49. [CrossRef]
40. Monastyrnaya, M.; Peigneur, S.; Zelepuga, E.; Sintsova, O.; Gladkikh, I.; Leychenko, E.; Isaeva, M.; Tytgat, J.; Kozlovskaya, E. Kunitz-Type Peptide HCRG21 from the Sea Anemone *Heteractis crispa* Is a Full Antagonist of the TRPV1 Receptor. *Mar. Drugs* **2016**, *14*, 229. [CrossRef]
41. Logashina, Y.A.; Mosharova, I.V.; Korolkova, Y.V.; Shelukhina, I.V.; Dyachenko, I.A.; Palikov, V.A.; Palikova, Y.A.; Murashev, A.N.; Kozlov, S.A.; Stensvåg, K.; et al. Peptide from sea anemone *Metridium senile* affects transient receptor potential ankyrin-repeat 1 (TRPA1) function and produces analgesic effect. *J. Biol. Chem.* **2017**, *292*, 2992–3004. [CrossRef]
42. Moran, Y.; Weinberger, H.; Sullivan, J.C.; Reitzel, A.M.; Finnerty, J.R.; Gurevitz, M. Concerted Evolution of Sea Anemone Neurotoxin Genes Is Revealed through Analysis of the *Nematostella vectensis* Genome. *Mol. Biol. Evol.* **2008**, *25*, 737–747. [CrossRef]
43. García-Fernández, R.; Peigneur, S.; Pons, T.; Alvarez, C.; González, L.; Chávez, M.A.; Tytgat, J. The kunitz-type protein ShPI-1 inhibits serine proteases and voltage-gated potassium channels. *Toxins* **2016**, *8*, 1–17. [CrossRef]
44. Norton, R.S.; Chandy, K.G. Venom-derived peptide inhibitors of voltage-gated potassium channels. *Neuropharmacology* **2017**. [CrossRef]
45. Prentis, P.; Pavasovic, A.; Norton, R. Sea Anemones: Quiet Achievers in the Field of Peptide Toxins. *Toxins* **2018**, *10*, 36. [CrossRef]
46. Mitchell, M.L.; Shafee, T.; Papenfuss, A.T.; Norton, R.S. Evolution of cnidarian trans-defensins: Sequence, structure and exploration of chemical space. *Proteins Struct. Funct. Bioinform.* **2019**, *87*, 551–560. [CrossRef]
47. Diochot, S.; Baron, A.; Rash, L.D.; Deval, E.; Escoubas, P.; Scarzello, S.; Salinas, M.; Lazdunski, M. A new sea anemone peptide, APETx2, inhibits ASIC3, a major acid-sensitive channel in sensory neurons. *EMBO J.* **2004**, *23*, 1516–1525. [CrossRef]
48. Diochot, S.; Loret, E.; Bruhn, T.; Béress, L.; Lazdunski, M. APETx1, a new toxin from the sea anemone *Anthopleura elegantissima*, blocks voltage-gated human ether-a-go-go-related gene potassium channels. *Mol. Pharmacol.* **2003**, *64*, 59–69. [CrossRef]
49. Diochot, S.; Schweitz, H.; Béress, L.; Lazdunski, M. Sea anemone peptides with a specific blocking activity against the fast inactivating potassium channel Kv3.4. *J. Biol. Chem.* **1998**, *273*, 6744–6749. [CrossRef]
50. Sachkova, M.Y.; Singer, S.A.; Macrander, J.; Reitzel, A.M.; Peigneur, S.; Tytgat, J.; Moran, Y. The birth and death of toxins with distinct functions: A case study in the sea anemone *Nematostella*. *Mol. Biol. Evol.* **2019**. [CrossRef]
51. Wilcoxss, G.R.; Foghsli, H.; Nortonsgii, R.S. Refined Structure in Solution of the Sea Anemone Neurotoxin ShI. *J. Biol. Chem.* **1993**, *268*, 24707–24719.
52. Gwynn, J.P.; Douglas, C.W.I. Comparison of amylase-binding proteins in oral streptococci. *FEMS Microbiol. Lett.* **1994**, *124*, 373–379. [CrossRef]
53. Homoki, J.; Gyémánt, G.; Balogh, P.; Stündl, L.; Bíró-Molnár, P.; Paholcsek, M.; Váradi, J.; Ferenc, F.; Kelentey, B.; Nemes, J.; et al. Sour cherry extract inhibits human salivary α-amylase and growth of *Streptococcus mutans* (a pilot clinical study). *Food Funct.* **2018**, *9*, 4008–4016. [CrossRef]
54. Forester, S.C.; Gu, Y.; Lambert, J.D. Inhibition of starch digestion by the green tea polyphenol, (-)-epigallocatechin-3-gallate. *Mol. Nutr. Food Res.* **2012**, *56*, 1647–1654. [CrossRef]
55. Barroso, H.; Ramalhete, R.; Domingues, A.; Maci, S. Inhibitory activity of a green and black tea blend on *Streptococcus mutans*. *J. Oral Microbiol.* **2018**, *10*, 1481322. [CrossRef]

56. Gladkikh, I.; Monastyrnaya, M.; Leychenko, E.; Zelepuga, E.; Chausova, V.; Isaeva, M.; Anastyuk, S.; Andreev, Y.; Peigneur, S.; Tytgat, J.; et al. Atypical reactive center Kunitz-type inhibitor from the sea anemone *Heteractis crispa*. *Mar. Drugs* **2012**, *10*, 1545–1565. [CrossRef]
57. Sreerama, N.; Woody, R.W. Estimation of Protein Secondary Structure from Circular Dichroism Spectra: Comparison of CONTIN, SELCON, and CDSSTR Methods with an Expanded Reference Set. *Anal. Biochem.* **2000**, *287*, 252–260. [CrossRef]
58. Liman, E.R.; Tytgat, J.; Hess, P. Subunit stoichiometry of a mammalian K+ channel determined by construction of multimeric cDNAs. *Neuron* **1992**, *9*, 861–871. [CrossRef]
59. Kuzmic, P.; Elrod, K.C.; Cregar, L.M.; Sideris, S.; Rai, R.; Janc, J.W. High-Throughput Screening of Enzyme Inhibitors: Simultaneous Determination of Tight-Binding Inhibition Constants and Enzyme Concentration. *Anal. Biochem.* **2000**, *50*, 45–50. [CrossRef]

marine drugs

Article

Echinochrome A Promotes Ex Vivo Expansion of Peripheral Blood-Derived CD34$^+$ Cells, Potentially through Downregulation of ROS Production and Activation of the Src-Lyn-p110δ Pathway

Ga-Bin Park [1], Min-Jung Kim [1], Elena A. Vasileva [2], Natalia P. Mishchenko [2], Sergey A. Fedoreyev [2], Valentin A. Stonik [2], Jin Han [3], Ho Sup Lee [4], Daejin Kim [5,*] and Jee-Yeong Jeong [1,*]

1 Department of Biochemistry, Cancer Research Institute, Kosin University College of Medicine, Busan 49267, Korea
2 G.B. Elyakov Pacific Institute of Bioorganic Chemistry, Far-Eastern Branch of the Russian Academy of Science, Vladivostok 690022, Russia
3 National Research Laboratory for Mitochondrial Signaling, Department of Physiology, Cardiovascular and Metabolic Disease Center, Inje University College of Medicine, Busan 47392, Korea
4 Department of Internal Medicine, Kosin University College of Medicine, Busan 49267, Korea
5 Department of Anatomy, Inje University College of Medicine, Busan 47392, Korea
* Correspondence: jyjeong@kosin.ac.kr (J.Y.J.); kimdj@inje.ac.kr (D.K.); Tel.: +82-51-990-5425 (J.Y.J.); +82-51-890-8651 (D.K.)

Received: 21 August 2019; Accepted: 6 September 2019; Published: 9 September 2019

Abstract: Intracellular reactive oxygen species (ROS) play an important role in the proliferation and differentiation of hematopoietic stem and progenitor cells (HSPCs). HSPCs are difficult to be expanded ex vivo while maintaining their stemness when they are exposed to oxidative damage after being released from the bone marrow. There have been efforts to overcome this limitation by using various cytokine cocktails and antioxidants. In this study, we investigated the effects of echinochrome A (Ech A)-a well-established and non-toxic antioxidant-on the ex vivo expansion of HSPCs by analyzing a CD34$^+$ cell population and their biological functions. We observed that Ech A-induced suppression of ROS generation and p38-MAPK/JNK phosphorylation causes increased expansion of CD34$^+$ cells. Moreover, p38-MAPK/JNK inhibitors SB203580 and SP600125 promoted ex vivo expansion of CD34$^+$ cells. We also demonstrated that the activation of Lyn kinase and p110δ is a novel mechanism for Ech A to enhance ex vivo expansion of CD34$^+$ cells. Ech A upregulated phospho-Src, phospho-Lyn, and p110δ expression. Furthermore, the Ech A-induced ex vivo expansion of CD34$^+$ cells was inhibited by pretreatment with the Src family inhibitor PP1 and p110δ inhibitor CAL-101; PP1 blocked p110δ upregulation and PI3K/Akt activation, whereas CAL-101 and PI3K/Akt pathway inhibitor LY294002 did not block Src/Lyn activation. These results suggest that Ech A initially induces Src/Lyn activation, upregulates p110δ expression, and finally activates the PI3K/Akt pathway. CD34$^+$ cells expanded in the presence of Ech A produced equal or more hematopoietic colony-forming cells than unexpanded CD34$^+$ cells. In conclusion, Ech A promotes the ex vivo expansion of CD34$^+$ cells through Src/Lyn-mediated p110δ expression, suppression of ROS generation, and p38-MAPK/JNK activation. Hence, Ech A is a potential candidate modality for the ex vivo, and possibly in vivo, expansion of CD34$^+$ cells.

Keywords: hematopoietic stem and progenitor cells; CD34$^+$ cells; ex vivo expansion; Lyn; Src; p110δ; ROS

1. Introduction

Hematopoietic stem and progenitor cell (HSPC) transplantation is widely used for the treatment of various hereditary diseases and blood-related malignancies, such as leukemia, and to promote hematologic recovery following anticancer therapy [1]. HSPCs can be harvested from bone marrow, umbilical cord blood (UCB), or mobilized peripheral blood (PB) using granulocyte colony-stimulating factor (G-CSF) administration for autologous and allogeneic transplantation [2]. Currently, PB-HSPC transplantation accounts for more than 60% of total HSPC transplantation worldwide, mainly due to the less invasive collection procedures [3]. However, the insufficient number of HSPCs, even after multiple days of collection, is a limiting factor for their clinical application of transplantation [4]. Several researchers are exploring ex vivo expansion of HSPCs to overcome this limitation; however, ex vivo expansion remains a difficult challenge for HSPC-based therapies.

Reactive oxygen species (ROS) are generated in the mitochondria; they regulate proliferation, differentiation, motility, and quiescence in many cell types, including HSPCs [5,6]. A previous study using a mouse model showed that increased levels of ROS can promote the differentiation of stem cells [7]. Quiescent HSPCs reside in a hypoxic niche in the bone marrow microenvironment that protects them from oxidative stress caused by excessive ROS production, mitochondrial dysfunction, or a combination of both [7,8]. HSPCs can proliferate and differentiate in the oxygen-rich vascular niche, resulting in increased intracellular ROS levels. ROS can regulate HSPC activity and various levels of ROS accumulation may affect the fate of HSPCs. High levels of ROS can trigger HSPC dysfunction, aging, and DNA damage. On the contrary, moderate levels of ROS are necessary for the proliferation, mobilization, and differentiation of HSPCs, and low-ROS cells have been shown to retain long-term self-renewal ability [7,9–11]. Culture media with appropriate cytokines are usually required for ex vivo cultures of HSPCs. However, it is still important to regulate the levels of ROS, as cytokine treatment itself triggers intracellular ROS generation [12]. Antioxidants can effectively remove excess ROS and maintain the redox balance of cells [13,14]. A recent study showed that N-acetyl cysteine (NAC) can reduce ROS levels to enhance ex vivo expansion of HSPCs [15].

Src family kinases (SFKs), including Lyn, Fyn, Fgr, Yes, Lck, Hck, Blk, and Trk, are well known for their contribution to malignant transformation and oncogenesis, and control downstream targets to regulate cell proliferation, differentiation, adhesion, migration, and the cell cycle [16]. Because of their role in cancer development and progression, SFKs have become critical targets for cancer therapy [17]. In the immune system, the most well-known function of SFKS is their role in integrin signaling [16]. Fyn and Lck kinases are also found in T cells and natural killer (NK) cells [18]. Lyn is a non-receptor tyrosine kinase that is predominantly found in the hematopoietic cells of myeloid and B lymphocyte lineages [19]. Lyn was originally identified as a hematopoietic-specific kinase; it is expressed in multiple tissues and is involved in the signaling of the B-cell receptor [20], GM-CSF receptor [21], erythropoietin (EPO) receptor [22], and c-kit [23]. Lyn phosphorylates several signaling molecules, including PI3K, FAK [24], ras-GAP, and Stat5 [25]. Lyn also plays an important role in acute myeloid leukemia (AML) cell proliferation [26], and the silencing of Lyn in imatinib-resistant chronic myelogenous leukemia (CML) cells can induce apoptosis [27]. Lyn activation induces p110 expression, whereas Lyn inhibition decreased migration in ovarian cancer cells exposed to cigarette smoke [28]. Colon cancer cells use Lyn for activation of the anti-apoptotic PI3K p110/Akt pathway and the induction of epithelial-mesenchymal transition (EMT) [29]. Therefore, several pieces of evidence show an important association of Lyn in both leukemia and solid tumor development. However, the exact roles and Lyn/Src activation in the relationship with ROS during the ex vivo expansion of HSPCs are still unclear.

Echinochrome A (Ech A) is a dark red pigment that is isolated from eggs, spines, and larvae of sea urchins [30]. Ech A is known to possess antioxidant, antiviral, antialgal, and antimicrobial activities [31,32]. Importantly, Ech A was shown to exhibit diverse intracellular antioxidant mechanisms, including the elimination of free radicals [33], inhibition of pulmonary fibrosis [34], and chelation of metal ions [35]. In this study, we demonstrate that Ech A is an effective agent to promote the ex vivo expansion of G-CSF-mobilized PB-derived CD34$^+$ HSPCs through Src/Lyn-mediated p110δ upregulation, the suppression of ROS generation, and p38-MAPK/JNK activation.

2. Results

2.1. Ech A Suppresses ROS Production and Promotes Expansion of PBMC-Derived CD34$^+$ Cells

HSPCs reside in a hypoxic niche in the bone marrow, suggesting that HSPCs need to adopt unique metabolic properties, including intracellular ROS levels. We found that PB-derived CD34$^+$ cells (PB-CD34$^+$ cells) exhibit higher ROS levels than BM-derived CD34$^+$ cells (Figure 1A). We then examined whether Ech A can modulate ROS levels to cause an ex vivo expansion of PB-CD34$^+$ cells. To determine the optimal concentration of Ech A, G-CSF-mobilized PB mononuclear cells (PBMCs) were treated with different concentrations of Ech A (0, 1, 10, 20, 50, and 100 μM) for 24 h, and the CD34$^+$ cell number was analyzed by flow cytometry. Cells treated with 10 μM Ech A for 24 h showed approximately two-fold higher CD34$^+$ cell number than those in the control group (Figure S1A); therefore, we chose that condition for subsequent experiments. The effect of Ech A on the ex vivo expansion of PBMCs containing CD34$^+$ or purified PB-CD34$^+$ was investigated after 1 day or 4 days of culture, respectively (Figure 1B). The toxic reagent N-acetyl cysteine (NAC)—a well-known potent antioxidant—was used as the positive control. Immunophenotypic analysis showed a significantly higher percentage of CD34$^+$ cells and the CD34+ cell number in Ech A-treated group (PBMCs, 12.91% ± 3.22%, 2.05 ± 0.66-fold; PB-CD34$^+$ cells, 73.37% ± 1.11%, 4.95 ± 0.28-fold) than that in the control group (PBMCs, 7.07 ± 0.66%, 0.87 ± 0.08-fold; PB-CD34$^+$ cells, 67.27 ± 1.79%, 3.71 ± 0.18-fold). As shown in Figure 1C, Ech A dramatically suppressed intracellular ROS production in PBMCs and PB-CD34$^+$ cells. Additionally, H_2O_2 treatment showed dramatic suppression of PB-CD34$^+$ cell expansion that was recovered by Ech A treatment (Figure S2). These results suggest that Ech A promotes the ex vivo expansion of PBMC-derived CD34$^+$ cells by suppressing ROS levels.

2.2. Ech A Inhibits the Activation of p38-MAPK and JNK in PB-CD34$^+$ Cells

After 1 or 4 days of culture, the levels of phosphorylated p38-MAPK and JNK were significantly increased in the expanded cells (Figure 2A; negative control). However, the phosphorylation of p38-MAPK and JNK was dramatically suppressed upon the treatment of Ech A or NAC (Figure 2A). On the other hand, ERK1/2 phosphorylation remained unchanged in the cells. To examine whether p38-MAPK/JNK activation inhibits the ex vivo expansion of human PB-CD34$^+$ cells, cells were cultured in the presence of vehicle (0.1% DMSO), SB203580 (SB; 5 μM), or SP600125 (SP; 5 μM) for 1 or 4 days. The expanded cells were harvested for cell counts, and the analysis of CD34 expression by flow cytometry. As illustrated in Figure 2B, the total number of PBMCs was comparable irrespective of whether cells were incubated with or without SB or SP. Cell cultures with SB or SP showed a considerable increase in the number of CD34$^+$ cells compared to the DMSO control group. In particular, the number of CD34$^+$ cells was approximately 1.5-fold higher in the presence of SB (PBMCs, 2.17% ± 0.06%, 1.45 ± 0.05-fold; PB-CD34$^+$ cells, 72.27% ± 5.01%, 6.38 ± 0.27-fold) or SP (PBMCs, 2.33% ± 0.31%, 1.51 ± 0.22-fold; PB-CD34$^+$ cells, 71.27% ± 7.83%, 6.34 ± 0.61-fold) than that in the DMSO control group (PBMCs, 1.33% ± 0.06%, 0.85 ± 0.07-fold; PB-CD34$^+$ cells, 55.00% ± 0.56%, 4.43 ± 0.05-fold). However, ROS levels in PB-CD34$^+$ cells were unaffected by SB or SP (Figure 2C). These results suggest that p38-MAPK/JNK inhibition increases the ex vivo expansion of CD34$^+$ cells, even at high ROS levels.

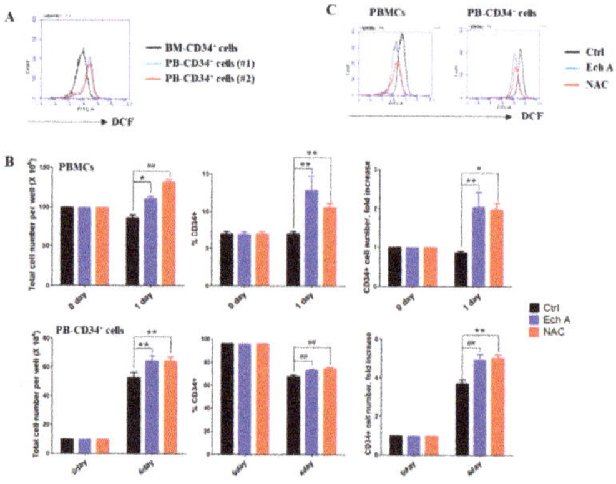

Figure 1. Ech A increases PB-CD34$^+$ cell expansion by inhibiting reactive oxygen species' (ROS) generation. (**A**) Cells were treated with 10 μM 2′7′-dichlorodihydro-fluorescein diacetate for 30 min. The values in the 2′7′-dichlorofluorescein histograms indicate MFI (mean fluorescence intensity). (**B**,**C**) Cells were treated with 10 μM Ech A for 1 day (PB mononuclear cells, PBMCs) or 4 days (PB-CD34$^+$ cells). For NAC treatment, cells were treated with 5 mM NAC for 4 h, washed, suspended in complete medium, and incubated for an additional 1 day (PBMCs) or 4 days (PB-CD34$^+$ cells). (**B**) Total cell number was measured using the ADAM-MC automated mammalian cell counter (NanoEntech, Seoul, Korea). For flow cytometric immunophenotypic analysis, cells were stained with CD34-PE, CD38-FITC, CD45-APC, and 7-AAD. Each value was expressed as the mean ± SEM of three independent experiments. (**C**) Cells were treated with 10 μM 2′7′-dichlorodihydro-fluorescein diacetate for 30 min and ROS levels were subsequently measured usingthe flow cytometer.

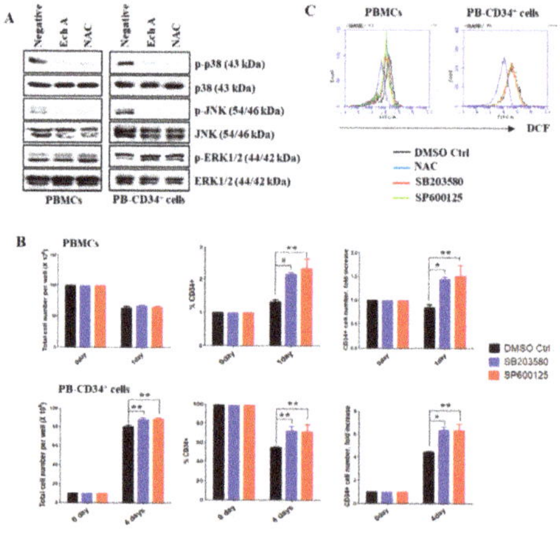

Figure 2. Ech A enhances PB-CD34$^+$ cell expansion by suppressing the activation of p38-MAPK and JNK. Cells were treated with 10 μM Ech A for 1 day (PBMCs) or 4 days (PB-CD34$^+$ cells). For NAC treatment, cells were treated with 5 mM NAC for 4 h, washed, suspended in complete medium, and incubated for an additional 1 day (PBMCs) or 4 days (PB-CD34$^+$ cells). (**A**) Total protein was subjected to western blot analysis with the indicated antibodies. β-actin served as the loading control. (B, C) Cells were pretreated with SB203580 (10 μM) or SP600125 (10 μM) for 4 hr. (**B**) Total cell number was measured using the ADAM-MC automated mammalian cell counter. For flow cytometric immunophenotypic analysis, cells were stained with CD34-PE, CD38-FITC, CD45-APC, and 7-AAD. Each value was expressed as the mean ± SEM of three independent experiments. (**C**) Cells were treated with 10 μM 2′7′-dichlorodihydro-fluorescein diacetate for 30 min. The values in the 2′7′-dichlorofluorescein histograms indicate MFI.

2.3. *Ech A Regulates PB-CD34$^+$ Cell Expansion via PI3K/Akt Pathway*

We further assessed the possible molecular mechanisms underlying Ech A-mediated ex vivo expansion of PB-CD34$^+$ cells. Our results showed that phosphorylation of PI3K-p85 and Akt was enhanced to a greater extent in Ech A- or NAC-treated cells than that in untreated cells (Figure 3A); however, phospho-PTEN level were reduced. To verify the requirement of PI3K/Akt signaling activation for PB-CD34$^+$ cell expansion, we used the PI3K/Akt inhibitor LY294002. As shown in Figure 3B, pretreatment of the Ech A or NAC treatment group with LY294002 (PBMCs, 7.83 ± 1.31%, 3.29 ± 0.73-fold; PB-CD34$^+$ cells, 71.43 ± 6.45%, 9.55 ± 1.41-fold) substantially reduced the percentage of CD34$^+$ cells as well as CD34$^+$ cell number compared to Ech A or NAC single treatment group (PBMCs, 23.63 ± 1.7%, 14.43 ± 2.42-fold; PB-CD34$^+$ cells, 84.43 ± 0.93%, 22.33 ± 1.49-fold).

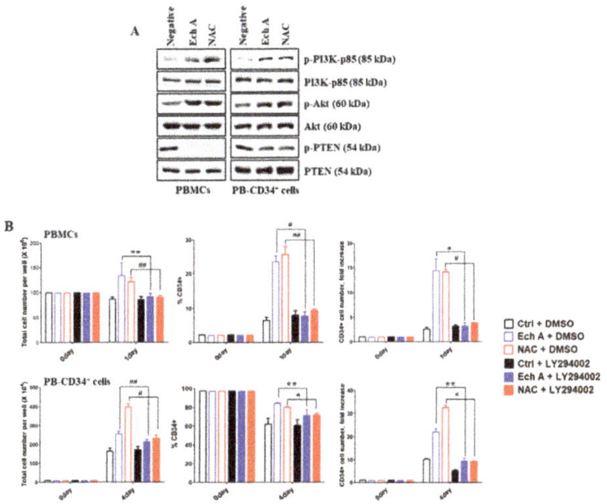

Figure 3. Echinochrome A (Ech A) upregulates PB-CD34$^+$ cell expansion by activating PI3K/Akt pathway. Cells were treated with 10 μM Ech A for 1 day (PBMCs) or 4 days (PB-CD34$^+$ cells). For NAC treatment, cells were treated with 5 mM NAC for 4 h, washed, suspended in complete medium, and incubated for an additional 1 day (PBMCs) or 4 days (PB-CD34$^+$ cells). (**A**) Total cell lysates for each condition were immunoblotted with the indicated antibodies. (**B**) Cell were pretreated with LY294002 (10 μM) for 4 h. Total cell number was determined using the ADAM-MC automated mammalian cell counter. For flow cytometric immunophenotypic analysis, cells were stained with CD34-PE, CD38-FITC, CD45-APC, and 7-AAD. Each value was expressed as the mean ± SEM of three independent experiments.

2.4. *The PI3K p110δ Isoform Is Required for Ech A-Induced CD34$^+$ Cell Expansion*

Next, we examined which p110 isoforms were associated with the expansion of PB-CD34$^+$ cells, following Ech A or NAC treatment using antibodies, each specific for different p110 isoforms of PI3K. Ech A- or NAC-treated PBMCs or PB-CD34$^+$ cells showed a higher expression of p110δ than untreated PB-CD34$^+$ cells; however, p110α, p110β, and p110γ expression was not affected by Ech A or NAC treatment (Figure 4A). To identify the role of p110δ in Ech A- or NAC-induced PB-CD34$^+$ cell expansion, cells were treated with Ech A or NAC in the presence or absence of the p110δ specific inhibitor, CAL-101. The percentage of CD34$^+$ cells and the CD34$^+$ cell number in the Ech A or NAC single treatment group (PBMCs, 23.63% ± 1.7%, 15.32 ± 1.27-fold; PB-CD34$^+$ cells, 82.07% ± 0.32%, 18.55 ± 1.12-fold) were remarkably decreased by CAL-101 pretreatment (PBMCs, 7.57% ± 1.99%, 3.37 ± 0.74-fold; PB-CD34$^+$ cells, 70.67% ± 2.73%, 7.93 ± 1.23-fold) (Figure 4B).

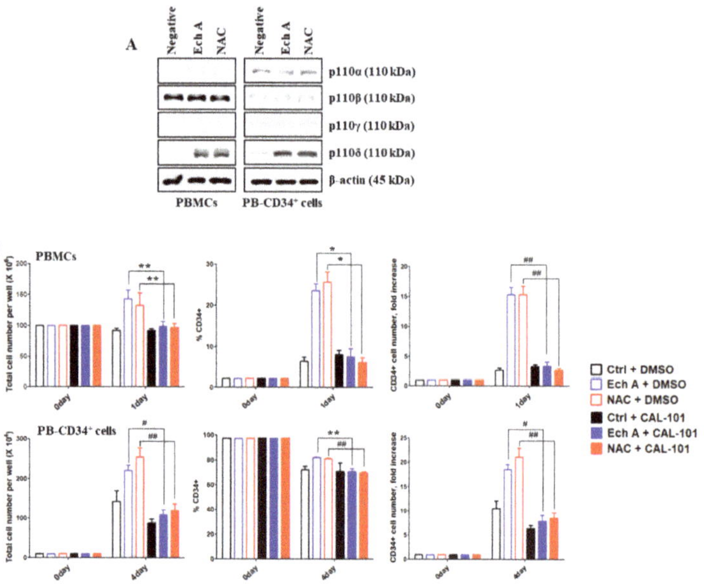

Figure 4. Ech A induces the activation of the PI3K p110δ isoform for PB-CD34$^+$ cell expansion. Cells were treated with 10 μM Ech A for 1 day (PBMCs) or 4 days (PB-CD34$^+$ cells). For NAC treatment, cells were treated with 5 mM NAC for 4 h, washed, suspended in complete medium, and incubated for an additional 1 day (PBMCs) or 4 days (PB-CD34$^+$ cells). (**A**) Total protein was subjected to western blot analysis with the indicated antibodies. (**B**) Cells were pretreated with CAL-101 (20 μM) for 4 h. Total cell number was determined using the ADAM-MC automated mammalian cell counter. For flow cytometric immunophenotypic analysis, cells were stained with CD34-PE, CD38-FITC, CD45-APC, and 7-AAD. Each value was expressed as the mean ± SEM of three independent experiments.

2.5. Src/Lyn Is a Major Upstream Signal for Ech A-Induced p110δ-Mediated CD34$^+$ Cell Expansion

We also investigated Src family kinases associated with the increased expression of p110δ upon Ech A or NAC treatment in PB-CD34$^+$ cells. Compared with untreated controls, treatment with Ech A or NAC increased Src phosphorylation levels, but produced little effect on Fyn phosphorylation. Interestingly, Lyn was significantly phosphorylated only by Ech A treatment, but not by NAC (Figure 5A). To identify the requirement for the Src/Lyn pathway in Ech A- or NAC-induced p110δ expression, we used the Src/Lyn inhibitor PP1. The percentages of CD34$^+$ cells and the CD34+ cell number in the Ech A or NAC single treatment group (PBMCs, 14.2% ± 1.39%, 8.37 ± 0.13-fold; PB-CD34$^+$ cells, 81.57% ± 1.88%, 9.43 ± 0.55-fold) were significantly lower than that in the PP1 pretreatment group (PBMCs, 8.63% ± 2.65%, 4.41 ± 1.40-fold; PB-CD34$^+$ cells, 70.27% ± 1.54%, 6.84 ± 0.11-fold) (Figure 5B). To establish a possible link between Ech A- and NAC-induced Src/Lyn phosphorylation and PI3K activation during the ex vivo expansion of CD34$^+$ cells, we treated cells with PP1, LY294002, or CAL-101. First, we confirmed the activity of various inhibitors used in this study on each target molecule (Figure S3). As shown in Figure 5C, PP1 dramatically suppressed Ech A or NAC-mediated expression of p110δ and PI3K/Akt activation. On the other hand, LY294002 and CAL-101 did not inhibit Ech A- or NAC-induced Src/Lyn activation (Figure 5D,E). These results suggest that Lyn is activated prior to p110δ and PI3K/Akt and plays a critical role as an upstream regulatory molecule in Ech A-induced ex vivo expansion of PB-CD34$^+$ cells.

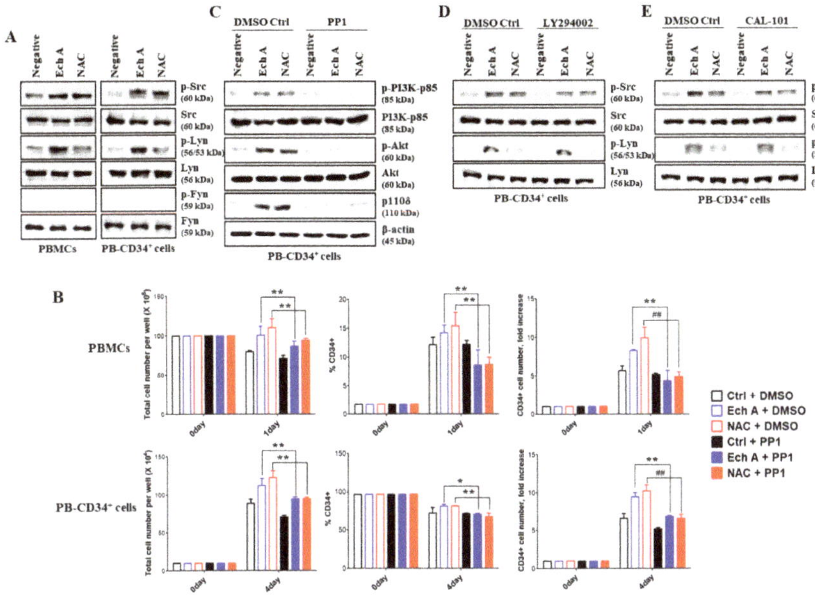

Figure 5. Src/Lyn is major upstream signal for p110δ-mediated $CD34^+$ cell expansion by Ech A. Cells were treated with 10 μM Ech A for 1 day (PBMCs) or 4 days (PB-$CD34^+$ cells). For NAC treatment, cells were treated with 5 mM NAC for 4 h, washed, suspended in complete medium, and incubated for an additional 1 day (PBMCs) or 4 days (PB-$CD34^+$ cells). (**A**,**C**–**E**) Total cell lysates for each condition were harvested and immunoblotted with the indicated antibodies. (**B**–**E**) Cells were pretreated with PP1 (10 μM), LY294002 (10 μM), or CAL-101 (20 μM) for 4 h. (**B**) Total cell number was determined using the ADAM-MC automated mammalian cell counter. For flow cytometric immunophenotypic analysis, cells were stained with CD34-PE, CD38-FITC, CD45-APC, and 7-AAD. Each value was expressed as the mean ± SEM of three independent experiments.

2.6. Ex Vivo Expanded $CD34^+$ Cells Maintain Their Colony-Forming Capacity

As CFU indicates the presence of HSPCs, the colony forming potential (colony-forming unit/burst-forming unit-erythroid (CFU/BFU-E), CFU-granulocyte/macrophage (CFU-GM), and CFU-granulocyte/erythroid/macrophage/megakaryocytes (CFU-GEMM), and total CFU) of freshly isolated $CD34^+$ cells or $CD34^+$ cells, expanded in the absence or presence of Ech A (10 μM) or NAC (5 mM), was investigated (Figure 6). The frequency of CFU/BFU-E (Ech A, 173.3 ± 3.51; NAC, 181.7 ± 0.58) and total CFU (Ech A, 248.0 ± 5; NAC, 262.7 ± 1.53) in the 10 μM Ech A or 5 mM NAC group was significantly higher than that in the unexpanded (CFU/BFU-E, 91.3 ± 6.11; total CFU, 145.7 ± 6.03) or control expanded group (CFU/BFU-E, 99.3 ± 3.06; total CFU, 157.7 ± 3.06). The frequency of CFU-GM (Ech A, 73.33 ± 2.08; NAC, 80 ± 2) and CFU-GEMM (Ech A, 1.33 ± 0.58; NAC, 1 ± 0) was not vastly different from the unexpanded (CFU-GM, 52.67 ± 4.04; CFU-GEMM, 1.67 ± 0.58) or control group (CFU-GM, 57.3 ± 3.06; CFU-GEMM, 1 ± 0) (Figure 6A). Although the number of CFU/BFU-E was higher in the Ech A and NAC expanded groups, the size of CFU/BFU-E was larger in the unexpanded group (Figure 6B). Therefore, the addition of 10 μM Ech A certainly improved ex vivo expansion of HSPC numbers, but the potency may have slightly decreased.

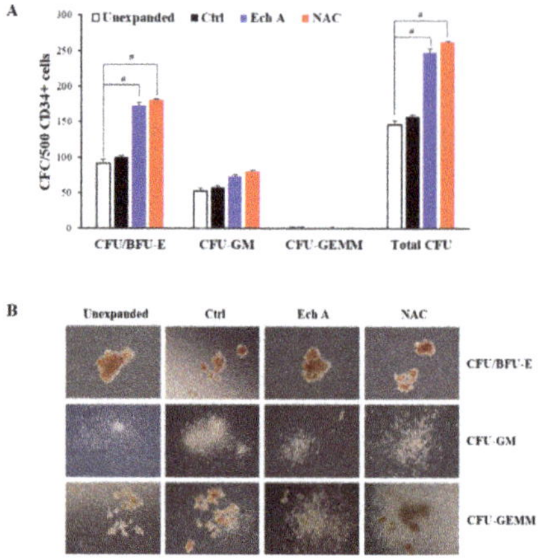

Figure 6. Ex vivo expanded CD34+ cells maintain their colony-forming capabilities. Purified PB-CD34$^+$ non-expanded cells, or cells expanded ex vivo in the presence or absence of NAC or Ech A for 4 days were evaluated for pluripotency using hematopoietic colony-forming assays in semi-solid methylcellulose media. (**A**) Colony-forming unit/burst-forming unit-erythroid (CFU/BFU-E), CFU-granulocyte/macrophage (CFU-GM), and CFU-granulocyte/erythroid/macrophage/megakaryocytes (CFU-GEMM) per 500 CD34$^+$ cells plated were enumerated after 14 days of culture. (**B**) Representative images of CFU/BFU-E, CFU-GM, and CFU-GEMM for each experimental condition. Magnification: ×200.

3. Discussion

HSPCs with self-renewal and multipotent capacity offer a valuable source for cell-based therapy and regenerative medicine [36]. Many limitations facing during HSPC transplantations would have been overcome if ex vivo HSPC expansion and maintenance become possible. However, the characteristics of the HSPCs are often altered once they leave the hypoxic bone marrow niche, affecting the quality and quantity of the cultured HSPCs. Studies have shown that the fate of HSPCs is regulated by the microenvironment of the so-called "stem cell niches" that contain oxygen saturations of approximately 5% [7]. The increased oxygen tension in normoxic cultures causes the stem cells to lose their stemness [37]. Various attempts have been carried out to maintain the stemness of HSPCs and to overcome the limitations associated with ex vivo culturing. These include the utility of transcription factors, co-culturing with feeder cells [38], the addition of cytokine cocktails [39], and genetic modification [40]. However, these approaches have some drawbacks, especially when used in a clinical setting. A few previous studies have suggested that the use of antioxidants can ameliorate oxidative stress-mediated damage in cultured HSPCs [41]. In this study, we investigated whether PB-CD34$^+$ cells can be efficiently expanded ex vivo by utilizing Ech A, which has been demonstrated as an antioxidant in previous studies [32,34].

HSPCs remain quiescent in the osteoblastic niche—the lowest end of the oxygen gradient in the bone marrow. However, in the oxygen-rich vascular niche, stem cells can proliferate and differentiate closer to blood circulation, resulting in increased intracellular ROS levels. However, an extremely low or high level of ROS would cause impaired repopulation capacity or trigger exhaustion of HSPCs [9]. Physiologically, with the aid of intracellular antioxidant enzyme systems and endogenous antioxidants, HSPCs are able to cope with the damage caused by cumulative ROS [42]. However, the damage is overwhelmed when HSPCs are subjected to ex vivo expansion, wherein a sharp increase in ROS levels is often experienced. It is, therefore, critical to regulate the intracellular ROS levels during ex vivo culturing for the better expansion and maintenance of HSPCs. It has been previously demonstrated that a reduction in intracellular ROS levels by supplementing antioxidants or lowering oxygen tension in cell cultures could improve HSPC expansion, and their engraftment and hematopoietic reconstitution abilities in non-obese diabetic/severe combined immunodeficiency (NOD/SCID) mice [43]. Consistent with this finding, PB-CD34$^+$ cells provoked aberrant ROS generation in the normoxic culture (Figure 1A). PB-CD34$^+$ cells exhibited higher ROS levels than BM-CD34$^+$ cells (Figure 1A). ROS is a critical mediator of HSPC quiescence with p38-MAPK. Higher ROS levels can activate the p38-MAPK pathway, which in turn can promote phosphorylation of p38-MAPK [44]. Our results also showed that PB-CD34$^+$ cells can upregulate phospho-p38-MAPK and phospho-JNK, likely due to high ROS levels (Figure 2A). p38-MAPK plays a role in hematopoiesis regulation, particularly in erythropoiesis and granule formation [45]. Recently, p38-MAPK was identified as an intrinsic modulator that can negatively regulate HSPC self-renewal [46]. Therefore, both ROS and p38-MAPK have been shown to play an important role in maintaining HSPC quiescence. Several studies have indicated that HSPCs lose their ability to regenerate due to elevated ROS levels and specific phosphorylation of p38-MAPK. Pharmacological inhibition of ROS or p38-MAPK activity can restore HSPC function in the ROS^{high} mouse population and rescue these mice from bone marrow damage [7]. Treatment of Ech A and NAC potently suppressed the activation of p38-MAPK and JNK, and the p38-MAPK inhibitor SB203580 and the JNK inhibitor SP600125 promoted CD34$^+$ cell expansion, potentially by inhibiting differentiation (Figure 2). It is noteworthy that the suppression of ROS by Ech A ameliorated the activation of p38-MAPK and JNK, suggesting that Ech A acts as an efficient antioxidant in the ex vivo culture of PB-CD34$^+$ cells, and subsequently promotes CD34$^+$ cell expansion.

SFKs in hematopoietic tissues can function as primary regulatory factors, as described in the first *p60-Src* gene perturbation experiment to confirm its role in osteopetrosis development [47]. Subsequent studies revealed SFK activities in B cells, bone marrow, obese cell lines, and Lyn-expressing HSPCs in all blood cell lines except T cells [19]. In some studies, Lyn was shown to play negative roles in monocyte production and plasma cell function, as revealed in *Lyn*$^{-/-}$ mice by M-phi tumorigenesis [48] and IgM hyperglobulinemia [20]. Although not widely studied, SFKs have also been suggested as important regulators of erythropoiesis. Avian Src was originally discovered as an oncogene that promotes sarcoma and erythroleukemia [49]. Interestingly, *Lyn*$^{-/-}$ mice among the SFK gene-deficient mice showed an age-dependent increase in the production of splenic erythroblasts [50]. In BM-derived cultures, early-stage *Lyn*$^{-/-}$ erythroblasts exhibited a reduced ability to expand and develop beyond the Kit$^+$CD71$^+$ stage [51]. Therefore, SFKs, such as Lyn and Src, are major signaling mediators that modulate diverse stimuli to regulate differentiation, migration, proliferation, apoptosis, and metabolism. However, there is limited information regarding the precise role Lyn/Src and their underlying molecular mechanisms in the ex vivo expansion of PB-CD34$^+$ cells. PI3K/Akt signaling can be activated by the downregulation of PTEN by BCR–ABL2. PTEN is a lipid phosphatase that interferes with PI3K signaling by dephosphorylating phosphatidylinositol-3,4,5-trisphosphate. Class I PI3Ks consist of four different catalytic isoforms (p110α, p110β, p110γ, and p110δ) and two standard regulatory subunits (p85 and p101) [52]. PI3K plays an important role in HSPC maintenance and regulation of lineage development [53]. In this study, we found, for the first time to our knowledge, that Ech A activates Lyn, which in turn upregulates p110δ expression, and suppresses ROS production and p38-MAPK/JNK phosphorylation, resulting in enhanced ex vivo expansion of PB-CD34$^+$ cells (Figures 4 and 5). Furthermore, the addition of Ech A increased CFU/BFU-E producing cell numbers (Figure 6), which suggests that an appropriate use of Ech A is advantageous for CD34$^+$ cells to maintain self-renewal potential during ex vivo expansion.

Our findings, as summarized in Figure 7, demonstrate that Ech A can effectively inhibit ROS production in PB-CD34$^+$ cells. ROS-mediated p38-MAPK/JNK activation can reduce the number of CD34$^+$ cells, and decrease the self-renewal of PB-CD34$^+$ cells, which was reversed by Ech A treatment. Our results also demonstrate a novel Lyn-mediated p110δ expression by Ech A in PB-CD34$^+$ cells, although the precise molecular mechanism of Ech A-induced ex vivo expansion, especially how Lyn and p110δ are coordinated in PB-CD34$^+$ cells in response to Ech A, remains unclear. Taken together, Ech A was found to be an effective agent for promoting cell proliferation and maintaining the stemness of HSPCs. Ech A is beneficial for CD34$^+$ cells to maintain their self-renewal potential and function during the ex vivo expansion, and possibly during in vivo expansion of HSPCs.

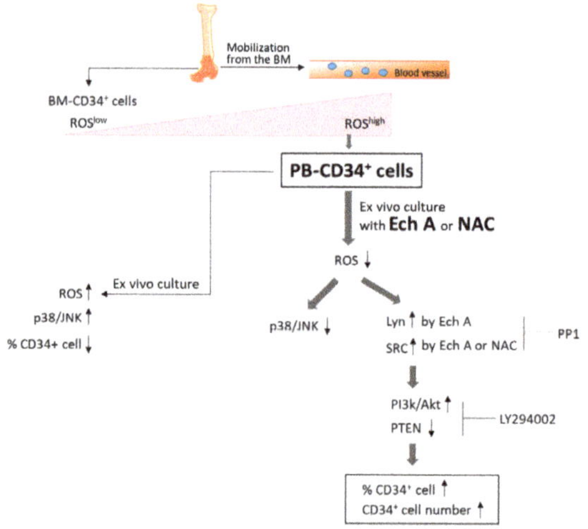

Figure 7. Schematic representation of Ech A and NAC in the ex vivo expansion of PB-CD34$^+$ cells. Mobilized PB-CD34$^+$ cells showed higher ROS levels than BM-CD34$^+$ cells. Ech A suppressed intracellular ROS production in PB-CD34$^+$ cells. Ech A also increased Lyn/Src phosphorylation and PI3K/Akt activation. Our results suggest that Ech A promotes ex vivo expansion of CD34$^+$ cells through Lyn/Src-mediated p110δ expression.

4. Materials and Methods

4.1. Isolation of PBMCs and Purification of PB-CD34$^+$ Cells

This study was conducted using samples from healthy donors and patients, and the study protocol was approved by the Institutional Review Board at the Kosin University College of Medicine. Informed consent for the study was obtained from all donors. Purified BM- or PB-CD34$^+$ cells were obtained either from BM (Lonza, Basel, Swizerland) or from small aliquots of mobilized PB from healthy donors and patients. CD34$^+$ cells from PBMCs were immunoselected using the MACS CD34 MicroBead kit UltraPure (Miltenyi Biotec, Bergisch Gladbach, Germany). Human CD34$^+$ cells were enriched from PBMCs by magnetic bead positive selection using Miltenyi immunomagnetically activated cell sorter (MACS; Miltenyi Biotec). PB-CD34$^+$ cells were then stained for CD45, and the CD34$^+$ purity of greater than 95% was reanalyzed by flow cytometry. PB-CD34$^+$ cells were expanded in serum-free medium (SFEM) (Stem Cell Technologies, Vancouver, Canada) supplemented with 50 ng/mL rhSCF (PeproTech, Rocky Hill, NJ, USA), 10 ng/mL rhIL3 (PeproTech), and 25 μg/mL LDL (Stem Cell Technologies).

4.2. Chemicals and Reagents

Ech A was received as a gift from G.B. Elyakov, Pacific Institute of Bioorganic Chemistry, Vladivostok, Russia. PPI, SP600125, SB203580, LY294002, and CAL-101 were purchased from Selleck Chemicals (Houston, TX, USA). NAC was obtained from Sigma-Aldrich (St. Louis, MO, USA).

4.3. Immunophenotypic Analysis by Flow Cytometry

PBMCs, PB-CD34$^+$ cells, and BM-CD34$^+$ cells were tested for cell surface antigen expression by immunofluorescence and flow cytometric analysis. Cells were harvested and rinsed with PBS, following which CD34-PE (Miltenyi Biotec, #130-113-179, 1:50), CD38-FITC (Miltenyi Biotec, #130-113-426, 1:50), CD45RA-APC (Miltenyi Biotec, #130-117-742, 1:50), and 7-AAD (eBioscience, Waltham, MA, USA,

3 μL/10^5 cells) were added. Thereafter, cells were incubated at 4 °C for 10 min in the dark. Finally, the stained cells were analyzed using a BD Accuri™ C6 (BD Biosciences).

4.4. Determination of Intracellular ROS Production

The intracellular accumulation of ROS was determined by flow cytometry after staining with the fluorescent probe DCFH-DA (10 μM, 2′,7′-dichlorodihydro-fluorescein diacetate; Molecular Probes, Invitrogen, Milan, Italy). DCFH-DA was deacetylated in cells by esterase to a nonfluorescent compound DCFH, which remains trapped within the cell and is cleaved and oxidized by ROS in the presence of endogenous peroxidase to a highly fluorescent compound DCF (2′,7′-dichlorofluorescein). Cells were incubated with 10 μM DCFH-DA for 30 min at 37 °C, washed, and resuspended in PBS. ROS levels were monitored using a BD Accuri™ C6 (BD Biosciences).

4.5. Immunoblotting

Cells were lysed in RIPA (radioimmunoprecipitation assay) buffer (Elpis Biotech, Daejeon, Korea) supplemented with a protease inhibitor cocktail (Calbiochem, La Jolla, CA, USA) and protein phosphatase inhibitors (Calbiochem). Protein concentrations were determined using a BCA assay kit (Pierce, Rockford, IL, USA). Proteins (10 μg/sample) were resolved in an SDS-PAGE gel and transferred to a nitrocellulose membrane (Millipore Corp., Billerica, MA, USA). Membranes were blocked with 5% skim milk prior to western blot analysis. Chemiluminescence was detected using an ECL kit (Advansta Corp., Menlo Park, CA, USA) and the Amersham Imager 600 (GE Healthcare Life Sciences, Little Chalfont, UK). The following primary antibodies were used on fresh individual membranes to minimize interference by stripping and reprobing: phospho-JNK (Thr^{183}/Tyr^{185}), JNK, phospho-p38 MAPK (Thr^{180}/Tyr^{182}), p38 MAPK, phospho-ERK1/2 (Thr^{202}/Tyr^{204}), ERK1/2, phospho-Src (Tyr^{416}), Src, phospho-Lyn (Tyr^{507}), Lyn, phospho-Akt (Ser^{473}), Akt, phospho-PI3K p85 (Tyr^{458}/Tyr^{199}), PI3K p85, PI3K p110α, PI3K p110β, PI3K p110γ, PI3K p110δ, phospho-PTEN (Ser^{380}/$Thr^{382/383}$), PTEN, and Fyn (Cell Signaling Technology, Beverly, MA, USA); and β-actin and phospho-Fyn (Santa Cruz Biotechnology, Santa Cruz, CA, USA). All the raw data from immunoblotting experiments are presented in Figure S4.

4.6. Colony-Forming Cell (CFC) Assay

$CD34^+$ cells (500 cells/dish) were plated in methylcellulose medium (Methocult H4100, STEMCELL Technologies, Inc., Canada) supplemented with SCF (50 ng/mL), IL-3 (10 ng/mL), GM-CSF (10 ng/mL) (PeproTech), and EPO (1 U/mL) in 35-mm culture dishes and incubated at 37 °C in a 5% CO_2 chamber for 14 days. Colonies were counted and analyzed using a scoring grid and an inverted microscope (Olympus, Japan). Colonies were classified based on their morphology as colony-forming unit/burst-forming unit-erythroid (CFU/BFU-E), CFU-granulocyte/macrophage (CFU-GM), and CFU-granulocyte/erythroid/macrophage/megakaryocytes (CFU-GEMM).

4.7. Statistical Analysis

The data were analyzed using Student's *t*-tests and one-way analyses of variance (ANOVA) with GraphPad Prism software, and are presented as standard error of the mean (SEM), unless otherwise stated. Statistical significance was defined as * $p < 0.01$, ** $p < 0.05$, # $p < 0.001$, and ## $p < 0.005$.

Supplementary Materials: The following are available online at http://www.mdpi.com/1660-3397/17/9/526/s1, Figure S1: Dose-dependent effect of Ech A or NAC on ex vivo expansion of PBMCs; Figure S2: Ech A recovered PB-$CD34^+$ cell expansion that was suppressed by H_2O_2 treatment; Figure S3: Each inhibitor was confirmed to work as expected; Figure S4: Raw data from immunoblotting experiments.

Author Contributions: Conceptualization, J.H. and J.-Y.J.; funding acquisition, J.-Y.J.; investigation, G.-B.P., M.-J.K., and H.S.L.; methodology, G.-B.P. and J.-Y.J.; resources, E.A.V., N.P.M., S.A.F., V.A.S., and J.H.; supervision, J.-Y.J.; writing—original draft, G.-B.P., D.K., and J.-Y.J.

Funding: This study was supported by the Korean National Research Foundation (KNRF) grants 2015M3A9B6073646, 2017M3A9G7072564 (both to J.Y.J.), and 2017K1A3A1A49070056 (to J.H.). The study was also supported by the Ministry of Education and Science of the Russian Federation (RFMEFI61317X0076).

Conflicts of Interest: The authors declare that they have no competing interests.

References

1. Gratwohl, A.; Baldomero, H.; Schwendener, A.; Rocha, V.; Apperley, J.; Frauendorfer, K.; Niederwieser, D. The EBMT activity survey 2007 with focus on allogeneic HSCT for AML and novel cellular therapies. *Bone Marrow Transpl.* **2009**, *43*, 257–291. [CrossRef] [PubMed]
2. Verfaillie, C.M. Hematopoietic stem cells for transplantation. *Nat. Immunol.* **2002**, *3*, 314–317. [CrossRef] [PubMed]
3. D'Souza, A.; Lee, S.; Zhu, A.; Pasquini, M. Current use and trends in hematopoietic cell transplantation in the united states. *Biol. Blood Marrow Transpl.* **2017**, *23*, 1417–1421. [CrossRef] [PubMed]
4. Kallinikou, K.; Anjos-Afonso, F.; Blundell, M.P.; Ings, S.J.; Watts, M.J.; Thrasher, A.J.; Limch, D.C.; Bonnet, D.; Yong, K.L. Engraftment defect of cytokine-cultured adult human mobilized CD34(+) cells is related to reduced adhesion to bone marrow niche elements. *Br. J. Haematol.* **2012**, *158*, 778–787. [CrossRef]
5. Kobayashi, C.I.; Suda, T. Regulation of reactive oxygen species in stem cells and cancer stem cell. *J. Cell Physiol.* **2012**, *227*, 421–430. [CrossRef]
6. Kim, S.M.; Hwang, K.A.; Choi, K.C. Potential roles of reactive oxygen species derived from chemical substances involved in cancer development in the female reproductive system. *BMB Rep.* **2018**, *51*, 557–562. [CrossRef]
7. Jang, Y.Y.; Sharkis, S.J. A low level of reactive oxygen species selects for primitive hematopoietic stem cells that may reside in the low-oxygenic niche. *Blood* **2007**, *110*, 3058–3063. [CrossRef]
8. Suda, T.; Takubo, K.; Semenza, G.L. Metabolic regulation of hematopoietic stem cells in the hypoxic niche. *Cell Stem Cell* **2011**, *9*, 298–310. [CrossRef]
9. Ludin, A.; Gur-Cohen, S.; Golan, K.; Kaufmann, K.B.; Itkin, T.; Medaglia, C.; Lu, X.J.; Ledergor, G.; Kollet, O.; Lapidot, T. Reactive oxygen species regulate hematopoietic stem cell self-renewal, migration and development, as well as their bone marrow microenvironment. *Antioxid. Redox Signal.* **2014**, *21*, 1605–1619. [CrossRef]
10. Ergen, A.V.; Goodell, M.A. Mechanisms of hematopoietic stem cell aging. *Exp. Gerontol.* **2010**, *45*, 286–290. [CrossRef]
11. Tasdogan, A.; Kumar, S.; Allies, G.; Bausinger, J.; Beckel, F.; Hofemeister, H.; Mulaw, M.; Madan, V.; Scharffetter-Kochanek, K.; Feuring-Buske, M.; et al. DNA damage-induced HSPC malfunction depends on ROS accumulation downstream of IFN-1 signaling and bid mobilization. *Cell Stem Cell* **2016**, *19*, 752–767. [PubMed]
12. Pervaiz, S.; Taneja, R.; Ghaffari, S. Oxidative stress regulation of stem and progenitor cells. *Antioxid. Redox Signal.* **2009**, *11*, 2777–2789. [CrossRef] [PubMed]
13. Fan, J.; Cai, H.; Li, Q.; Du, Z.; Tan, W. The effects of ROS-mediating oxygen tension on human CD34(+)CD38(−) cells induced into mature dendritic cells. *J. Biotechnol.* **2012**, *158*, 104–111. [CrossRef] [PubMed]
14. Lee, S.J.; Jang, H.K.; Choi, Y.J.; Eum, W.S.; Park, J.; Choi, S.Y.; Kwon, H.Y. PEP-1-paraoxonase 1 fusion protein prevents cytokine-induced cell destruction and impaired insulin secretion in rat insulinoma cells. *BMB Rep.* **2018**, *51*, 538–543. [CrossRef] [PubMed]
15. Chan, C.Y.; Zyriyantey, A.H.; Taib, I.S.; Tan, H.Y.; Muhd, K.A.W.H.; Chow, P.W. Effects of n-acetyl-cysteine supplementation on ex-vivo clonogenicity and oxdative profile of lineage-committed hematopoietic stem/progenitor cells. *J. Teknologi.* **2018**, *80*, 1–8.
16. Parsons, S.J.; Parsons, J.T. Src family kinases, key regulators of signal transduction. *Oncogene* **2004**, *23*, 7906–7909. [CrossRef] [PubMed]
17. Zhang, S.; Yu, D. Targeting Src family kinases in anti-cancer therapies: Turning promise into triumph. *Trends Pharmacol. Sci.* **2012**, *33*, 122–128. [CrossRef]
18. Lowell, C.A. Src-family kinases: Rheostats of immune cell signaling. *Mol. Immunol.* **2004**, *41*, 631–643. [CrossRef]

19. Yamanashi, Y.; Mori, S.; Yoshida, M.; Kishinoto, T.; Yamamoto, T.; Toyoshima, K. Selective expression of a protein-tyrosine kinase, p56lyn, in hematopoietic cells and association with production of human T-cell lymphotropic virus type I. *Proc. Natl Acad. Sci. USA* **1989**, *86*, 6538–6542. [CrossRef]
20. Hibbs, M.L.; Tarlinton, D.M.; Armes, J.; Grail, D.; Hodgson, G.; Maglitto, R.; Stacker, S.A.; Dunn, A.R. Multiple defects in the immune system of Lun-deficient mice, culminating in autoimmune disease. *Cell* **1995**, *83*, 301–311. [CrossRef]
21. Scapini, P.; Pereira, S.; Zhang, H.; Lowell, C.A. Multiple roles of Lyn kinase in myeloid cell signaling and function. *Immunol. Rev.* **2009**, *228*, 23–40. [CrossRef] [PubMed]
22. Tilbrook, P.A.; Ingley, E.; Williams, J.H.; Hibbs, M.L.; Klinken, S.P. Lyn tyrosine kinase is essential for erythropoietin-induced differentiation of J2E erythroid cells. *EMBO J.* **1997**, *16*, 1610–1619. [CrossRef] [PubMed]
23. Linnekin, D.; DeBerry, C.S.; Mou, S. Lyn associates with the juxtamembrane region of c-kit and is activated by stem cell factor in hematopoietic cell lines and normal progenitor cells. *J. Biol. Chem.* **1997**, *272*, 27450–27455. [CrossRef] [PubMed]
24. Ingley, E.; Sarna, M.K.; Beaumont, J.G.; Tilbrook, P.A.; Tsai, S.; Takemoto, Y.; Williams, J.H.; Klinken, S.P. HS1 interacts with Lyn and is critical for erythropoietin-induced differentiation of erythroid cells. *J. Biol. Chem.* **2000**, *275*, 7887–7893. [CrossRef] [PubMed]
25. Chin, H.; Arai, A.; Wakao, H.; Kamiyama, R.; Miyasaka, N.; Miura, O. Lyn physically associates with the erythropoietin receptor and may play a role in activation of the Stat5 pathway. *Blood* **1998**, *91*, 3734–3745. [PubMed]
26. Dos Santos, C.; Demur, C.; Bardet, V.; Prade-Houdellier, N.; Payrastre, B.; Recher, C. A critical role for Lyn in acute myeloid leukemia. *Blood* **2008**, *111*, 2269–2279. [CrossRef] [PubMed]
27. Ptasznik, A.; Nakata, Y.; Kalota, A.; Emerson, S.G.; Gewirtz, A.M. Short interfering RNA (siRNA) targeting the Lyn kinase induces apoptosis in primary, and drug-resistant, BCR-ABL1(+) leukemia cells. *Nat. Med.* **2004**, *10*, 1187–1189. [CrossRef]
28. Park, G.B.; Kim, D. PI3K catalytic isoform alteration promotes the LIMK1-related metastasis through the PAK1 or ROCK1/2 activation in cigarette smoke-exposed ovarian cancer cells. *Anticancer Res.* **2017**, *37*, 1805–1818.
29. Park, G.B.; Kim, D. Insulin-like growth factor-1 activates different catalytic subunits p110 of PI3K in a cell-type-dependent manner to induce lipogenesis-dependent epithelial-mesenchymal transition through the regulation of ADAM10 and ADAM17. *Mol. Cell Biochem.* **2018**, *439*, 199–211. [CrossRef]
30. Anderson, H.A.; Mathieson, J.W.; Thomson, R.H. Distribution of spinochrome pigments in echinoids. *Comp. Biochem. Physiol.* **1969**, *28*, 333–345. [CrossRef]
31. Pozharitskaya, O.N.; Shikov, A.N.; Laakso, I.; Seppänen-Laakso, T.; Makarenko, I.E.; Faustova, N.M.; Makarova, M.N.; Makarov, V.G. Bioactivity and chemical characterization of gonads of green sea urchin Strongylocentrotus droebachiensis from Barents Sea. *J. Funct. Foods* **2015**, *17*, 227–234. [CrossRef]
32. Fedoreyev, S.A.; Krylova, N.V.; Mishchenko, N.P.; Vasileva, E.A.; Pislyagin, E.A.; Lunikhina, O.V.; Lavrov, V.F.; Svitich, O.A.; Ebralidze, L.K.; Leonova, G.N. Antiviral and antioxidant properties of Echinochrome A. *Mar. Drugs* **2018**, *16*, 509. [CrossRef] [PubMed]
33. Ultkina, N.K.; Pokhilo, N.D. Free radical scavenging activities of naturally occurring and synthetic analogues of sea urchin naphthazarin pigments. *Nat. Prod. Commun.* **2012**, *7*, 901–904.
34. Lebed'ko, O.A.; Ryzhavskii, B.Y.; Demidova, O.V. Effect of antioxidant Echinochrome A on bleomycin-induced pulmonary fibrosis. *Bull. Exp. Biol. Med.* **2015**, *159*, 351–354. [CrossRef] [PubMed]
35. Lebedev, A.V.; Ivanova, M.V.; Levitsky, D.O. Iron chelators and free radical scavengers in naturally occurring polyhydroxylated 1,4-naphthoquinones. *Hemoglobin* **2008**, *32*, 165–179. [CrossRef] [PubMed]
36. Abdul Hamid, Z.; Lin Lin, W.H.; Abdalla, B.J.; Bee Yuen, O.; Latif, E.S.; Mohamed, J.; Rajab, N.F.; Paik Wah, C.; Wak Harto, M.K.A.; Budin, S.B. The role of *Hibiscus sabdariffa* L. (Roselle) in maintenance of ex vivo murine bone marrow-derived hematopoietic stem cells. *Sci. World J.* **2014**, 1–10. [CrossRef]
37. Liu, A.M.; Qu, W.W.; Liu, X.; Qu, C.K. Chromosomal instability in in vitro cultured mouse hematopoietic cells associated with oxidative stress. *Am. J. Blood Res.* **2012**, *2*, 71–76.
38. Rausch, O.; Marshall, C.J. Cooperation of p38 and extracellular signal-regulated kinase mitogen-activated protein kinase pathways during granulocyte colony-stimulating factor-induced hemopoietic cell proliferation. *J. Biol. Chem.* **1999**, *274*, 4096–4105. [CrossRef]

39. Katsoulidis, E.; Li, Y.; Yoon, P.; Sassano, A.; Altman, J.; Kannan-Thulasiraman, P.; Balasubramanian, L.; Parmar, S.; Varga, J.; Tallman, M.S.; et al. Role of the p38 mitogen-activated protein kinase pathway in cytokine-mediated hematopoietic suppression in myelodysplastic syndromes. *Cancer Res.* **2005**, *65*, 9029–9037. [CrossRef]
40. Verma, A.; Deb, D.K.; Sassano, A.; Kambhampati, S.; Wickrema, A.; Uddin, S.; Mohindru, M.; Van Besien, K.; Platanias, L.C. Cutting edge: Activation of the p38 mitogen-activated protein kinase signaling pathway mediates cytokine-induced hemopoietic suppression in aplastic anemia. *J. Immunol.* **2002**, *168*, 5984–5988. [CrossRef]
41. Miyamato, K.; Araki, K.Y.; Naka, K.; Arai, F.; Takubo, K.; Yamazaki, S.; Matsuoka, S.; Miyamoto, T.; Ito, K.; Ohmura, M.; et al. FOXO3a is essential for maintenance of the hematopoietic stem cell pool. *Cell Stem Cell* **2007**, *1*, 101–112. [CrossRef] [PubMed]
42. Parmar, K.; Mauch, P.; Vergilio, J.A.; Sackstein, R.; Down, J.D. Distribution of hematopoietic stem cells in the bone marrow according to regional hypoxia. *Proc. Natl. Acad. Sci. USA* **2007**, *104*, 5431–5436. [CrossRef] [PubMed]
43. Wang, Z.; Du, Z.; Cai, H.; Ye, Z.; Fan, J.; Tan, W.S. Low oxygen tension favored expansion and hematopoietic reconstitution of CD34(+) CD38(−) cells expanded from human cord blood-derived CD34(+) cells. *Biotechonol. J.* **2016**, *11*, 945–953. [CrossRef]
44. Shao, L.; Li, H.; Pazhanisamy, S.K.; Meng, A.; Wang, Y.; Zhou, D. Reactive oxygen species and hematopoietic stem cell senescence. *Int. J. Hematol.* **2011**, *94*, 24–32. [CrossRef] [PubMed]
45. Geest, C.R.; Coffer, P.J. MAPK signaling pathways in the regulation of hematopoiesis. *J. Luekoc. Biol.* **2009**, *86*, 237–250. [CrossRef] [PubMed]
46. Hinge, A.; Xu, J.; Javier, J.; Mose, E.; Kumar, S.; Kapur, R.; Srour, E.F.; Malik, P.; Aronow, B.J.; Filippi, M.D. p190-B RhoGAP and intracellular cytokine signals balance hematopoietic stem and progenitor cell self-renewal and differentiation. *Nat. Commun.* **2017**, *8*, 14382. [CrossRef] [PubMed]
47. Soriano, P.; Montgomery, C.; Geske, R.; Bradley, A. Targeted disruption of the c-src proto-oncogene leads to osteopetrosis in mice. *Cell* **1991**, *64*, 693–702. [CrossRef]
48. Harder, K.W.; Parsons, L.M.; Armes, J.; Evans, N.; Kountouri, N.; Clark, R.; Quilici, C.; Grail, D.; Hodgson, G.S.; Dunn, A.R.; et al. Gain-and loss-of-function Lyn mutant mice define a critical inhibitory role for Lyn in the myeloid lineage. *Immunity* **2001**, *15*, 603–615. [CrossRef]
49. Debuire, B.; Henry, C.; Bernissa, M.; Bierte, G.; Claverie, J.M.; Saule, S.; Martin, P.; Stehelin, D. Sequencing the erbA gene of avian erythroblastosis virus reveals a new type of oncogene. *Science* **1984**, *224*, 1456–1459. [CrossRef]
50. Satterthwaite, A.B.; Lowell, C.A.; Khan, W.N.; Sideras, P.; Alt, F.W.; Witte, O.N. Independent and opposing roles for Btk and lyn in B and myeloid signaling pathways. *J. Exp. Med.* **1998**, *188*, 833–844. [CrossRef]
51. Karur, V.G.; Lowell, C.A.; Besmer, P.; Aqosti, V.; Wojchowski, D.M. Lyn kinase promotes erythroblast expansion and late-stage development. *Blood* **2006**, *108*, 1524–1532. [CrossRef] [PubMed]
52. Polak, R.; Buitenhuis, M. The PI3K/PKB signaling module as key regulator of hematopoiesis: Implications for therapeutic strategies in leukemia. *Blood* **2012**, *119*, 911–923. [CrossRef] [PubMed]
53. Thorpe, L.M.; Yuzugullu, H.; Zhao, J.J. PI3K in cancer: Divergent roles of isoforms, modes of activation and therapeutic targeting. *Nat. Rev. Cancer* **2015**, *15*, 7–24. [CrossRef] [PubMed]

marine drugs

MDPI

Article

Therapeutic Cell Protective Role of Histochrome under Oxidative Stress in Human Cardiac Progenitor Cells

Ji Hye Park [1,2], Na-Kyung Lee [1,2], Hye Ji Lim [1,2], Sinthia Mazumder [1,2], Vinoth Kumar Rethineswaran [1,2], Yeon-Ju Kim [1,2], Woong Bi Jang [1,2], Seung Taek Ji [1,2], Songhwa Kang [1,2], Da Yeon Kim [1,2], Le Thi Hong Van [1,2], Ly Thanh Truong Giang [1,2], Dong Hwan Kim [3], Jong Seong Ha [1,2], Jisoo Yun [1,2], Hyungtae Kim [4], Jin Han [5], Natalia P. Mishchenko [6], Sergey A. Fedoreyev [6], Elena A. Vasileva [6], Sang Mo Kwon [1,2,*] and Sang Hong Baek [7,*]

1 Laboratory of Regenerative Medicine and Stem Cell Biology, Department of Physiology, Medical Research Institute, School of Medicine, Pusan National University, Yangsan 50612, Korea; siwonvin@naver.com (J.H.P.); ahlng2005@naver.com (N.-K.L.); dla9612@naver.com (H.J.L.); sinthiambbs@gmail.com (S.M.); vinrebha@gmail.com (V.K.R.); twou1234@nate.com (Y.-J.K.); jangwoongbi@naver.com (W.B.J.); jst5396@hanmail.net (S.T.J.); songhwa.kang@gmail.com (S.K.); ekdus0258@gmail.com (D.Y.K.); lethihongvan25121978@gmail.com (L.T.H.V.); lythanhtruonggiang@gmail.com (L.T.T.G.); jongseong@pusan.ac.kr (J.S.H.); jsyun14@hanmail.net (J.Y.)

2 Research Institute of Convergence Biomedical Science and Technology, Pusan National University School of Medicine, Yangsan 50612, Korea

3 Department of Neurosurgery & Medical Research Institute, Pusan National University Hospital, Busan 49241, Korea; smile0402@hanmail.net

4 Department of Thoracic and Cardiovascular Surgery, Pusan National University Yangsan Hospital, Yangsan 50612, Korea; 2719k@naver.com

5 National Research Laboratory for Mitochondrial Signaling, Department of Physiology, Department of Health Sciences and Technology, BK21 Plus Project Team, Cardiovascular and Metabolic Disease Center, Inje University College of Medicine, Busan 47392, Korea; phyhanj@gmail.com

6 G.B. Elyakov Pacific Institute of Bioorganic Chemistry, Far-Eastern Branch of the Russian Academy of Science, Vladivostok 690022, Russia; mischenkonp@mail.ru (N.P.M.); fedoreev-s@mail.ru (S.A.F.); vasilieva_el_an@mail.ru (E.A.V.)

7 Division of Cardiology, Seoul St. Mary's Hospital, School of Medicine, The Catholic University of Korea, Seoul 06591, Korea

* Correspondence: smkwon323@hotmail.com or smkwon323@pusan.ac.kr (S.M.K.); whitesh@catholic.ac.kr (S.H.B.); Tel.: +82-51-510-8070 (S.M.K.); +82-2-2258-6030 (S.H.B.); Fax: +82-51-510-8076 (S.M.K.); +82-2-591-3614 (S.H.B.)

Received: 3 June 2019; Accepted: 18 June 2019; Published: 21 June 2019

Abstract: Cardiac progenitor cells (CPCs) are resident stem cells present in a small portion of ischemic hearts and function in repairing the damaged heart tissue. Intense oxidative stress impairs cell metabolism thereby decreasing cell viability. Protecting CPCs from undergoing cellular apoptosis during oxidative stress is crucial in optimizing CPC-based therapy. Histochrome (sodium salt of echinochrome A—a common sea urchin pigment) is an antioxidant drug that has been clinically used as a pharmacologic agent for ischemia/reperfusion injury in Russia. However, the mechanistic effect of histochrome on CPCs has never been reported. We investigated the protective effect of histochrome pretreatment on human CPCs (hCPCs) against hydrogen peroxide (H_2O_2)-induced oxidative stress. Annexin V/7-aminoactinomycin D (7-AAD) assay revealed that histochrome-treated CPCs showed significant protective effects against H_2O_2-induced cell death. The anti-apoptotic proteins B-cell lymphoma 2 (Bcl-2) and Bcl-xL were significantly upregulated, whereas the pro-apoptotic proteins BCL2-associated X (Bax), H_2O_2-induced cleaved caspase-3, and the DNA damage marker, phosphorylated histone (γH2A.X) foci, were significantly downregulated upon histochrome treatment of hCPCs in vitro. Further, prolonged incubation with histochrome alleviated the replicative cellular senescence of hCPCs. In conclusion, we report the protective effect of histochrome against oxidative stress and present the use of a potent and bio-safe cell priming agent as a potential therapeutic strategy in patient-derived hCPCs to treat heart disease.

Keywords: cardiac progenitor cells; histochrome; echinochrome A; oxidative stress; cell therapy

---

1. Introduction

Stem cells have been reported to recover damaged hearts from myocardial infarction and have been investigated for use in myocardial regeneration [1–3]. Cardiac progenitor cells (CPCs) were first identified by Anversa et al. [4]. CPCs are classified as a prevailing stem cell population in the heart and have crucial roles in cardiac homeostasis [5,6]. CPCs can differentiate into multiple cell lineages of the heart, and thus, are a promising cell resource for regenerating ischemic hearts [7]. Recent preclinical studies suggest that transplantation of CPCs into the ischemic myocardium can significantly improve cardiac regeneration via the formation of vasculature and new myocytes [8–10]. Furthermore, CPCs have the potential to produce and remodel extracellular matrix (ECM) proteins [11], trigger CPC proliferation, and stimulate growth factor secretion [12]. According to these positive results, CPC might be a promising stem cell source in cardiovascular regeneration. However, current evidence suggests that poor viability of engrafted CPCs in the infarcted myocardium primarily restricts the therapeutic efficacy of CPCs [13,14]. Thus, increasing the survival of CPCs can be a beneficial strategy to enhance the therapeutic effect in ischemic heart disease.

Reactive oxygen species (ROS), such as hydrogen peroxide (H_2O_2), superoxide radicals, and hydroxyl radicals, are produced during infarction or reperfusion of ischemic hearts [15]. ROS involvement has been reported in various important development processes, cell signaling, and regulation of homeostasis [16]. Low levels of ROS are involved in the regulation of stem cell fate decision, stem cell proliferation, differentiation, and survival [17]. However, excessive ROS production leads to impaired cell metabolism and decreased cell viability [18], thereby inhibiting transplanted CPCs to regenerate the damaged heart [19]. Consequently, protecting CPCs from undergoing apoptosis and enhancing their ability to survive under oxidative stress is crucial in optimizing CPC-based therapy.

Echinochrome A is a common sea urchin pigment [20] that has a chemical structure of 6-ethyl-2,3,5,7,8-pentahydroxy-1,4-naphthoquinone (Figure 1A) and exhibits antioxidant, anti-viral [21], anti-inflammatory [22], and anti-diabetic activities [23]. Echinochrome A prevents mitochondrial dysfunction and activation of mitogen-activated protein kinase (MAPK) cell death signaling pathways caused by cardiotoxic drug treatment [24]. Echinochrome A regulates mitochondrial biogenesis in cardiomyocytes by upregulating the transcription of mitochondrial regulatory genes, such as mitochondrial transcriptional factor A (TFAM), nuclear respiratory factor (NRF-1), and proliferator-activated receptor gamma co-activator (PGC-1α) [25]. Echinochrome A inhibits the phosphorylation of serine-16 and threonine-17, located in the active center of phospholamban (membrane phosphoprotein and main regulator of the SERCA2A receptor responsible for the transfer of calcium ions from the cytosol to the sarcoplasmic reticulum), preventing ischemic myocardial damage by reducing the infarction zone [26].

Echinochrome A is insoluble in water, however, its water-soluble sodium salt is used for medical applications, which is manufactured under inert conditions in ampoules and is known as the Histochrome® drug. Histochrome has been used in Russia in ophtalmological and cardiological clinical practice. In ophthalmology, histochrome is used for the treatment of degenerative diseases of the retina and cornea, macular degeneration, primary open-angle glaucoma, diabetic retinopathy, hemorrhage in the vitreous body, retina, and anterior chamber, and dyscirculatory disorder in the central artery and vein of the retina [27]. An overview of clinical applications of histochrome in cardiology is presented in monography [28]. In the first place, histochrome has been used for the treatment of myocardial ischemia/reperfusion injury. Even a single injection of histochrome immediately after reperfusion recovered the ECG signs of myocardial necrosis and significantly (up to 30%) reduces the necrosis zone after a 10-day course. The use of histochrome prevented lipid peroxidation, reduced the frequency of left ventricular failure, did not affect the level of blood pressure and heart rate, and decreased the frequency of post-infarction angina pectoris. Practical experience of histochrome treatment confirmed the absence of any adverse effects and the safety of its application [28].

The cardioprotective effect of histochrome on patient-derived CPCs has never been reported. Thus, we investigated whether pretreatment of CPCs with histochrome promotes cell survival against oxidative stress during cardiac regeneration.

2. Results

2.1. Histochrome Does Not Affect Surface Expression Markers of Human Cardiac Progenitor Cells (hCPCs)

To evaluate the cytotoxicity of histochrome in human CPCs (hCPCs), hCPCs were treated with different concentrations of histochrome for 24 h. Cell survival was found to be significantly increased for 0.5 μM to 10 μM of histochrome and significantly decreased at concentrations above 100 μM ($p < 0.01$ versus 0 μM; Figure 1B). Based on the data obtained, we determined that histochrome concentration under 50 μM used for the further experiments. No change in the morphology of hCPCs was observed on pretreatment with 0 μM, 5 μM, 10 μM, and 20 μM concentrations of histochrome (Figure 1C). To eliminate the possibility of change in CPC characteristics on pretreatment with histochrome, we investigated typical surface expression markers of hCPCs using fluorescence-activated cell sorting (FACS) analysis. As shown in Figure 1D, histochrome-treated CPCs showed positive expression of cardiac stem cell markers such as mast/stem cell growth factor receptor kit (c-kit), cluster of differentiation 66 (CD166), CD29, CD105, and CD44. However, negative expression was observed for hematopoietic markers, such as CD45 and CD34, in pretreated hCPCs compared to that in control cells.

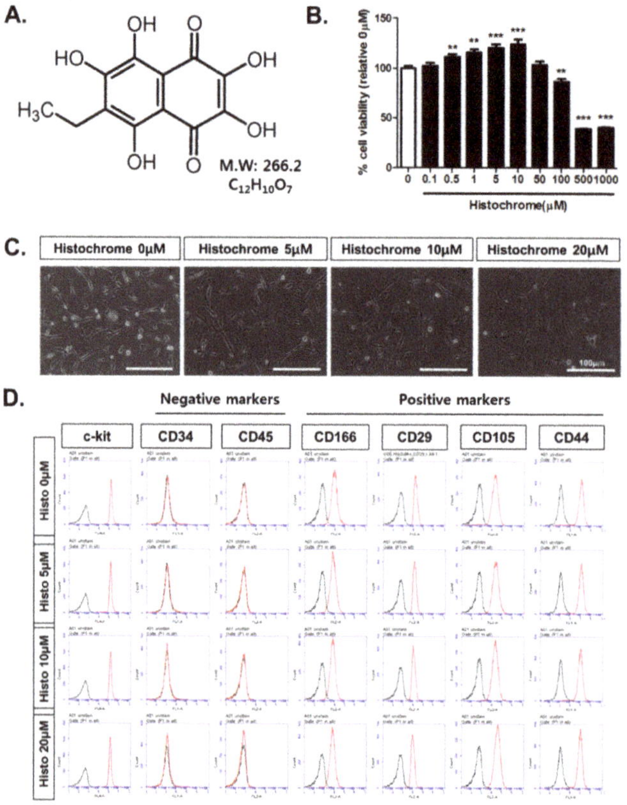

Figure 1. Effects of histochrome treatment on human cardiac progenitor cells (hCPCs) characterization. (**A**) Chemical structure of echinochrome A—active substance of the histochrome drug. (**B**) hCPCs were treated with different concentrations of histochrome for 24 h and viability was measured using cell viability, Proliferation & Cytotoxicity assay (CCK assay). Data are presented as the mean ± standard deviation (SD). **, $p < 0.01$ versus 0 μM, ***, $p < 0.001$ versus 0 μM. $n = 6$ (**C**) Morphological analysis of hCPCs pretreated with histochrome. Scale bar = 100 μm, (**D**) Expression of stem cell marker by flow cytometric analysis, $n = 3$. Error bars indicate standard effort of the mean (S.E.M)

2.2. Histochrome Reduced Cellular and Mitochondrial Reactive Oxygen Species (ROS) Levels in hCPCs during H_2O_2-Induced Oxidative Stress

To investigate whether pretreating hCPCs with histochrome protects them against oxidative stress, we performed a cellular ROS staining assay. Cellular ROS-tagged green intensity was found to be significantly increased upon exposure to H_2O_2 (Figure 2A). We observed that pretreatment with histochrome decreased the cellular ROS levels in a dose-dependent manner. The 2′,7′–difluorofluorescin diacetate (H_2-DFFDA) assay revealed that pretreatment with 10 μM of histochrome significantly decreased cellular ROS levels (Figure 2B). Furthermore, we investigated the effects of pretreatment with histochrome on mitochondrial superoxide production in hCPCs. The increased production of mitochondrial superoxide caused by H_2O_2 addition was found to be significantly reduced in histochrome-treated hCPCs (Figure 2C). Our data suggested that histochrome has intracellular ROS scavenging activity in hCPCs under oxidative stress.

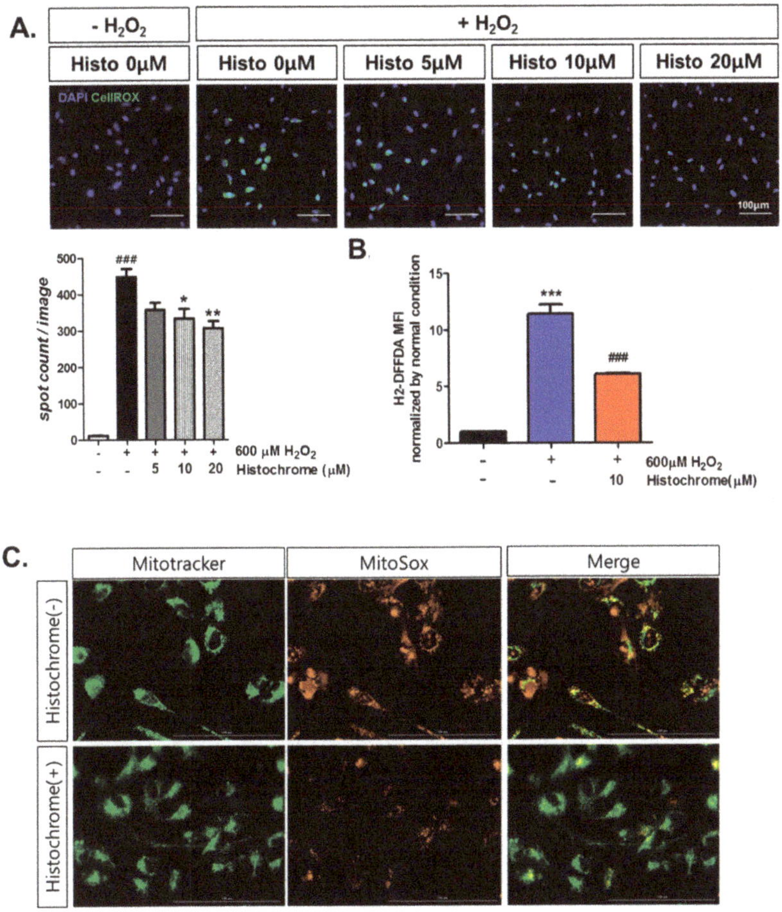

Figure 2. Intracellular reactive oxygen species (ROS) and mitochondrial ROS scavenging activity of histochrome in hCPCs. (**A**) hCPCs were pretreated with histochrome at 0 μM, 5 μM, 10 μM, and 20 μM for 24 h followed by the addition of 600 μM H_2O_2 for 1 h. Intracellular ROS scavenging activity was measured using CellRox staining. Representative image of increased intensity of CellRox produced by ROS and decreased intensity on pretreating with histochrome. Data are presented as the mean ± SD of three independent experiments. Scale bar = 100 μm, ### $p < 0.01$ versus -H_2O_2 -histochrome; * $p < 0.05$; ** $p < 0.01$ versus +H_2O_2 -histochrome, $n = 3$. Error bars indicate S.E.M. (**B**) 2′,7′–difluorofluorescin diacetate (H_2-DFFDA)assay was used to measure cellular ROS production. *** $p < 0.001$ versus -H_2O_2 -histochrome; ###, $p < 0.001$ versus +H_2O_2 -histochrome, $n = 3$. Error bars indicate S.E.M. (**C**) After pretreatment with histochrome for 24 h, hCPCs were exposed to H_2O_2 for 1 h and mitochondrial superoxide production was measured with MitoSOX staining. Representative image of the increased intensity of MitoSOX and decreased intensity on pretreatment with histochrome. Scale bar = 100 μm.

2.3. *Anti-Apoptotic Effect of Histochrome against H_2O_2-Induced Cell Death*

To investigate the anti-apoptotic effects of histochrome in hCPCs, cells were treated with 1 mM H_2O_2 for 4 h and cell apoptosis was evaluated using flow cytometry by staining with Annexin V and 7-aminoactinomycin D (7-AAD). Annexin V/7-AAD assay revealed that treatment with H_2O_2 significantly increased the percentage of apoptotic cells (+H_2O_2, -Histochrome; 14.3% ± 2.36%) compared to the percentage of apoptotic cells in the non-treated control group (-H_2O_2, -Histochrome;

-8.7% ± 0.84%, -H_2O_2, +Histochrome; 5.6% ± 0.40%, Figure 3A). In contrast, pretreatment of hCPCs with 10 μM of histochrome significantly increased the percentage of viable cells (+H_2O_2, +Histochrome; 95.2% ± 0.40%, Figure 3A) while decreasing the number of apoptotic cells (+H_2O_2, +Histochrome; 2.4% ± 0.49%, Figure 3A). We also investigated the effect of histochrome on cell morphology using phase contrast microscopy (Figure 3B). H_2O_2 treatment caused abnormal morphology and reduced cell viability. However, pretreatment with histochrome attenuated the morphological change induced by H_2O_2. In addition, live cell imaging analysis suggested that pretreatment with histochrome under the H_2O_2-induced oxidative stress condition significantly increased the number of live cells in a dose-dependent manner (Figure 3C).

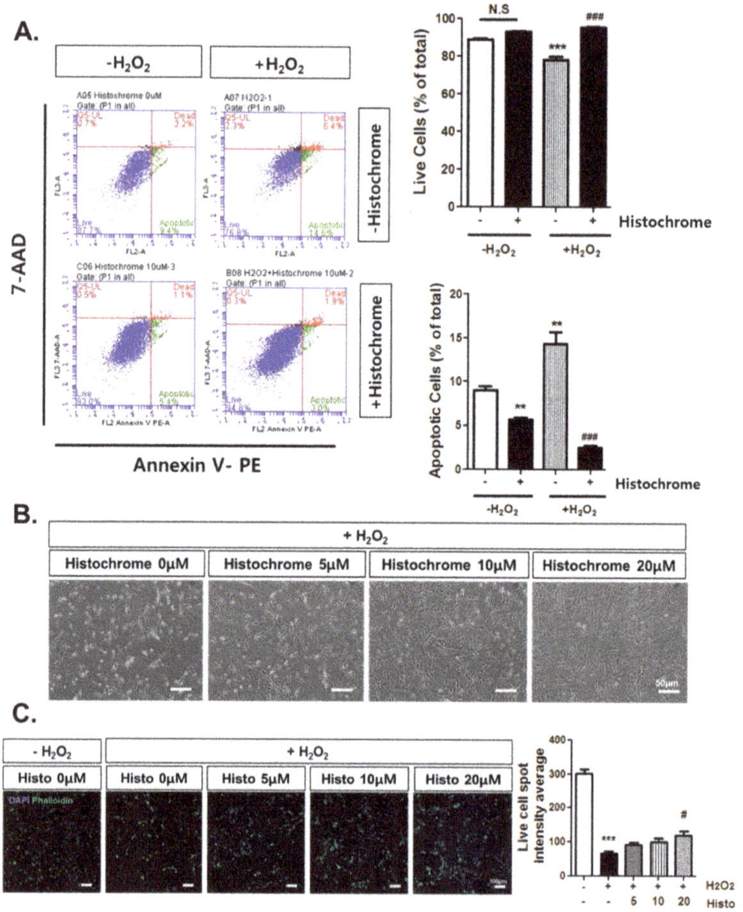

Figure 3. Anti-apoptotic effect of histochrome against H_2O_2-induced cell death. (**A**) hCPCs were pretreated with 10 μM of histochrome for 24 h and then exposed to 1 mM H_2O_2 for 4 h. Apoptotic cells were quantified by fluorescence-activated cell sorting (FACS) analysis with Annexin V / 7-AAD staining. ** $p < 0.01$; *** $p < 0.001$ versus -H_2O_2 -histochrome; ### $p < 0.001$ versus +H_2O_2 -histochrome. (**B**) Representative images showing the morphology of hCPCs pretreated with histochrome (0 μM, 5 μM, 10 μM, and 20 μM) in the presence of H_2O_2-induced oxidative stress. Morphology of hCPCs was observed by phase contrast microscope. Scale bar = 50 μm (**C**) Live cells were quantified by phalloidin (green fluorescence) intensity. *** $p < 0.001$ versus -H_2O_2 -histochrome; # $p < 0.05$ versus +H_2O_2 -histochrome. Scale bar = 100 μm, $n = 3$. Error bars indicate S.E.M.

2.4. Histochrome Protects hCPCs against Oxidative Stress through Downregulation of Pro-Apoptotic Signals and Upregulation of Anti-Apoptotic Signals

Further, we investigated the expression of apoptosis-related proteins by western blotting. Pretreatment with histochrome was observed to reduce expression of pro-apoptotic protein, Bcl-2 associated X (Bax) while promoting the expression of anti-apoptotic proteins, B-cell lymphoma 2 (Bcl-2), and Bcl-xL. In addition, pretreatment with histochrome remarkably decreased the expression levels of cytochrome C and cleaved-caspase-3 (Figure 4A). Our data suggested that histochrome protects hCPCs against oxidative stress through decreased pro-apoptotic signals and increased anti-apoptotic signals. Further, we checked DNA damage marker, phosphorylated histone (γH2A.X) foci by immunocytochemistry (Figure 4B). We found that pretreatment of hCPCs with histochrome prevented DNA damage caused by oxidative stress. Overall, our results suggested that pretreatment with histochrome regulates cell apoptosis by altering cell survival signals and inhibiting ROS-induced DNA damage.

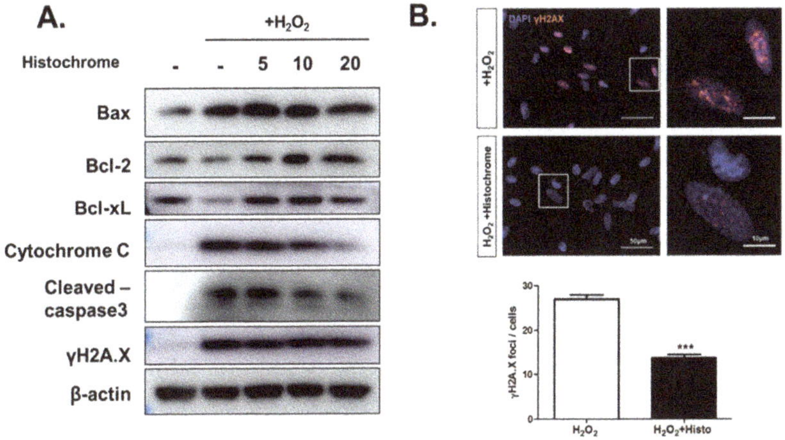

Figure 4. hCPCs pretreated with histochrome show downregulation of pro-apoptotic signals and upregulation of anti-apoptotic signals under the oxidative stress condition. (**A**) hCPCs were pretreated with histochrome for 24 h, oxidative stress was induced in hCPCs by 1 mM H_2O_2. Expression of apoptosis signaling-related proteins was determined by western blotting. (**B**) Immunofluorescence was performed with the DNA damage marker γH2A.X to quantify DNA damage of hCPCs. Images were captured using a LionHeart FX automated microscope (Biotek, Winooski, VT, USA). *** $p < 0.001$ versus $+H_2O_2$, $n = 5$. Error bars indicate S.E.M.

2.5. Prolonged Treatment with Histochrome Attenuates Cellular Senescence in hCPCs

Several antioxidants have been reported to be associated with inhibition of cellular senescence [29–31]. To examine whether histochrome affects cellular senescence, we investigated the long-term effect of histochrome treatment on an in vitro culture of hCPCs. Evaluation of senescence-associated β galactosidase (SA-β-gal) activity in senescent hCPCs (passage 13) revealed a significant increase in the number of SA-β-gal positive cells (sene; 40.7% ± 3.07%) (Figure 5). However, increased SA-β-gal positive cells were significantly downregulated (sene+Histochrome; 31.3% ± 2.87%) on prolong treatment of hCPCs with histochrome. This suggested that long-term treatment of histochrome alleviates replicative cellular senescence in hCPCs.

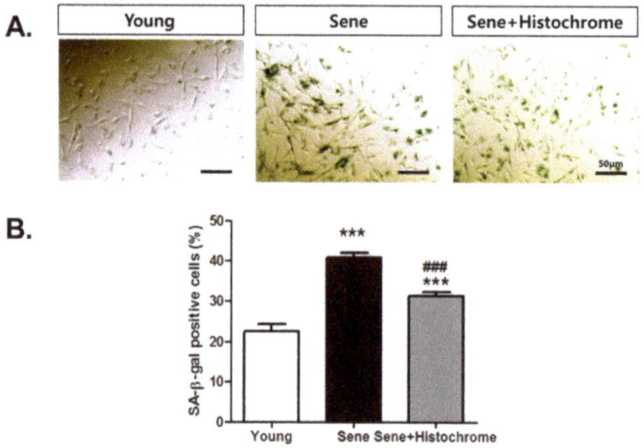

Figure 5. Effect of prolonged treatment with histochrome on hCPCs senescence. (**A**) Representing images of senescence-β-galactosidase (SA- β-gal) stained hCPCs (Scalebar = 50 μm). (**B**) SA- β-gal positive cells were quantified and presented as a graph (*** $p < 0.001$, versus Young; ### $p < 0.001$, versus Sene) Error bars indicate S.E.M. Abbreviation: Sene, senescent hCPCs (passage 13); sene + histochrome, prolonged treatment with histochrome (till passage 13).

3. Discussion

To enhance the engraftment rate of transplanted cells, several studies have been performed focusing on cell priming, using physical stimulations such as heat shock, and chemical stimulations using natural products and growth factors. Recently, stem cell priming using natural products has been proposed as a new strategy to enhance the cell activity and promote stable and efficient cell functioning. In our previous study, we demonstrated that pretreatment with fucoidan, a marine-sulfated polysaccharide derived from seaweeds, inhibits cellular senescence and promotes neo-vasculogenic potential [32].

In this study, we identified a novel priming factor for enhancing cell therapy potentials against oxidative stress. A recent study has revealed that echinochrome A promotes cardiomyocyte differentiation of mouse embryonic stem cells via direct binding to serine-threonine kinase PKCι and inhibition of its activity [33]. We are the first to report the effects of histochrome on hCPCs. In the present study, we demonstrated that pretreatment with histochrome enhanced the survival of hCPCs against oxidative stress. Further, pretreatment with different concentrations (0 μM, 5 μM, 10 μM, 15 μM, and 20 μM) of histochrome did not alter the expression of multipotent cardiac stem cell markers such as c-kit (Histo 0 μM; 99.9% ± 0.1%, Histo 5 μM; 99.9% ± 0.1%, Histo 10 μM; 99.8% ± 0.1%, and Histo 20 μM; 99.9% ± 0.1%, respectively); CD29 (Histo 0 μM; 99.9% ± 0.1%, Histo 5 μM; 99.6% ± 0.1%, Histo 10 μM; 99.1% ± 0.2%, and Histo 20 μM; 93.7% ± 5.6%, respectively); CD166 (Histo 0 μM; 88.9% ± 1.5%, Histo 5 μM; 80.2% ± 2.7%, Histo 10 μM; 80.9% ± 1.5%, and Histo 20 μM; 79.8% ± 2.1%, respectively); CD105 (Histo 0 μM; 95.0% ± 0.8%, Histo 5 μM; 98.5% ± 0.1%, Histo 10 μM; 97.8% ± 0.1%, and Histo 20 μM; 99.7% ± 0.1%, respectively); and CD44 (Histo 0 μM; 97.8% ± 1.0%, Histo 5 μM; 99.5% ± 0.1%, Histo 10 μM; 99.4% ± 0.2%, and Histo 20 μM; 99.6% ± 0.1%, respectively). In contrast, histochrome-treated hCPCs showed negative expression of hematopoietic markers such as CD34 (Histo 0 μM; 0.7% ± 0.01%, Histo 5 μM; 1.1% ± 0.1%, Histo 10 μM; 0.6% ± 0.1%, and Histo 20 μM; 1.0% ± 0.2%, respectively) and CD45 (Histo 0 μM; 0.1% ± 0.1%, Histo 5 μM; 0.1% ± 0.06%, Histo 10 μM; 0%, and Histo 20 μM; 0%, respectively).

In ischemic heart disease, ROS is produced upon reperfusion [34]. Excessive ROS formation promotes cell death which induces development and progression of cardiovascular disease [35].

The generation of ROS is associated with alteration in electrophysiology leading to myocardial ischemia [36]. In addition, mitochondrial ROS scavenging has been reported for its potential to prevent cardiac failure [37]. It is necessary to target intracellular ROS and mitochondrial ROS to prevent cell death caused by oxidative stress. Histochrome showed high intracellular ROS scavenging activity and reduced production of mitochondrial superoxide in hCPCs. Furthermore, pretreatment with histochrome revealed an anti-apoptotic effect against H_2O_2-induced cell death.

The Bcl-2-family members (Bcl-2, Bcl-xL, Bax) are predominant regulators of cell cycle progression and apoptosis [38]. Specifically, Bcl-2 and Bcl-xL are well-known negative regulators of apoptosis which promote cell survival [39]. On the other hand, the apoptosis regulator Bax inhibits cell survival [40] and cell cycle progression [41]. In this study, pretreatment with histochrome upregulated the expression of Bcl-2 and Bcl-xl and downregulated that of Bax under the H_2O_2-induced oxidative stress condition. DNA damage induces the formation of double stranded breaks (DSBs) and stimulates phosphorylation of histone H2AX [42]. Subsequently, γ-H2A.X is used as a reference marker for DNA damage. In our study, pretreatment of hCPCs with histochrome reduced the expression of the DNA damage marker, γH2A.X foci under the oxidative stress condition. Thus, we concluded that histochrome prevents ROS-mediated DNA damage in hCPCs (Figure 6).

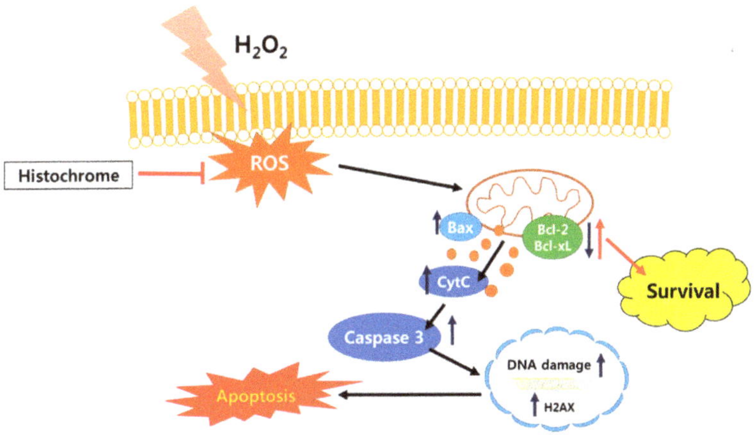

Figure 6. Schematic representation of cytoprotective effects of histochrome against H_2O_2-induced cell death via reduction of DNA damage and activation of survival signaling.

Any cell undergoes a limited number of divisions and thus, following a certain number of cell cycles, it enters an irreversible cell cycle arrest which is referred to as cellular senescence [43]. Stem cell therapy for regeneration of tissues requires over hundreds of millions of cells [44]. Repetitive in vitro cultures are essential and cellular senescence is a major threat in such stem cell therapies. Thus, preventing cellular senescence is a promising strategy in stem cell therapy. SA-β-gal assay revealed that histochrome delayed the progression of cellular senescence in hCPCs. Thus, our study suggests that histochrome can be a potential effective strategy to overcome cellular senescence.

Overall, our present study demonstrated that histochrome protects hCPCs against oxidative stress by regulating cell survival signaling. Furthermore, histochrome prevents cellular senescence of hCPCs. Thus, our study presents a simple and effective strategy to improve cell survival in post-transplanted CPCs under ischemic oxidative stress conditions and improve the efficiency in myocardial regeneration.

4. Materials and Methods

4.1. Cell Cultures and Treatment

Human fetal right auricle(RA) tissue was received from Pusan National University YangSan Hospital and the study was approved by the Institutional Review Board (IRB) (IRB No. 05-2015-133). C-kit positive hCPCs were isolated and cultured, as previously reported [45,46]. hCPCs were maintained at 37 °C with 5% CO_2 in Ham's Nutrient Mixture F-12 (Hyclone, GE Healthcare, Chicago, IL, USA) and supplemented with 10% Fetal bovine serum (FBS; Gibco#16000-044, Thermo Fisher Scientific, Carlsbad, CA, USA), 1% penicillin-streptomycin (PS; Welgene, Daegu, Republic of Korea), 0.005 unit/mL of human erythropoietin (hEPO, R&D systems, Minneapolis, MN, USA), 10 ng/mL of recombinant human basic fibroblast growth factor (rb-FGF, Peprotech, Rocky Hill, NJ, USA), and 2 mM of glutathione (Sigma-Aldrich, St. Louis, CA, USA). Passages 4–10 were utilized for the experiments as passage 13 was found to be senescent cells. hCPCs were treated with different concentrations of H_2O_2 (Sigma-Aldrich, St. Louis, CA, USA) and a final concentration of 600 μM (to investigate the antioxidant effect), 1 mM (to confirm anti-apoptotic effect) was used.

The standardized substance echinochrome A (registration number in Russian Federation is P N002362/01) was isolated from the sea urchin *Scaphechinus mirabilis* by a previously described method [47]. The purity of echinochrome A (99.0%) was confirmed using LC-MS data (Shimadzu LCMS-2020, Kyoto, Japan). Purified echinochrome A appeared as red–brown needles, had a melting point of 221 °C, and similar nuclear magnetic resonance (NMR) spectra to that reported previously [47]. We used a solution of echinochrome A sodium salts in ampoules with trade name Histochrome®. Histochrome was generated by combining echinochrome A (1 g) with sodium carbonate (0.4 g) in a water solution heated in inert gas until CO_2 was completely removed. This solution at a concentration of 0.2 mg/mL echinochrome A (750 μM) was sealed in ampoules in inert gas. After opening of the ampoule, histochrome was used as a stock solution to be diluted with appropriate solvents or culture media.

4.2. Cell Cytotoxicity Assay

To determine cell cytotoxicity, hCPCs were seeded at 5000 cells/well in a 96-well plate. The following day, cells were pretreated with different concentrations of histochrome and incubated for 24 h. Cell viability was evaluated using a cell-counting kit (CCK) cell viability assay kit (#CCK-3000, DonginLS, Seoul, Republic of Korea), following the manufacturer's instructions [48,49]. The cell viability was measured by incubating cells with the CCK solution. The plates were incubated for 1 h, and the absorbance of each well was measured. Absorbance was measured at 450 nm using a microplate reader (TECAN, Mannedorf, Switzerland). Cell viability of the experimental group was represented as percentage to 0 μM.

4.3. Western Blot Analysis

For western blotting, hCPCs pretreated with different concentrations of histochrome were exposed to 1 mM H_2O_2 (Sigma-Aldrich, St. Louis, CA, USA) for 4 hours. Further, cells were lysed in the Radioimmunoprecipitation assay (RIPA) buffer containing protease inhibitor and phosphatase inhibitor. Equivalent concentration of proteins (20 μg) were separated on sodium dodecyl sulphate-polyacrylamide gel electrophoresis (SDS-PAGE) and transferred to 0.45 μm PVDF membrane (Millipore, Billerica, MA, USA). The membranes were blocked with 5% skim milk and incubated with primary antibodies overnight at 4 °C: cleaved-caspase 3 (Cell Signaling, Danvers, MA, USA), Bax, Bcl-2, Bcl-xL, cytochrome C, β-actin (Santa Cruz Biotechnology, Dallas, TX, USA), and γH2A.X (Abcam, Cambridge, UK). Further, the membranes were incubated with Horseradish peroxidase (HRP) -conjugated secondary antibody for 1 h at room temperature. The chemiluminescence signal were detected using enhanced chemiluminescence (ECL) reagent (Millipore, Billerica, MA, USA).

4.4. Immunocytochemistry

For immunocytochemistry, hCPCs were seeded at a density of 50,000 cells per well in a 2-well chamber slide (BioTek, Winooski, VT, USA). After pretreatment with histochrome for 24 h, cells were washed once with PBS and fixed in 4% paraformaldehyde (PFA) for 10 min. Cells were then permeabilized in 0.1% Triton X-100 + 0.01 M Glycine + Phosphate-buffered saline (PBS) solution for 30 min. Slides were blocked with 10% normal goat serum in PBST (0.1% Triton X-100 in PBS) and incubated for 1 h at room temperature. γH2A.X (phospho S139) antibody (#ab11174, 1:500 dilute in blocking buffer, Abcam, Cambridge, UK) was diluted in blocking solution and incubated overnight at 4 °C. The following day, slides were washed 3 times with PBS and incubated with Alexa Flour 488 goat IgG anti-rabbit antibody (1:200, Invitrogen, Carlsbad, CA, USA), and incubated for 1 hour in the dark. Following cell wash twice, cells were mounted using ProLong diamond anti-fade mountant with 4′,6-diamidino-2-phenylindole (DAPI). Slides were analyzed under a Lionheart FX automated microscope (BioTek, Winooski, VT, USA)

4.5. Flow Cytometry Analysis

To examine c-kit expression, hCPCs were fixed in 4% PFA for 10 min and washed with PBS. The cells were fixed and permeabilized as previously described [50]. The fixed cells were incubated with c-kit antibody (#130-091-733, Miltenyi Biotec, Bergisch Gladbach, Germany) for 30 min at 4 °C. For expression analysis of other stem cell markers, hCPCs were suspended in 100 μL FACS buffer (2 mM EDTA, 2% FBS in PBS solution) and incubated with CD34 (#55373, BD Bioscience, Franklin Lakes, NJ, USA), CD45 (#560839, BD Bioscience, Franklin Lakes, NJ, USA), CD166 (#559263, BD Bioscience, Franklin Lakes, NJ, USA), CD29 (#555443, BD Bioscience, Franklin Lakes, NJ, USA), CD105 (#560829, BD Bioscience, Franklin Lakes, NJ, USA), and CD90 (#130-097-930, Miltenyi Biotec, Bergisch Gladbach, Germany) FACS antibody. After incubation for 30 min, the cells were washed three times and resuspended in 100 μL FACS buffer. Expression of stem cell markers was analyzed on a BD Accuri flow cytometer (BD Bioscience, Franklin Lakes, NJ, USA).

4.6. ROS Measurement

Intracellular ROS levels were detected using CellROX green reagent (#C10444, Thermo Fisher Scientific, Carlsbad, CA, USA). Cells were stained according to the manufacturer's instructions. Imaging and quantification of cellular ROS levels were performed using the CX7 High-Content Screening (HCS) System (Thermo Fisher Scientific, Carlsbad, CA, USA). For H_2-DFFDA assay, hCPCs were harvested using Accutase (Sigma-Aldrich, St. Louis, CA, USA) and incubated with 10 μM carboxy-H_2-DFFDA at 37 °C in the dark. After washing with PBS, the cells were resuspended in 100 μL of FACS buffer. The intracellular ROS level was assessed based on the fluorescence intensity of the cells.

4.7. Mitochondrial Superoxide Measurement

hCPCs were plated on a confocal plate (50,000 cells per well) and incubated overnight. The following day, cells were pretreated with/without histochrome (in 2% Ham's F-12 medium) and incubated for 24 h. Cells were washed and incubated in low serum Ham's F-12 medium supplemented with 5 μM MitoSOX Red (#M36008, Thermo Fisher Scientific, Carlsbad, CA, USA) and 100 nM Mitotracker green (#M7514, Thermo Fisher Scientific, Carlsbad, CA, USA) for 30 min. Further, the cells were washed twice with PBS prior to analysis using a Lionheart FX automated microscope (BioTek, Winooski, VT, USA).

4.8. Cell Death Assay

hCPCs were pretreated with histochrome for 24 h in low serum (2% FBS) Ham's F-12 medium. After incubation, cells were washed with PBS and exposed to 1 mM H_2O_2 for 4 h in low serum medium. Further, cells were harvested and suspended in 1 × annexin binding buffer supplemented with Annexin

V (AnV; BD Pharminogen, #550475, San Diego, CA, USA) and 7-AAD(BD Pharminogen, San Diego, CA, USA).

4.9. Live Cell Imaging

For quantification of live cells in H_2O_2-induced oxidative stress, cells were stained with calcein (#R37601, Thermo Fisher Scientific, Carlsbad, CA, USA). Nuclei were stained with NucBlue Live Ready Probes Reagent (#R37605, Thermo Fisher Scientific, Carlsbad, CA, USA). Live cells were observed under the CX7 High-Content Screening (HCS) System (100×, Thermo Fisher Scientific, Carlsbad, CA, USA). Images were captured (25 images per well) and experiments were repeated four times. Green fluorescence indicated live cells.

4.10. Senescence Associated β-galactosidase Staining

Senescent cells were quantified by SA-β-gal assay kit (#9860, Cell Signaling Technology, Beverly, MA, USA) according to the manufacturer's instructions. After X-gal staining, images were captured using an Olympus microscope (OLYMPUS, Tokyo, Japan). Each experiment was repeated three times.

4.11. Statistical Analysis

Data are presented as means ± standard deviation (SD). Statistical significance was assessed by student's *t*-test to compare between the two groups. $p < 0.05$ was considered statically significant.

5. Conclusions

Pretreatment with histochrome (sodium salt of echinochrome A—a common sea urchin pigment) enhances cell survival under oxidative stress conditions by regulating the apoptosis signaling pathway and preventing DNA damage. Furthermore, histochrome attenuates cellular senescence in hCPCs. Our results suggest that pretreating c-kit-positive hCPCs with histochrome before transplantation might be a potential therapeutic strategy in treating ischemic heart disease.

Author Contributions: J.H.P. conception and design, conducted the experiments, data analysis and manuscript writing; N.-K.L., H.J.L., S.M., conducted the experiments, V.K.R., Y.-J.K., W.B.J., S.T.J., S.K., D.Y.K., L.T.H.V., L.T.T.G., D.H.K., J.S.H., J.Y. data analysis, H.T.K., provide cardiac tissue, N.P.M., S.A.F., E.A.V., J.H. prepared histochrome, S.H.B. and S.M.K. financial support, manuscript writing, and final approval of manuscript.

Funding: This research was funded by the National Research Foundation (NRF - 2018R1A2B6006380, NRF - 2015M3A9B4066493, NRF – 2015R1A5A2009656), the Korean Health Technology R&D Project, Ministry of Health and Welfare (HI18C2459, HI18C2458, HI17C1662) funded by the Korean government, and the Ministry of Science and Higher Education of the Russian Federation (RFMEFI61317X0076).

Acknowledgments: We thanks the students, Jun Bum Heo, Chae Ra Ahn, Hee Jeen Kim, and Geon Uk Ha, who participated in the experiment.

Conflicts of Interest: The authors declare no conflict of interest.

References

1. Joo, H.J.; Kim, J.H.; Hong, S.J. Adipose Tissue-Derived Stem Cells for Myocardial Regeneration. *Korean Circ. J.* **2017**, *47*, 151–159. [CrossRef] [PubMed]
2. Madigan, M.; Atoui, R. Therapeutic Use of Stem Cells for Myocardial Infarction. *Bioengineering (Basel)* **2018**, *5*, 28. [CrossRef] [PubMed]
3. Zhu, W.; Gao, L.; Zhang, J. Pluripotent Stem Cell Derived Cardiac Cells for Myocardial Repair. *J. Vis. Exp.* **2017**. [CrossRef] [PubMed]
4. Beltrami, A.P.; Barlucchi, L.; Torella, D.; Baker, M.; Limana, F.; Chimenti, S.; Kasahara, H.; Rota, M.; Musso, E.; Urbanek, K.; et al. Adult cardiac stem cells are multipotent and support myocardial regeneration. *Cell* **2003**, *114*, 763–776. [CrossRef]

5. Bearzi, C.; Rota, M.; Hosoda, T.; Tillmanns, J.; Nascimbene, A.; De Angelis, A.; Yasuzawa-Amano, S.; Trofimova, I.; Siggins, R.W.; Lecapitaine, N.; et al. Human cardiac stem cells. *Proc. Natl. Acad. Sci. USA* **2007**, *104*, 14068–14073. [CrossRef] [PubMed]
6. Leri, A.; Rota, M.; Hosoda, T.; Goichberg, P.; Anversa, P. Cardiac stem cell niches. *Stem Cell Res.* **2014**, *13*, 631–646. [CrossRef]
7. Anversa, P.; Kajstura, J.; Rota, M.; Leri, A. Regenerating new heart with stem cells. *J. Clin. Investig.* **2013**, *123*, 62–70. [CrossRef]
8. Ellison, G.M.; Vicinanza, C.; Smith, A.J.; Aquila, I.; Leone, A.; Waring, C.D.; Henning, B.J.; Stirparo, G.G.; Papait, R.; Scarfo, M.; et al. Adult c-kit(pos) cardiac stem cells are necessary and sufficient for functional cardiac regeneration and repair. *Cell* **2013**, *154*, 827–842. [CrossRef]
9. Li, Z.; Lee, A.; Huang, M.; Chun, H.; Chung, J.; Chu, P.; Hoyt, G.; Yang, P.; Rosenberg, J.; Robbins, R.C.; et al. Imaging survival and function of transplanted cardiac resident stem cells. *J. Am. Coll. Cardiol.* **2009**, *53*, 1229–1240. [CrossRef]
10. Smith, R.R.; Barile, L.; Cho, H.C.; Leppo, M.K.; Hare, J.M.; Messina, E.; Giacomello, A.; Abraham, M.R.; Marban, E. Regenerative potential of cardiosphere-derived cells expanded from percutaneous endomyocardial biopsy specimens. *Circulation* **2007**, *115*, 896–908. [CrossRef]
11. Bax, N.A.; van Marion, M.H.; Shah, B.; Goumans, M.J.; Bouten, C.V.; van der Schaft, D.W. Matrix production and remodeling capacity of cardiomyocyte progenitor cells during in vitro differentiation. *J. Mol. Cell Cardiol.* **2012**, *53*, 497–508. [CrossRef] [PubMed]
12. Al-Daccak, R.; Charron, D. Allogenic benefit in stem cell therapy: Cardiac repair and regeneration. *Tissue Antigens* **2015**, *86*, 155–162. [CrossRef] [PubMed]
13. Li, Q.; Guo, Y.; Ou, Q.; Chen, N.; Wu, W.J.; Yuan, F.; O'Brien, E.; Wang, T.; Luo, L.; Hunt, G.N.; et al. Intracoronary administration of cardiac stem cells in mice: A new, improved technique for cell therapy in murine models. *Basic Res. Cardiol.* **2011**, *106*, 849–864. [CrossRef] [PubMed]
14. Teng, L.; Bennett, E.; Cai, C. Preconditioning c-Kit-positive Human Cardiac Stem Cells with a Nitric Oxide Donor Enhances Cell Survival through Activation of Survival Signaling Pathways. *J. Biol. Chem.* **2016**, *291*, 9733–9747. [CrossRef] [PubMed]
15. Sawyer, D.B.; Siwik, D.A.; Xiao, L.; Pimentel, D.R.; Singh, K.; Colucci, W.S. Role of oxidative stress in myocardial hypertrophy and failure. *J. Mol. Cell Cardiol.* **2002**, *34*, 379–388. [CrossRef]
16. Cieslar-Pobuda, A.; Yue, J.; Lee, H.C.; Skonieczna, M.; Wei, Y.H. ROS and Oxidative Stress in Stem Cells. *Oxid. Med. Cell. Longev.* **2017**, *2017*. [CrossRef]
17. Maraldi, T.; Angeloni, C.; Giannoni, E.; Sell, C. Reactive Oxygen Species in Stem Cells. *Oxid. Med. Cell. Longev.* **2015**, *2015*. [CrossRef]
18. Kwon, S.H.; Pimentel, D.R.; Remondino, A.; Sawyer, D.B.; Colucci, W.S. H(2)O(2) regulates cardiac myocyte phenotype via concentration-dependent activation of distinct kinase pathways. *J. Mol. Cell. Cardiol.* **2003**, *35*, 615–621. [CrossRef]
19. Rosdah, A.A.; Bond, S.T.; Sivakumaran, P.; Hoque, A.; Oakhill, J.S.; Drew, B.G.; Delbridge, L.M.D.; Lim, S.Y. Mdivi-1 Protects Human W8B^{2+} Cardiac Stem Cells from Oxidative Stress and Simulated Ischemia-Reperfusion Injury. *Stem Cells Dev.* **2017**, *26*, 1771–1780. [CrossRef]
20. Anderson, H.A.; Mathieson, J.W.; Thomson, R.H. Distribution of spinochrome pigments in echinoids. *Comp. Biochem. Physiol.* **1969**, *28*, 333–345. [CrossRef]
21. Fedoreyev, S.A.; Krylova, N.V.; Mishchenko, N.P.; Vasileva, E.A.; Pislyagin, E.A.; Iunikhina, O.V.; Lavrov, V.F.; Svitich, O.A.; Ebralidze, L.K.; Leonova, G.N.; et al. Antiviral and Antioxidant Properties of Echinochrome A. *Mar. Drugs* **2018**, *16*, 509. [CrossRef] [PubMed]
22. Lennikov, A.; Kitaichi, N.; Noda, K.; Mizuuchi, K.; Ando, R.; Dong, Z.; Fukuhara, J.; Kinoshita, S.; Namba, K.; Ohno, S.; et al. Amelioration of endotoxin-induced uveitis treated with the sea urchin pigment echinochrome in rats. *Mol. Vis.* **2014**, *20*, 171–177. [PubMed]
23. Mohamed, A.S.; Soliman, A.M.; Marie, M.A.S. Mechanisms of echinochrome potency in modulating diabetic complications in liver. *Life Sci.* **2016**, *151*, 41–49. [CrossRef] [PubMed]
24. Jeong, S.H.; Kim, H.K.; Song, I.S.; Lee, S.J.; Ko, K.S.; Rhee, B.D.; Kim, N.; Mishchenko, N.P.; Fedoryev, S.A.; Stonik, V.A.; et al. Echinochrome A protects mitochondrial function in cardiomyocytes against cardiotoxic drugs. *Mar. Drugs* **2014**, *12*, 2922–2936. [CrossRef] [PubMed]

25. Jeong, S.H.; Kim, H.K.; Song, I.S.; Noh, S.J.; Marquez, J.; Ko, K.S.; Rhee, B.D.; Kim, N.; Mishchenko, N.P.; Fedoreyev, S.A.; et al. Echinochrome a increases mitochondrial mass and function by modulating mitochondrial biogenesis regulatory genes. *Mar. Drugs* **2014**, *12*, 4602–4615. [CrossRef] [PubMed]
26. Kim, H.K.; Youm, J.B.; Jeong, S.H.; Lee, S.R.; Song, I.S.; Ko, T.H.; Pronto, J.R.; Ko, K.S.; Rhee, B.D.; Kim, N.; et al. Echinochrome A regulates phosphorylation of phospholamban Ser16 and Thr17 suppressing cardiac SERCA2A Ca^{2+} reuptake. *Pflugers Arch.* **2015**, *467*, 2151–2163. [CrossRef] [PubMed]
27. Egorov, E.A.; Alekhina, V.A.; Volobueva, T.M.; Fedoreev, S.A.; Mishchenko, N.P.; Kol'tsova, E.A. [Histochrome, a new antioxidant, in the treatment of ocular diseases]. *Vestn. Oftalmol.* **1999**, *115*, 34–35. [PubMed]
28. Afanas'ev, S.A.; Vecherskii, Y.; Maksimov, I.V.; Markov, V.A.; Rebrova, T. *Cardioprotective Effect of Antioxidant Histochrome in Cardiology and Cardiac Surgery Practice*; STT: Tomsk, Russia, 2012; 150p. (In Russian)
29. Han, X.M.; Wu, S.X.; Wu, M.F.; Yang, X.F. Antioxidant effect of peony seed oil on aging mice. *Food Sci. Biotechnol.* **2017**, *26*, 1703–1708. [CrossRef]
30. Kim, J.E.; Jin, D.H.; Lee, S.D.; Hong, S.W.; Shin, J.S.; Lee, S.K.; Jung, D.J.; Kang, J.S.; Lee, W.J. Vitamin C inhibits p53-induced replicative senescence through suppression of ROS production and p38 MAPK activity. *Int. J. Mol. Med.* **2008**, *22*, 651–655.
31. Suh, N.; Lee, E.B. Antioxidant effects of selenocysteine on replicative senescence in human adipose-derived mesenchymal stem cells. *BMB Rep.* **2017**, *50*, 572–577. [CrossRef]
32. Lee, J.H.; Lee, S.H.; Choi, S.H.; Asahara, T.; Kwon, S.M. The sulfated polysaccharide fucoidan rescues senescence of endothelial colony-forming cells for ischemic repair. *Stem Cells* **2015**, *33*, 1939–1951. [CrossRef] [PubMed]
33. Kim, H.K.; Cho, S.W.; Heo, H.J.; Jeong, S.H.; Kim, M.; Ko, K.S.; Rhee, B.D.; Mishchenko, N.P.; Vasileva, E.A.; Fedoreyev, S.A.; et al. A Novel Atypical PKC-Iota Inhibitor, Echinochrome A, Enhances Cardiomyocyte Differentiation from Mouse Embryonic Stem Cells. *Mar. Drugs* **2018**, *16*, 192. [CrossRef] [PubMed]
34. Kukielka, G.L.; Smith, C.W.; Manning, A.M.; Youker, K.A.; Michael, L.H.; Entman, M.L. Induction of interleukin-6 synthesis in the myocardium. Potential role in postreperfusion inflammatory injury. *Circulation* **1995**, *92*, 1866–1875. [CrossRef] [PubMed]
35. Hori, M.; Nishida, K. Oxidative stress and left ventricular remodelling after myocardial infarction. *Cardiovasc. Res.* **2009**, *81*, 457–464. [CrossRef]
36. Sedova, K.; Bernikova, O.; Azarov, J.; Shmakov, D.; Vityazev, V.; Kharin, S. Effects of echinochrome on ventricular repolarization in acute ischemia. *J. Electrocardiol.* **2015**, *48*, 181–186. [CrossRef] [PubMed]
37. Dey, S.; DeMazumder, D.; Sidor, A.; Foster, D.B.; O'Rourke, B. Mitochondrial ROS Drive Sudden Cardiac Death and Chronic Proteome Remodeling in Heart Failure. *Circ. Res.* **2018**, *123*, 356–371. [CrossRef] [PubMed]
38. Maddika, S.; Ande, S.R.; Panigrahi, S.; Paranjothy, T.; Weglarczyk, K.; Zuse, A.; Eshraghi, M.; Manda, K.D.; Wiechec, E.; Los, M.; et al. Cell survival, cell death and cell cycle pathways are interconnected: Implications for cancer therapy. *Drug Resist. Updat.* **2007**, *10*, 13–29. [CrossRef]
39. Cory, S.; Adams, J.M. The Bcl2 family: Regulators of the cellular life-or-death switch. *Nat. Rev. Cancer* **2002**, *2*, 647–656. [CrossRef]
40. Antonsson, B.; Martinou, J.C. The Bcl-2 protein family. *Exp. Cell Res.* **2000**, *256*, 50–57. [CrossRef]
41. Zinkel, S.; Gross, A.; Yang, E. BCL2 family in DNA damage and cell cycle control. *Cell Death Differ.* **2006**, *13*, 1351–1359. [CrossRef]
42. Kuo, L.J.; Yang, L.X. Gamma-H2AX—A novel biomarker for DNA double-strand breaks. *In Vivo* **2008**, *22*, 305–309. [PubMed]
43. Shay, J.W.; Wright, W.E. Hayflick, his limit, and cellular ageing. *Nat. Rev. Mol. Cell Biol.* **2000**, *1*, 72–76. [CrossRef] [PubMed]
44. Turinetto, V.; Vitale, E.; Giachino, C. Senescence in Human Mesenchymal Stem Cells: Functional Changes and Implications in Stem Cell-Based Therapy. *Int. J. Mol. Sci.* **2016**, *17*, 1164. [CrossRef] [PubMed]
45. Choi, S.H.; Jung, S.Y.; Suh, W.; Baek, S.H.; Kwon, S.M. Establishment of isolation and expansion protocols for human cardiac C-kit-positive progenitor cells for stem cell therapy. *Transplant. Proc.* **2013**, *45*, 420–426. [CrossRef] [PubMed]
46. Park, J.H.; Choi, S.H.; Kim, H.; Ji, S.T.; Jang, W.B.; Kim, J.H.; Baek, S.H.; Kwon, S.M. Doxorubicin Regulates Autophagy Signals via Accumulation of Cytosolic Ca^{2+} in Human Cardiac Progenitor Cells. *Int. J. Mol. Sci.* **2016**, *17*, 1680. [CrossRef] [PubMed]

47. Mischenko, N.P.; Fedoreyev, S.A.; Pokhilo, N.D.; Anufriev, V.P.; Denisenko, V.A.; Glazunov, V.P. Echinamines A and B, first aminated hydroxynaphthazarins from the sea urchin Scaphechinus mirabilis. *J. Nat. Prod.* **2005**, *68*, 1390–1393. [CrossRef]
48. Kim, D.; Kim, H.J.; Cha, S.H.; Jun, H.S. Protective Effects of Broussonetia kazinoki Siebold Fruit Extract against Palmitate-Induced Lipotoxicity in Mesangial Cells. *Evid Based Complement Altern. Med.* **2019**, *2019*, 4509403. [CrossRef]
49. Kim, J.; Shin, S.H.; Kang, J.K.; Kim, J.W. HX-1171 attenuates pancreatic beta-cell apoptosis and hyperglycemia-mediated oxidative stress via Nrf2 activation in streptozotocin-induced diabetic model. *Oncotarget* **2018**, *9*, 24260–24271. [CrossRef]
50. Monsanto, M.M.; White, K.S.; Kim, T.; Wang, B.J.; Fisher, K.; Ilves, K.; Khalafalla, F.G.; Casillas, A.; Broughton, K.; Mohsin, S.; et al. Concurrent Isolation of 3 Distinct Cardiac Stem Cell Populations from a Single Human Heart Biopsy. *Circ. Res.* **2017**, *121*, 113–124. [CrossRef]

marine drugs

MDPI

Article

Echinochrome A Attenuates Cerebral Ischemic Injury through Regulation of Cell Survival after Middle Cerebral Artery Occlusion in Rat

Ran Kim [1], Daeun Hur [1], Hyoung Kyu Kim [2], Jin Han [2], Natalia P. Mishchenko [3], Sergey A. Fedoreyev [3], Valentin A. Stonik [3] and Woochul Chang [1,*]

1 Department of Biology Education, College of Education, Pusan National University, Busan 46241, Korea
2 National Research Laboratory for Mitochondrial Signaling, Department of Physiology, College of Medicine, Cardiovascular and Metabolic Disease Center (CMDC), Inje University, Busan 614-735, Korea
3 G.B. Elyakov Pacific Institute of Bioorganic Chemistry, Far-Eastern Branch of the Russian Academy of Science, Vladivostok 690022, Russia
* Correspondence: wchang1975@pusan.ac.kr; Tel.: +82-51-510-3124; Fax: +82-514-8576

Received: 10 July 2019; Accepted: 23 August 2019; Published: 28 August 2019

Abstract: Of late, researchers have taken interest in alternative medicines for the treatment of brain ischemic stroke, where full recovery is rarely seen despite advanced medical technologies. Due to its antioxidant activity, Echinochrome A (Ech A), a natural compound found in sea urchins, has acquired attention as an alternative clinical trial source for the treatment of ischemic stroke. The current study demonstrates considerable potential of Ech A as a medication for cerebral ischemic injury. To confirm the effects of Ech A on the recovery of the injured region and behavioral decline, Ech A was administered through the external carotid artery in a rat middle cerebral artery occlusion model after reperfusion. The expression level of cell viability-related factors was also examined to confirm the mechanism of brain physiological restoration. Based on the results obtained, we propose that Ech A ameliorates the physiological deterioration by its antioxidant effect which plays a protective role against cell death, subsequent to post cerebral ischemic stroke.

Keywords: echinochrome A; brain ischemic stroke; cell survival

1. Introduction

Although medical knowledge and technology have advanced considerably, cerebral ischemic stroke patients experience pain with severe disabilities and high mortality due to brain damage resulting from middle cerebral artery occlusion (MCAo) [1,2]. The progression of pathological changes in acute ischemic stroke includes oxidative stress, free radical production, brain edema, neuronal apoptosis, and finally death [3,4]. Intravenous recombinant tissue plasminogen activator (rtPA) or other agents such as anti-cytokines, calcium channel blockers, and free radical scavengers for therapeutic thrombolysis are the generally applied treatments in the early stage of the disease [5]. However, there is rarely a complete recovery of ischemia neuronal damage. Therefore, in recent years, researchers have recognized the importance of finding inventive strategies for the restoration of brain injury.

Natural derived products, including molecules from marine organisms, have gained recognition as alternative therapeutic sources. The past decade has seen a rise in the application of various compounds from isolated marine species as a popular and promising therapeutic approach for human diseases [6]. Marine organisms are capable of overcoming some insuperable conditions such as light, temperature, pressure, and oxygen and ion concentration due to their distinct habitat environment [7]. Echinochrome A (Ech A), a dark red pigment, is most commonly extracted from the shells, spines, and eggs of sea urchins [8]. The biologically active compound possesses antiviral, antialgal, and antioxidant properties [8,9]. Ech A is an active substance in the cardioprotective drug Histochrome, registered in Russia (P N002363/01). It presented a positive outcome in animal disease model with experimental hemorrhagic stroke as previously described [10]. Histochrome accelerates the alleviation of neurological symptoms and edema, which are mainly caused by the release of free iron and oxidative stress. The effects of Ech A on ischemic stroke have not been previously studied. In particular, the high antioxidant efficacy exerts a beneficial advantage in the research of stroke [11]. Oxidative stress contributes to irreversible pathophysiological cellular damages during the initial and later phases of ischemic stroke [11]. Despite the restoration of blood flow to rescue the ischemic brain, reperfusion is known to aggravate oxidative stress damage and generate reactive oxygen species (ROS) [12]. Ech A neutralizes the iron cations that accumulate in the region of ischemic damaged tissue [12]. However, researchers have rarely considered Ech A as a therapeutic candidate to overcome brain ischemic stroke.

Based on the results obtained using an experimental rat MCAo model, we demonstrate the potential of Ech A for treating brain ischemic stroke. In the present study, the therapeutic effects of Ech A were evaluated. The administration of Ech A recovered the brain region and alleviated the repressed behaviors in the rat MCAo model. Our results indicate that the administration of Ech A influences the expression of cell viability related factors, thereby confirming its effect on physiological improvements.

2. Results and Discussion

2.1. Ech A Mitigates Cerebral Ischemic Injury

To confirm the mitigative effect of Ech A on cerebral ischemic disease, rat MCAo models were exposed to 10 μM Ech A and subsequently assessed for brain infarct volume and water content. We used 2,3,5-triphenyltetrazolium chloride (TTC) staining, one of the most conventional methods, to visualize the infarct region of the ischemic cerebrum. Ech A substantially shows the visual recovery reducing the brain infarct volumes at 7 days after reperfusion (Figure 1A). Alleviation of the injured area after exposure to Ech A was confirmed by comparing the percentage of white region in the control brain with the Ech A treatment group through TTC staining (Sham: 0.0%, control group: 52.7%, 10 μM Ech A: 21.9%) (Figure 1B). Next, we investigated the water content of rat MCAo model brain tissue, which is a marker of severe ischemic injury [13]. The water content is used to signify the ischemic brain edema in the infarct hemisphere [14], and to examine the effect of Ech A treatment on the blood–brain barrier (BBB) leakage in this study. Cerebral edema plays a key role in fatal outcomes associated with numerous neurological conditions, including ischemic stroke [15]. The percentage of water content in the control group was increased, as compared to the sham group. The Ech A-treated group revealed decreased water content as compared to the control group (sham: 79.4%, control: 81.7%, 10 μM Ech A: 80.3%) (Figure 1C). Taken together, we construe that Ech A presents the visual restoration in the infarct cerebrum of rat MCAo models. However, the functional recovery and the reparative mechanism by Ech A treatment on brain ischemic disease remain to be identified.

2.2. Ech A Encourages Affirmative Behavioral Changes after Ischemic Stroke

Functional assessments were applied to determine behavioral changes in the rat model for aggressive central nervous damage [16]. Two methods, namely, the cylinder test and swim test, were adopted and modified. The cylinder test evaluates the frequency of forelimb use and asymmetric movement in postural weight support [17]. In the cylinder test, cerebrally injured rats (control group) exhibited increased asymmetry use, especially practical use of the unaffected forelimb, when compared to the sham group. Furthermore, the 10 μM Ech A-treated group showed behavioral recovery with increased use of both forelimbs and decreased use of the unaffected forelimb, as compared to the control group (simultaneous use: sham 38.0%, control 26.0%, 10 μM Ech A 35.0%; unaffected use: sham 26.0%, control 39.0%, 10 μM Ech A 32.0%) (Figure 2A).

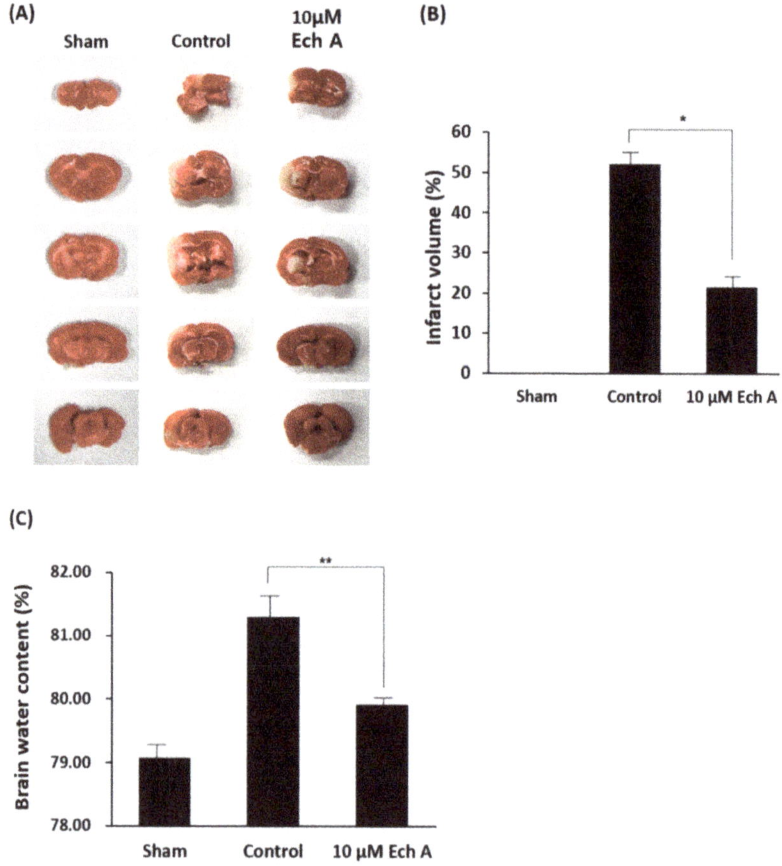

Figure 1. Echinochrome A (Ech A) alleviates the infarcted brain region of rat middle cerebral artery occlusion (MCAo). (**A**) Representative TTC staining of brain sections of the damaged area in the sham, control and 10 μM Ech A treatment groups of a rat MCAo/reperfusion model. (* $p < 0.05$). (**B**) Quantification of size in the infarcted brain region from each experimental group. (**C**) Quantification of water content in infarcted brain region from each experimental group (** $p < 0.01$).

Stroke results in the reduction of predominant activities such as mobility, climbing, and swimming [18]. Since the forced swim test (FST) is frequently used to confirm these activities, this method was applied to assess the antidepressant-like behavior in MCAo models [18]. In this test, while brain infarct rats showed increasing immobility, the behavioral recovered rats (after 10 μM Ech A treatment) show alleviated immobility time during the FST (sham: 33 s, control: 81 s, 10 μM Ech A: 51 s) (Figure 2B). Our results indicate that treatment with an appropriate amount of Ech A enhances the motor ability in brain ischemic disease.

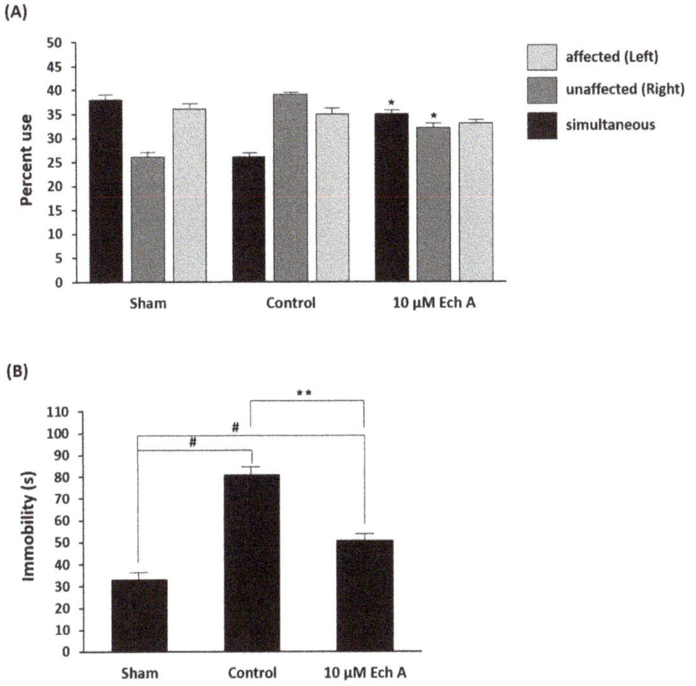

Figure 2. Declined movements are restored after Ech A treatment following ischemic stroke. (**A**) Assessment of percent use of affected (left), unaffected (right), and simultaneous (both) forelimbs on the wall of the cylinder (* $p < 0.05$). (**B**) Total amount of immobility time in the forced swim test (# $p < 0.01$ compared with the values of the sham group; ** $p < 0.01$ compared with the values of the control group).

2.3. Ech A Affects the Expression of Cell Survival-Related Molecules of Rat Ischemic Stroke Brain

To demonstrate the mechanism of physiological improvements, which include the restoration of the damaged brain region and the intensification of attenuated behavior after Ech A treatment, we focused on the occurrences after ischemia reperfusion injury. Ischemia reperfusion-injured brain suffers from oxidative stress and induces the cell death regulating pathway [19]. Considering this, we investigated the expression levels of cell viability-related factors in our experimental animal model, including Bcl-2, Caspase-3, Bax (Figure 3A), p-ERK/ERK, p-AKT/AKT (Figure 3B), and brain-derived neurotrophic factor (BDNF) (Figure 3C). The effect of Ech A treatment on the expression of these regulators was estimated in the brain tissue of MCAo rats. Bcl-2, caspase-3, and Bax work as major mediators for cell survival and death and are activated by various stimuli [18,19]. Bcl-2, an apoptosis inhibitor, is a key player in the mechanism of anti-apoptosis [20,21]. In contrast, caspase-3 and Bax are pro-apoptosis molecules which signify the onset of apoptosis [21]. Compared to the control group, Ech A treatment in the MCAo rat model significantly increased the expression level of Bcl-2 and decreases the levels of caspase-3 and Bax. The extracellular signal-related kinases (ERK) are essential regulators associated with vital cellular functions, including cell proliferation, differentiation, migration, senescence, and apoptosis in the generic mitogen-activated protein kinase (MAPK) signaling pathway [22]. Furthermore, in the PI3K/AKT/mTOR signaling pathway, AKT is also a core component of various processes of cellular activities, including nutrient uptake, anabolic reactions, metabolism, cell growth, proliferation, differentiation, apoptosis, and survival [23]. Our results indicate an increase in the expression levels of p-ERK/ERK and p-AKT/AKT in the Ech A-treated MCAo rat model as compared to the control group. The brain-derived neurotrophic factor (BDNF) significantly supports neuronal differentiation and survival, synaptic formation and plasticity, and neurogenesis, and has been widely researched in various neurological conditions [24]. Our studies reveal increased BDNF expression in the brain of MCAo rat model after exposure to Ech A, as compared to the control group. Taken together, these findings confirm that Ech A relieves the physiological decline in the MCAo rat model by increasing and supporting cell survival in the injured brain region.

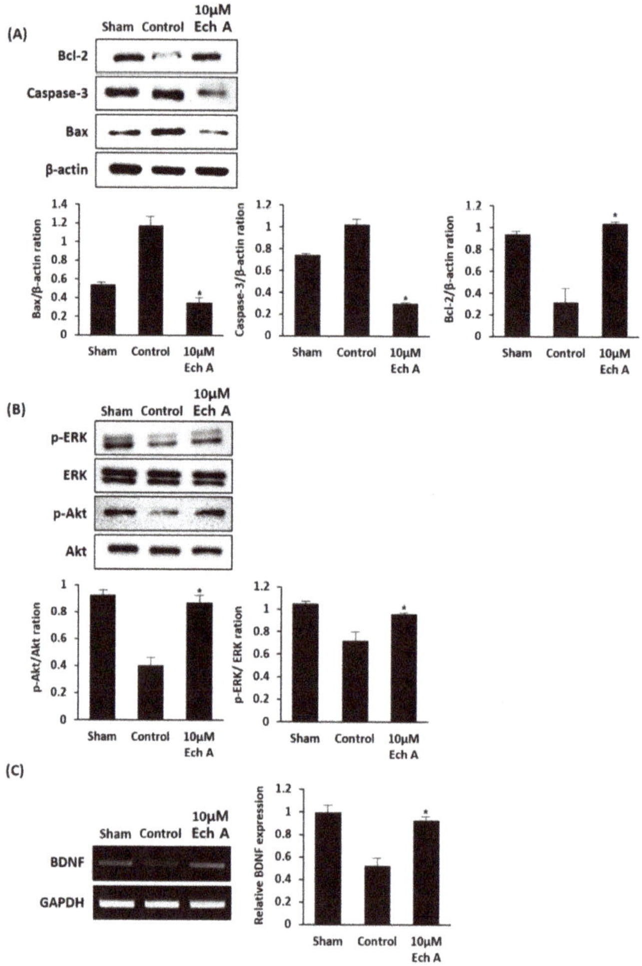

Figure 3. Ech A treatment in cerebral injured brain alters the expression levels of cell viability-related factors. (**A**) The protein expression levels of cell survival and death regulators, such as Bcl-2, caspase-3, and Bax. (**B**) The protein expression levels of key players in vital cellular function regulation pathways, such as ERK and AKT. (**C**) The mRNA expression level of BDNF, supporting cell survival alteration in the injured brain region (* $p < 0.05$).

3. Experimental Section

3.1. Chemical

Ech A (6-ethyl-2,3,5,7,8-pentahydroxynaphthalene-1,4-dion) was isolated from the sand dollar *Scaphechinus mirabilis* using an extraction method as previously described [25]. The purity of Ech A

(>99%) was confirmed by liquid chromatography-mass spectrometry (Shimadzu LCMS-2020, Kyoto, Japan). We used 0.02% Ech A with saline solution.

3.2. Preparation of Ischemic Stroke Rat Models

3.2.1. Animals

Nine-week-old male Sprague Dawley (SD) rats (290–300 g; KOATECH, Gyeonggi-do, Korea) were handled in accordance with the animal welfare guidelines issued by the Korean National Institute of Health and the Korean Academy of Medical Sciences for the care and use of laboratory animals.

3.2.2. Middle Cerebral Artery Occlusion

We applied a modified surgical procedure of the standard method [26,27]. Briefly, rats were anesthetized with isoflurane in a mixture of 30% oxygen and 70% nitrous oxide. Using an operative microscope, a 3-0 nylon suture was inserted into the internal carotid artery (ICA) through the external carotid artery (ECA). After 90 min of occlusion, the suture was withdrawn for 7 days for reperfusion. The animals were randomly divided into three groups (n = 12 per group): group I, sham-operation (sham), group II, MCAo/reperfusion-induced ischemic group with saline treatment (control), group III, MCAo/reperfusion-induced ischemic group with 10 μM Ech A treatment.

3.3. Behavioral Test

We modified the FST and cylinder test to determine the motor ability of experimental animals. For the FST, at 7 days after reperfusion, rats were placed in an open cylinder (height: 60 cm, diameter: 20 cm) which was filled with water for 6 min, and their duration of immobility was measured for the last 4 min. In the cylinder test, rats were placed in a transparent cylinder (height: 30 cm, diameter: 20 cm) for 6 min. The use of their forelimbs was recorded for the last 4 min. The number of right and left forelimbs used independently, and both forelimbs use simultaneously, were observed and recorded. Each experiment was repeated five times.

3.4. Measurement of Brain Infarct Volume and Water Content

All animals were euthanized 7 days after MCAo operation. Brains were collected and sectioned into 2.0 mm coronal slices to assess the brain infarct volume. The brain sections were stained with TTC and the percentage of infarct volume was calculated by assessing the stained brain area using ImageJ software. To measure the brain water content, the pons and olfactory bulbs were removed and the wet weight (ww) of the brain was measured. The brains were subsequently dried at 110 °C for 24 h, and the dry weight (dw) of the brain was examined. The percentage water content in the brain was assessed using the following formula:

$$\text{Water content: } (\text{ww} - \text{dw})/\text{ww} \times 100\%$$

3.5. Western Blot

Brain tissues were homogenized in lysis buffer (Cell Signaling Technology, Beverly, MA, USA) to collect the total proteins. Quantified proteins were separated by SDS-PAGE and transferred to polyvinylidene fluoride microporous membrane (Millipore, Temecula, CA, USA). The membranes were blocked with 0.1% Tween 20 in Tris-buffered saline containing 5% nonfat milk for 1 h at room temperature, and subsequently incubated with the primary antibody (Bcl-2, caspase-3, Bax, p-ERK, and ERK; Santa Cruz Biotechnology, Dallas, TX, USA; p-Akt, Akt, and β-actin; Cell Signaling Technology).

3.6. Polymerase Chain Reaction (PCR) Analysis

The total RNA of brain tissues was extracted using the Hybrid-R RNA purification kit (GeneAll, Seoul, Korea), and converted to cDNA using the cDNA synthesis kit (Thermo

Scientific, Vilnius, Lithuania). Amplification was performed in a DNA thermal cycler using the following synthesized primers: 5′-GATGAGGACCAGAAGGTTCG-3′ (forward) and 5′-GATTGGGTA GTTCGGCATTG-3′ (reverse) for BDNF; 5′-GCTGGGGCTCACCTGAAGGG-3′ (forward) and 5′-GGATGACCTTGCCCACAGCC-3′ (reverse) for GAPDH.

3.7. Statistical Analysis

All experimental data are presented as mean ± standard error of the mean (SEM). Comparisons between more than two groups were performed by one-way ANOVA using Bonferroni's correction. A p-value < 0.05 is considered significant.

4. Conclusions

Until recently, Ech A was rarely used for the treatment of brain ischemic stroke. Our findings indicate that Ech A as a novel therapeutic source from the ocean has considerable efficacy for cerebral ischemic injury. We demonstrate that Ech A restores the damaged brain area and strengthens the behavioral deterioration by supporting the expression of cell viability-related factors after brain ischemic stroke. Taken together, the results of this study propose a new application as a potential therapeutic agent for this marine drug.

Author Contributions: R.K. and D.H. conducted the experiments, tests, and data analyses. N.P.M. and S.A.F. provided echinochrome A. H.K.K., J.H., V.A.S., and W.C. summarized the work and wrote the manuscript.

Funding: This study was supported by the Basic Science Research Program through the National Research Foundation of Korea (NRF) funded by the Korea government (MSIT) (2018R1A2B6003158) and the Bio and Medical Technology Development Program of the National Research Foundation (NRF) funded by the Ministry of Science and ICT (NRF-2017M3A9G7072568), and the Ministry of Science and Higher Education of the Russian Federation (RFMEFI61317X0076).

Acknowledgments: This study was supported by a grant from the National Research Foundation of Korea (NRF). The study was carried out using the equipment of the Collective Facilities Center (The Far Eastern Center for Structural Molecular Research (NMR/MS) PIBOC FEB RAS).

Conflicts of Interest: The authors declare no conflict of interest.

References

1. Ai, J.; Wan, H.; Shu, M.; Zhou, H.; Zhao, T.; Fu, W.; He, Y. Guhong injection protects against focal cerebral ischemia-reperfusion injury via anti-inflammatory effects in rats. *Arch. Pharm. Res.* **2017**, *40*, 610–622. [CrossRef]
2. Yu, X.; Zhou, C.; Yang, H.; Huang, X.; Ma, H.; Qin, X.; Hu, J. Effect of ultrasonic treatment on the degradation and inhibition cancer cell lines of polysaccharides from *Porphyra yezoensis*. *Carbohydr. Polym.* **2015**, *117*, 650–656. [CrossRef]
3. Zhang, B.; Zhang, H.-X.; Shi, S.-T.; Bai, Y.-L.; Zhe, X.; Zhang, S.-J.; Li, Y.-J. Interleukin-11 treatment protected against cerebral ischemia/reperfusion injury. *Biomed. Pharmacother.* **2019**, *115*, 108816. [CrossRef]
4. Zhu, L.; He, D.; Han, L.; Cao, H. Stroke Research in China over the Past Decade: Analysis of NSFC Funding. *Transl. Stroke Res.* **2015**, *6*, 253–256. [CrossRef]
5. Baron, J.C.; Von Kummer, R.; Del Zoppo, G.J. Treatment of acute ischemic stroke. Challenging the concept of a rigid and universal time window. *Stroke* **1995**, *26*, 2219–2221. [CrossRef]
6. Martins, A.; Vieira, H.M.; Gaspar, H.; Santos, S. Marketed Marine Natural Products in the Pharmaceutical and Cosmeceutical Industries: Tips for Success. *Mar. Drugs* **2014**, *12*, 1066–1101. [CrossRef]
7. Dalmaso, G.Z.L.; Ferreira, D.; Vermelho, A.B. Marine Extremophiles: A Source of Hydrolases for Biotechnological Applications. *Mar. Drugs* **2015**, *13*, 1925–1965. [CrossRef]
8. Mohamed, A.S.; Soliman, A.M.; Marie, M.A.S. Mechanisms of echinochrome potency in modulating diabetic complications in liver. *Life Sci.* **2016**, *151*, 41–49. [CrossRef]
9. Sokolova, E.V.; Menzorova, N.I.; Davydova, V.N.; Kuz'Mich, A.S.; Kravchenko, A.O.; Mishchenko, N.P.; Yermak, I.M. Effects of Carrageenans on Biological Properties of Echinochrome. *Mar. Drugs* **2018**, *16*, 419. [CrossRef]

10. Stonik, V.A.; Gusev, E.; Martynov, M.Y.; Guseva, M.R.; Shchukin, I.A.; Agafonova, I.G.; Mishchenko, N.P.; Fedoreev, S.A. Development of medicines for hemorrhage stroke: The use of magnetic resonance tomography for estimating the effectiveness of histochrome. *Dokl. Biol. Sci.* **2005**, *405*, 421–423. [CrossRef]
11. Davis, S.M.; Pennypacker, K.R. Targeting antioxidant enzyme expression as a therapeutic strategy for ischemic stroke. *Neurochem. Int.* **2017**, *107*, 23–32. [CrossRef]
12. Strubakos, C.D.; Malik, M.; Wider, J.M.; Lee, I.; Reynolds, C.A.; Mitsias, P.; Przyklenk, K.; Hüttemann, M.; Sanderson, T.H. Non-invasive treatment with near-infrared light: A novel mechanisms-based strategy that evokes sustained reduction in brain injury after stroke. *Br. J. Pharmacol.* **2019**, *21*. [CrossRef]
13. Dzialowski, I.; Weber, J.; Doerfler, A.; Forsting, M. Brain Tissue Water Uptake after Middle Cerebral Artery Occlusion Assessed with CT. *J. Neuroimaging* **2004**, *14*, 42–48. [CrossRef]
14. Chen, M.; Li, X.; Zhang, X.; He, X.; Lai, L.; Liu, Y.; Zhu, G.; Li, W.; Li, H.; Fang, Q.; et al. The inhibitory effect of mesenchymal stem cell on blood-brain barrier disruption following intracerebral hemorrhage in rats: Contribution of TSG-6. *J. Neuroinflammation* **2015**, *12*, 61. [CrossRef]
15. Keep, R.F.; Hua, Y.; Xi, G. Brain water content. A misunderstood measurement? *Transl. Stroke Res.* **2012**, *3*, 263–265. [CrossRef]
16. Trueman, R.C.; Diaz, C.; Farr, T.D.; Harrison, D.J.; Fuller, A.; Tokarczuk, P.F.; Stewart, A.J.; Paisey, S.J.; Dunnett, S.B. Systematic and detailed analysis of behavioural tests in the rat middle cerebral artery occlusion model of stroke: Tests for long-term assessment. *J. Cereb. Blood Flow Metab.* **2017**, *37*, 1349–1361. [CrossRef]
17. Schallert, T.; Fleming, S.M.; Leasure, J.L.; Tillerson, J.L.; Bland, S.T. CNS plasticity and assessment of forelimb sensorimotor outcome in unilateral rat models of stroke, cortical ablation, parkinsonism and spinal cord injury. *Neuropharmacology* **2000**, *39*, 777–787. [CrossRef]
18. Buga, A.-M.; Ciobanu, O.; Bădescu, G.M.; Bogdan, C.; Weston, R.; Slevin, M.; Di Napoli, M.; Popa-Wagner, A. Up-regulation of serotonin receptor 2B mRNA and protein in the peri-infarcted area of aged rats and stroke patients. *Oncotarget* **2016**, *7*, 17415–17430. [CrossRef]
19. Sun, M.-S.; Jin, H.; Sun, X.; Huang, S.; Zhang, F.-L.; Guo, Z.-N.; Yang, Y. Free Radical Damage in Ischemia-Reperfusion Injury: An Obstacle in Acute Ischemic Stroke after Revascularization Therapy. *Oxidative Med. Cell. Longev.* **2018**, *2018*, 3804979. [CrossRef]
20. Tsujimoto, Y. Cell death regulation by the Bcl-2 protein family in the mitochondria. *J. Cell. Physiol.* **2003**, *195*, 158–167. [CrossRef]
21. Tian, X.; Shi, Y.; Liu, N.; Yan, Y.; Li, T.; Hua, P.; Liu, B. Upregulation of DAPK contributes to homocysteine-induced endothelial apoptosis via the modulation of Bcl2/Bax and activation of caspase 3. *Mol. Med. Rep.* **2016**, *14*, 4173–4179. [CrossRef] [PubMed]
22. Sun, Y.; Liu, W.-Z.; Liu, T.; Feng, X.; Yang, N.; Zhou, H.-F. Signaling pathway of MAPK/ERK in cell proliferation, differentiation, migration, senescence and apoptosis. *J. Recept. Signal Transduct.* **2015**, *35*, 600–604. [CrossRef] [PubMed]
23. Yu, J.S.L.; Cui, W. Proliferation, survival and metabolism: The role of PI3K/AKT/mTOR signalling in pluripotency and cell fate determination. *Development* **2016**, *143*, 3050–3060. [CrossRef] [PubMed]
24. Wurzelmann, M.; Romeika, J.; Sun, D. Therapeutic potential of brain-derived neurotrophic factor (BDNF) and a small molecular mimics of BDNF for traumatic brain injury. *Neural Regen. Res.* **2017**, *12*, 7–12. [PubMed]
25. Mischenko, N.P.; Fedoreyev, S.A.; Pokhilo, N.D.; Anufriev, V.P.; Denisenko, V.A.; Glazunov, V.P. Echinamines A and B, first aminated hydroxynaphthazarins from the sea urchin *Scaphechinus mirabilis*. *J. Nat. Prod.* **2005**, *68*, 1390–1393. [CrossRef] [PubMed]
26. Longa, E.Z.; Weinstein, P.R.; Carlson, S.; Cummins, R. Reversible middle cerebral artery occlusion without craniectomy in rats. *Stroke* **1989**, *20*, 84–91. [CrossRef] [PubMed]
27. Hill, J.W.; Nemoto, E.M. Transient middle cerebral artery occlusion with complete reperfusion in spontaneously hypertensive rats. *MethodsX* **2014**, *1*, 283–291. [CrossRef] [PubMed]

marine drugs

MDPI

Article

Echinochrome A Reduces Colitis in Mice and Induces In Vitro Generation of Regulatory Immune Cells

Su-Jeong Oh [1,†], Yoojin Seo [2,†], Ji-Su Ahn [1], Ye Young Shin [1], Ji Won Yang [2], Hyoung Kyu Kim [3], Jin Han [3], Natalia P. Mishchenko [4], Sergey A. Fedoreyev [4], Valentin A. Stonik [4] and Hyung-Sik Kim [1,2,*]

1 Department of Life Science in Dentistry, School of Dentistry, Pusan National University, Yangsan 50612, Korea; dhtnwjd26@naver.com (S.-J.O.); anjs08@naver.com (J.-S.A.); bubu3935@naver.com (Y.Y.S.)
2 Dental and Life Science Institute, Pusan National University, Yangsan 50612, Korea; amaicat24@naver.com (Y.S.); midnightnyou@naver.com (J.W.Y.)
3 National Research Laboratory for Mitochondrial Signaling, Department of Physiology, College of Medicine, Cardiovascular and Metabolic Disease Center (CMDC), Inje University, Busan 614-735, Korea; estrus74@gmail.com (H.K.K.); phyhanj@inje.ac.kr (J.H.)
4 G.B. Elyakov Pacific Institute of Bioorganic Chemistry, Far-Eastern Branch of the Russian Academy of Science, Vladivostok 690022, Russia; mischenkonp@mail.ru (N.P.M.); fedoreev-s@mail.ru (S.A.F.); stonik@piboc.dvo.ru (V.A.S.)
* Correspondence: hskimcell@pusan.ac.kr; Tel.: +82-51-510-8231
† These authors contributed equally to this work.

Received: 31 August 2019; Accepted: 26 October 2019; Published: 31 October 2019

Abstract: Echinochrome A (Ech A), a natural pigment extracted from sea urchins, is the active ingredient of a marine-derived pharmaceutical called 'histochrome'. Since it exhibits several biological activities including anti-oxidative and anti-inflammatory effects, it has been applied to the management of cardiac injury and ocular degenerative disorders in Russia and its protective role has been studied for other pathologic conditions. In the present study, we sought to investigate the therapeutic potential of Ech A for inflammatory bowel disease (IBD) using a murine model of experimental colitis. We found that intravenous injection of Ech A significantly prevented body weight loss and subsequent lethality in colitis-induced mice. Interestingly, T cell proliferation was significantly inhibited upon Ech A treatment in vitro. During the helper T (Th) cell differentiation process, Ech A stimulated the generation regulatory T (Treg) cells that modulate the inflammatory response and immune homeostasis. Moreover, Ech A treatment suppressed the in vitro activation of pro-inflammatory M1 type macrophages, while inducing the production of M2 type macrophages that promote the resolution of inflammation and initiate tissue repair. Based on these results, we suggest that Ech A could provide a beneficial impact on IBD by correcting the imbalance in the intestinal immune system.

Keywords: echinochrome A; marine drugs; inflammatory bowel disease; regulatory T cells; macrophages

1. Introduction

Echinochrome A (Ech A) is a dark red pigment separated from sea urchin shell and spine and has a chemical structure of 6-ethyl-2,3,5,7,8-pentahydroxy-1,4-naphthoquinone [1,2]. As a main active component of a commercial therapeutic agent called 'histochrome', Ech A has been used for the treatment of cardiovascular disorders and ophthalmopathic complications in Russia [3–5]. Among the several biological benefits of Ech A, anti-oxidant and anti-inflammatory capacity is proposed as a major underlying therapeutic mechanism. Indeed, Ech A has been shown to attenuate the oxidative stress caused by reactive oxygen species (ROS) and cardiac toxic drugs, providing mitochondrial protection of cardiomyocyte [6]. Park et al. have reported similar observations showing that Ech A reduced both cellular and mitochondrial ROS levels of patient-derived cardiac progenitors during the oxidative stress situation [7]. The anti-oxidative and anti-viral activity of Ech A has also been proved in vitro using a tick-borne encephalitis virus and herpes simplex virus type 1-infected cell models [8]. The therapeutic potential of Ech A was also evaluated in an experimental gastric ulcer model where Ech A provided anti-ulcerogenic effects by increasing endogenous enzymatic and non-enzymatic antioxidant levels in vivo [9]. In another study, Ech A treatment could reduce ROS production and pro-inflammatory tumor necrosis factor-α (TNF-α) secretion in a rat model of acute uveitis induced by lipopolysaccharide injection [10]. These previous findings imply that Ech A could exert a wide range of therapeutic impacts on other oxidative stress-related and inflammatory pathologic conditions; however, the cell-type specific regulation of Ech A on the immune system, which consists of various innate and adaptive immune cells, has not been elucidated yet.

Inflammatory bowel disease (IBD) is an intractable, chronic inflammatory disease of the digestive tract and Crohn's disease (CD) and ulcerative colitis (UC) are the major types of IBD [11,12]. The etiology and pathogenic mechanisms of IBD remain largely unknown and both environmental factors and genetic factors combined with immunological dysfunction seem to drive IBD development. To attenuate the excessive immune response, advanced immunotherapy using immune-modulators such as inflammatory cytokine blockers has been used recently; however, the presence of non-responder and uncontrolled side effects are the common challenging issues when using immunotherapy [13,14]. Therefore, there has been an unmet need to develop novel therapeutics for the effective management of IBD.

In this study, we investigated whether Ech A could exhibit a protective role in IBD progression using a chemical colitogen dextran sodium sulfate (DSS)-induced colitis mice model. To explore the therapeutic mechanism of Ech A, we also performed in vitro proliferation and polarization experiments with two major innate and adaptive immune cells, macrophage and $CD4^+$ helper T cells (Th cells), respectively. Our in vivo findings suggest that Ech A could attenuate the clinical signs, as well as histological improvement, for the first time in a colitis model which represents IBD. More importantly, in vitro results demonstrate that the anti-inflammatory function of Ech A is manifested by, in part, inducing immunomodulatory effector cells, such as M2 macrophages and Treg cells.

2. Results and Discussion

2.1. *Ech A Treatment Exerted a Protective Effect against DSS-Induced Colitis In Vivo*

To evaluate the therapeutic effects of Ech A on IBD, we gave a single intravenous (i.v) injection of Ech A or vehicle to DSS-induced colitis mice at day 1 and monitored the survival rate, body weight and disease activity index for 12 days. We found that a high dose (10 mg/kg; E10) of Ech A could significantly reduce body weight loss and increase the survival rate of colitis affected mice when compared with vehicle (+) and a low dose of Ech A (1 mg/kg; E1) treated groups (Figure 1A). According to the disease activity index score, clinical symptoms were also improved by Ech A treatment in a dose-dependent manner (Figure 1B). In the gross examination of the large intestine, pathologic shortening of the colon length due to colitis was reversed by the administration of Ech A (Figure 1C). H&E staining-based histopathological analysis revealed that typical pathologic signs of the colitis-affected damaged colon such as loss of epithelial structure and irregular morphology of crypts were ameliorated upon the administration of 10 mg/kg Ech A (Figure 1D). In addition, we found that excessive accumulation of immune cells within the epithelial and mesenchymal layer of the damaged colon was prevented upon Ech A treatment, suggesting that Ech A could exhibit anti-inflammatory roles in the in vivo mouse model (Figure 1D). Therefore, we concluded that Ech A could alleviate disease symptoms and play protective roles in DSS-induced colitis mice.

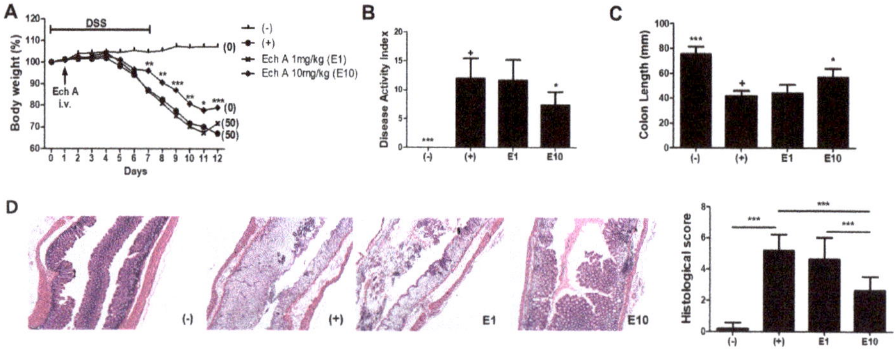

Figure 1. Echinochrome A (Ech A) administration provided therapeutic effects on DSS-induced colitis mice in a dose-dependent manner. (**A**) Body weight and survival rate monitoring results are shown. The body weight at day 0 considered was as 100%. Numbers in parentheses represent the percentage of dead mice. (**B**) Disease activity index score for colitis severity at day 12 was significantly reduced in the E10 group. (**C**) Colon length measurement results showing the protective role of Ech A against DSS-induced colonic damage. (**D**) The histopathological score of the colitis-affected and normal colon was evaluated with H&E stained tissue section. In total, six animals per group were used. Results are shown as mean ± SD. In (**B**) and (**C**), p-value significance was calculated by comparing other groups against the (+) group (marked as +). * $P < 0.05$, ** $P < 0.01$, *** $P < 0.001$.

2.2. Ech A Suppressed the Proliferation of Human MNCs and T Lymphocytes In Vitro

Based on the fact that excessive activation of the intestinal mucosal immune system triggered by increased epithelial permeability leads to aggravation of IBD progression [15,16], we next investigated whether Ech A could regulate the proliferation, differentiation and activation of various immune cells in vitro to explore the underlying therapeutic mechanisms of Ech A on the colitis model. First, we performed a mixed lymphocyte reaction (MLR) to evaluate the effect of Ech A on the expansion of human mononuclear cells (MNCs) and T lymphocytes. To stimulate in vitro proliferation, MNCs were treated with a non-specific mitogen concanavalin A (Con A) and cell proliferation capacity was evaluated using flow cytometry at day 5. Interestingly, the proliferation of Con A-treated MNCs was inhibited upon Ech A administration in a dose-dependent manner (Figure 2A,B). The percentage of proliferating cells in the control group was 60.4%, while it decreased to 49.3% and 37% upon 5 μM and 10 μM of Ech A treatment, respectively. Similarly, Ech A reduced the proliferation rate of CD3/CD28-stimulated T cells when compared with vehicle-treated samples (VC group: 72.2%; 5 μM Ech A group: 63.6%; 10 μM Ech A group: 54.9%) (Figure 2C,D), implying that Ech A could regulate immune cell proliferation in vitro.

2.3. Ech A Induced the Generation of Regulatory T Cells In Vitro

It is well known that naive Th (Th0) cells can differentiate into various subtypes of active Th cells such as Th1, Th2 and Treg cells upon specific cues and each type of mature Th cell plays a distinct and pivotal role in various disease developments including IBD [17,18]. Therefore, next we isolated $CD4^+$ naive Th0 cells from human cord blood then performed a differentiation experiment following the typical procedure with or without Ech A to evaluate the impact of Ech A on Th cell polarization. As shown in Figure 3, flow cytometry analysis on cell surface markers revealed that Ech A provided no significant impact on Th1/2 polarization in vitro (Figure 3A,B). On the other hand, Ech A treatment could stimulate the generation of Treg cells; indeed, approximately 10% of total Ech A-treated cells expressed the marker of the Treg cell marker Foxp3, while the spontaneous induction ratio of Treg cells were less than 1% on average (Figure 3C).

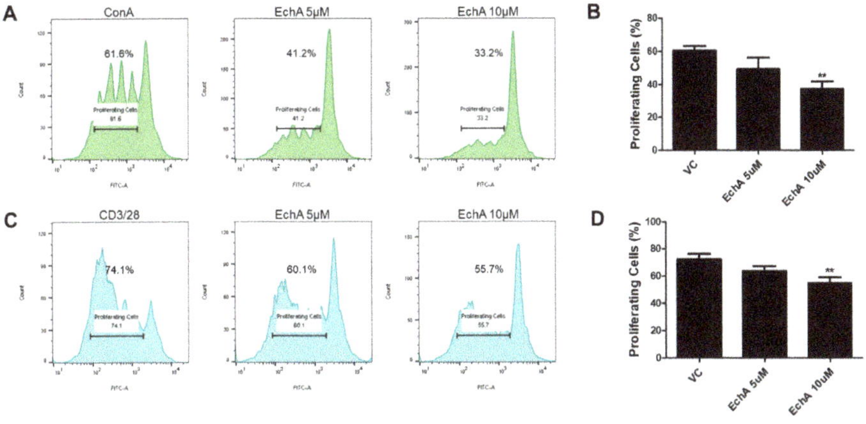

Figure 2. Ech A impact on mixed lymphocyte reaction (MLR) in vitro. CFSE-labeled human mononuclear cells (MNCs) were cultured for five days in the presence of mitogen or antibodies for CD3/28 with or without Ech A treatment, then the percentage of proliferated cells was evaluated using flow cytometry. The proliferation of both MNCs (**A**,**B**) and T cells (**C**,**D**) was reduced by Ech A treatment in a dose-dependent manner. VC, vehicle-treated control. ** $P < 0.01$. Results are shown as mean ± SD.

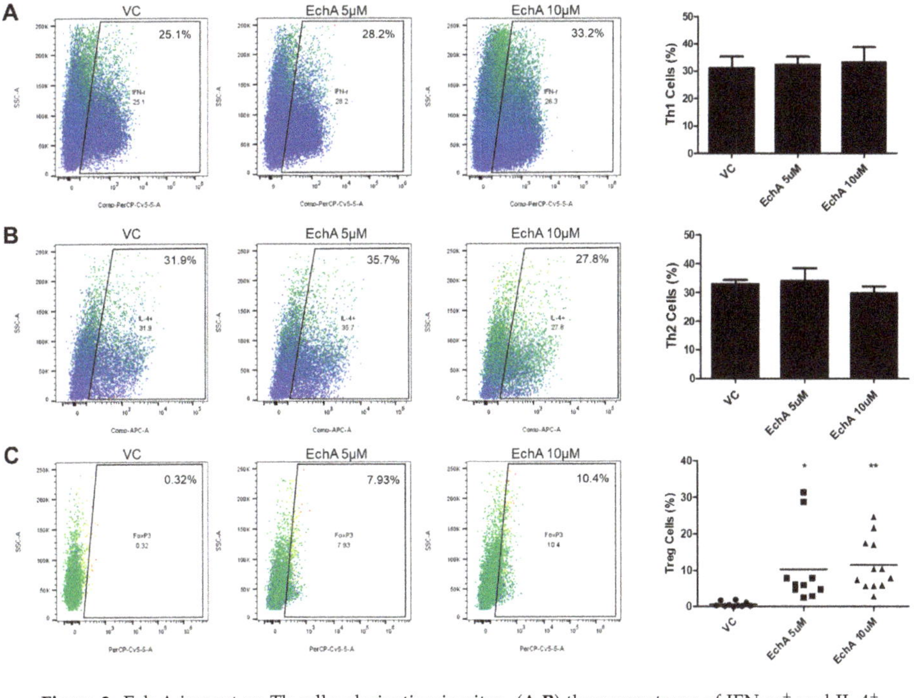

Figure 3. Ech A impact on Th cell polarization in vitro. (**A**,**B**) the percentages of IFN-γ $^{+}$ and IL-4^{+} cells among CD4^{+} Th cells were evaluated using flow cytometry to determine the induction ratio of Th1 and Th2 cells, respectively. No significant change was observed upon Ech A treatment. (**C**) Spontaneous generation of Foxp3^{+} Treg cells among CD4^{+} Th cells upon vehicle and Ech A treatment was assessed using flow cytometry. Ech A treatment led to an increase in Treg population compared to the vehicle-treated group. VC, vehicle-treated control. * $P < 0.05$, ** $P < 0.001$. Results are shown as mean ± SD.

2.4. Ech A Could Modulate the Polarization of Resting Macrophages into M1 and M2 Type In Vitro

As a key component of the innate immune system, macrophages play important roles in the host defense reaction by mediating acute inflammatory response against danger signals and promoting stimulation of the adaptive immune system [19]. Typically, two main subtypes of macrophages have been described after polarization: Classically activated M1 type (M1) and alternative M2 type (M2) [20]. In general, M1 macrophages tend to mediate the excessive and persistent pro-inflammatory responses, while M2 macrophages are known to contribute to tissue regeneration and resolution of inflammation. Given that chronic inflammation with the M1/M2 polarization balance skewed toward the M1 phenotype is the major characteristic of IBD progression [21,22], modulation of macrophage activity could be another therapeutic target. Thus, we conducted an in vitro experiment to evaluate the influence of Ech A on M1/M2 differentiation. For M1 type polarization, phorbol 12-myristate-13-acetate (PMA)-treated THP1 macrophages were further stimulated with LPS and IFN-γ. As expected, M1 macrophages produced a high level of tumor necrosis factor-alpha (TNF-α) upon stimulation (Figure 4A). It was noted that Ech A could reduce M1-derived TNF-α secretion in a dose-dependent manner (Figure 4A). On the contrary, the basal secretion level of interleukin 10 (IL-10) was increased in the presence of Ech A, indicating that Ech A could induce the spontaneous M2 polarization in vitro (Figure 4B).

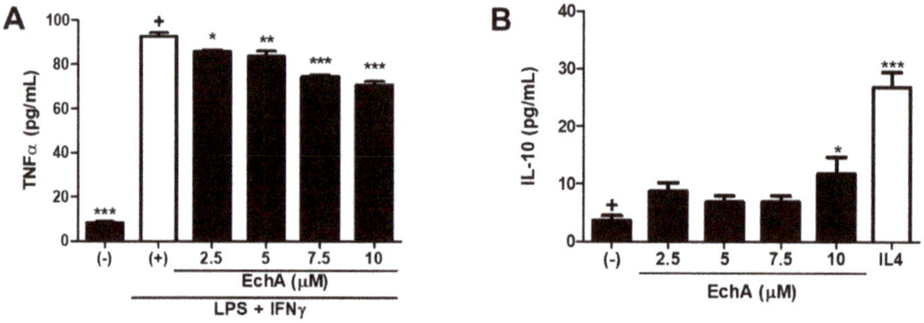

Figure 4. Ech A impact on M1/M2 macrophage polarization in vitro. (**A**) After five days of M1 induction, TNF-α concentration in the culture supernatant was measured by ELISA to estimate the M1 polarization efficiency. It is noted that Ech A prevented M1 polarization in vitro in a dose-dependent manner. (**B**) The IL-10 secretion level was determined using ELISA to evaluate the spontaneous M2 induction efficiency. Ech A treated macrophages were differentiated into M2 macrophages more effectively compared to vehicle-treated cells; (–), no induction control; (+), polarization induced control. The p-value significance was calculated by comparing other groups against the (+) and (–) groups (marked as +) in A and B, respectively. * $P < 0.05$, ** $P < 0.01$, *** $P < 0.001$. Results are shown as mean ± SD.

From the in vivo observation, Ech A provided significant protection against experimental colitis as it alleviated disease severity and increased the survival rate of mice. In the histomorphological analysis of the colon, marked loss of villus-crypt structure accompanied with edematous erosion and granulation tissue formation was attenuated by Ech A injection. Ech A also decreased the degree of inflammatory cell infiltrates in a dose-dependent manner, suggesting that Ech A could exhibit an anti-inflammatory capacity in the IBD status.

Importantly, following in vitro Th cell differentiation, the experiment revealed that Ech A treatment could promote Treg generation without affecting the Th1 or Th2 populations. Considering that Treg cells function as a key immunomodulator that regulates activation of other Th cells, Ech A could contribute to correct the immunological imbalance in vivo by inducing the Treg population, although it does not directly regulate Th1 or Th2 polarization. Indeed, Tsai et al. have reported that a member of the lectin family galectin-3 prevents colitis progression while galectin-3 knockout mice suffered from more severe symptoms than controls, and the therapeutic impact of galectin-3 was abrogated by CD25 neutralization, implying the importance of Treg cells in this context [23]. Here we also demonstrated that Ech A could regulate the direction of macrophagic polarization toward M2 differentiation. M1 suppression and/or M2 induction strategies have proven beneficial for IBD treatment. Abron et al. have reported that the soy bean-derived natural agent genistein reduced the severity of DSS-induced colitis by transforming M1 macrophages into M2 type followed by the reduction of pro-inflammatory cytokine levels [24]. In addition, adipose-tissue-derived mesenchymal stem cells could provide protection in colitis mice models via TNF-α-induced gene/protein 6-mediated M2 induction [25]. In particular, the TNF-α inhibitory effect of Ech A could be directly applicable for IBD therapeutics considering that TNF-α expressing immune cells are increased in the intestinal tract of IBD patients and TNF-α blockers, as well as anti-TNF-α agents, have been approved in clinic for IBD treatment [26].

To further highlight the benefits of Ech A application, the underlying mechanisms of Ech A mediated immune cell fate regulation should be explored for the fundamental understanding of the Ech A therapeutic function. According to a recent study, Ech A could stimulate ex vivo expansion of $CD34^+$ hematopoietic stem/progenitor cells (HSPC) with enhanced colony-forming capacity via suppression of intracellular ROS generation [27]. Mechanistically, ex vivo treatment of Ech A or anti-oxidant agent N-acetyl cysteine could not only inhibit oxidative stress-associated P38 MAPK activation but also increase Lyn/Src phosphorylation followed by activation of the PI3K-Akt signaling pathway, leading to high-quality HSPC expansion. Therefore, it would be worthwhile to investigate the therapeutic contribution of the anti-oxidative capacity of Ech A in IBD prevention in terms of HSPC-derived immune cell proliferation and differentiation. In addition, Ech A could bind directly to protein kinase C-iota (PKC i) and enhanced myocardial cell differentiation of mouse embryonic stem cells by antagonizing its activity [28]. Considering that the PKC family plays an important role in Th cell homeostasis [29,30], Ech A might regulate PKC activity to induce Treg population followed by M2 macrophagic activation.

In conclusion, we demonstrate the therapeutic potential of Ech A for IBD for the first time. We also emphasize that Ech A could induce immunomodulatory effector cell generation such as Treg cells and M2 macrophages along with suppression of pro-inflammatory M1 macrophage, leading to attenuation of excessive inflammation. These data suggest that Ech A could exert immune-cell type specific regulatory roles in vitro and possibly in vivo. Therefore, our findings not only suggest Ech A as a novel potent therapeutic agent for incurable IBD but also contribute to expanding the therapeutic utility of Ech A for various inflammatory diseases.

3. Materials and Methods

3.1. DSS-Induced Experimental Colitis Mice Modeling and Monitoring

All experiments were approved by and followed the regulations of the Institute of Laboratory Animals Resources (PNU-2018-2034, Pusan National University). Experimental colitis was induced in mice by the addition of 3% (wt/vol) DSS (MP Biochemicals, Solon, OH, USA) in drinking water for 7 days as previously described [31]. Four groups were designed as positive (DSS, n = 6) or negative (no DSS, n = 6) controls and a low-dose (1 mg/kg, n = 6) and a high dose (10 mg/kg, n = 6) of Ech A treated group. Ech A was administrated at day 1 via i.v injection, while a vehicle (0.1% DMSO in PBS) was given to negative control mice instead. Total 12 day-long daily monitoring for body weight and survival rate was conducted. On day 12, the disease activity index of surviving animals was scored by assessing stool consistency, rectal bleeding and coat roughness (grade from 0 to 4), general activity and bedding contamination with stool and blood (graded from 0 to 2). All subjects were then sacrificed for the evaluation of gross pathologic severity (measuring colon length) and further histological analysis using H&E staining.

3.2. *Mixed Leukocyte Reaction*

For MLR, human MNCs were labeled using the CellTrace CFSE cell labeling kit (Invitrogen, Grand Island, NY, USA) following the manufacturer's instructions. Cells were then seeded in a 6-well plate at a density of 5×10^4 /well and cultured in RPMI 1640 (Gibco, Grand Island, NY, USA) with supplement of 10% FBS (Gibco) and 100 U/mL penicillin/streptomycin (Gibco) in the presence of Con A (5 μg/mL for MNC proliferation) (Sigma, St. Lois, MO, USA) or anti-CD3/anti-CD28 (5 μg/mL and 2 μg/mL, respectively, for T cell proliferation) (eBioscience, San Diego, CA, USA) for 5 days. To assess the Ech A impact on cell proliferation, Ech A or vehicle was also treated during the culture period. After 5 days, cells were harvested and prepared for flow cytometry analysis.

3.3. *Isolation and Culture of Human CD4⁺ Naïve Th (Th0) Cells*

This study was approved by the Institutional Review Board of Pusan National University (II-1802-006-063). MNCs were isolated from human cord blood provided by Busan/Ulsan/Gyeongnam Cord Blood Bank using HetaSep (Stem Cell Technologies, British Columbia, Canada) and Lymphoprep (Stem Cell Technologies) as per the manufacturer's instructions. Total naive Th0 cells were then purified by negative selection with magnetic beads provided in the Human Naive $CD4^+$ T Cell Isolation Kit II (Miltenyi Biotec, Bergisch Gladbach, Germany). Purified cells were determined for their purity (more than 95% $CD4^+$ cells) and then plated in the density of 1×10^6 cells/well in a 12-well culture plate and cultured in expansion media consisting of the ImmunoCult-XF T Cell Expansion Medium (Stem Cell Technologies), ImmunoCult Human CD3/CD28/CD2 T Cell Activator (Stem Cell Technologies) and IL-2 (Peprotech, Rocky Hill, NJ, USA).

3.4. *Th1, Th2 and Treg Cell Differentiation*

For Th1 polarization, purified $CD4^+$ Th0 cells were cultured in expansion media supplemented with IL-12 (10 ng/mL) (Peprotech) and anti-IL-4 neutralizing antibodies (5 μg/mL) (BD Bioscience, San Jose, CA, USA) for 5 days. For Th2 induction, purified $CD4^+$ Th0 cells were cultured in expansion media with IL-4 (20 ng/mL) (Peprotech) and anti-IFN-γ neutralizing antibodies (5 μg/mL) (BioxCell, West Lebanon, NH, USA) for 5 days. To evaluate the spontaneous induction ratio of Treg cells, purified $CD4^+$ Th0 cells were cultured in expansion media for 5 days without any lineage-specific stimulants. To assess the Ech A impact on Th cell polarization, Ech A or vehicle was also treated during the culture period.

3.5. *Flow Cytometry Analysis*

To stimulate the production of lineage-specific markers, differentiated Th cells were treated with 50 ng/mL of PMA (Sigma) and 1 μM of Ionomycin (Sigma) with transport inhibitor GolgiStop (BD Biosciences) for 4 h. Cells were washed with PBS 4 times then incubated with FITC conjugated anti-human CD4 (BD Bioscience) at 4 °C for 30 min in the dark. After surface marker staining, cells were fixed and permeabilized using fixation and permeabilization buffer (BD Bioscience) then further stained with PerCP-Cy5.5-conjugated anti-human IFN-γ (BD Bioscience), APC-conjugated anti-human IL-4 (BD Bioscience), and PerCP-Cy5.5-conjugated anti-human FoxP3 (BD Bioscience) at 4 °C for 30 min in the dark. Nonspecific isotype-matched antibodies served as controls. Samples were analyzed with the BD FACS Verse flow cytometer (BD Biosciences) and data analysis was performed using FlowJo software.

3.6. *Macrophage Polarization*

THP1 cells were maintained in RPMI 1640 (Gibco, Grand Island, NY, USA) with a supplement of 10% FBS (Gibco) and 100 U/mL penicillin/streptomycin (Gibco). To induce monocytic differentiation, THP1 cells were plated at a density of 4×10^5 /well on 6-well culture plate and pre-treated with PMA (Sigma) for 48 h. After PMA treatment, cells were stabilized for another 24 h in the maintenance media. Macrophages were then polarized in M1 macrophages by incubation with 20 ng/mL of IFN-γ (Peprotech) and 10 μg/mL of LPS (Sigma) for 5 days. PMA-pretreated cells were cultured within the maintenance media for 5 days without any lineage-specific stimulants for the spontaneous polarization towards M2 macrophages. To assess the Ech A impact on macrophage polarization, Ech A or vehicle was also treated during the culture period. Five days later, the culture supernatant was collected and secreted cytokine levels were estimated using human TNF-α and the IL-10 Duoset ELISA kit (R&D system, Abingdon, UK).

3.7. Data Analysis

At least three individual experiments were conducted for in vitro experiments. Data are presented as mean ± standard error of the mean (SEM). All of the statistical comparisons were performed using one-way ANOVA followed by a Bonferroni post hoc test for multigroup comparisons using GraphPad Prism software (GraphPad Software, San Diego, CA, USA); p-values under 0.05 was considered statistically significant.

Author Contributions: Conceptualization; Y.S. and H.-S.K.; Methodology and data analysis, S.-J.O., Y.S., J.-S.A., Y.Y.S. and J.W.Y.; Providing material and supporting experiments, N.P.M., E.A.V., and S.A.F.; Writing-original draft preparation, S.-J.O. and Y.S.; Writing-review and editing, H.K.K., J.H., V.A.S. and H.-S.K.

Funding: This research was supported by the National Research Foundation of Korea (NRF) grant funded by the Korea government (MSIT) (No. NRF-2018R1A5A2023879 and NRF-2017R1E1A1A01074316) and partially supported by a clinical research grant from Pusan National University Hospital in 2018.

Conflicts of Interest: The authors declare no conflict of interest.

References

1. Lebedev, A.V.; Ivanova, M.V.; Levitsky, D.O. Echinochrome, a naturally occurring iron chelator and free radical scavenger in artificial and natural membrane systems. *Life Sci.* **2005**, *76*, 863–875. [CrossRef] [PubMed]
2. Lebedev, A.V.; Ivanova, M.V.; Levitsky, D.O. Iron chelators and free radical scavengers in naturally occurring polyhydroxylated 1,4-naphthoquinones. *Hemoglobin* **2008**, *32*, 165–179. [CrossRef] [PubMed]
3. Buimov, G.A.; Maksimov, I.V.; Perchatkin, V.A.; Repin, A.N.; Afanas'ev, S.A.; Markov, V.A.; Karpov, R.S. Effect of the bioantioxidant histochrome on myocardial injury in reperfusion therapy on patients with myocardial infarction. *Ter. Arkh.* **2002**, *74*, 12–16. [PubMed]
4. Zakirova, A.N.; Ivanova, M.V.; Golubiatnikov, V.B.; Mishchenko, N.P.; Kol'tsova, E.A.; Fedoreev, S.A.; Krasnovid, N.I.; Lebedev, A.V. Pharmacokinetics and clinical efficacy of histochrome in patients with acute myocardial infarction. *Eksp. Klin. Farmakol.* **1997**, *60*, 21–24.
5. Egorov, E.A.; Alekhina, V.A.; Volobueva, T.M.; Fedoreev, S.A.; Mishchenko, N.P.; Kol'tsova, E.A. Histochrome, a new antioxidant, in the treatment of ocular diseases. *Vestn. Oftalmol.* **1999**, *115*, 34–35.
6. Jeong, S.H.; Kim, H.K.; Song, I.S.; Lee, S.J.; Ko, K.S.; Rhee, B.D.; Kim, N.; Mishchenko, N.P.; Fedoryev, S.A.; Stonik, V.A.; et al. Echinochrome a protects mitochondrial function in cardiomyocytes against cardiotoxic drugs. *Mar. Drugs* **2014**, *12*, 2922–2936. [CrossRef]
7. Park, J.H.; Lee, N.K.; Lim, H.J.; Mazumder, S.; Kumar Rethineswaran, V.; Kim, Y.J.; Jang, W.B.; Ji, S.T.; Kang, S.; Kim, D.Y.; et al. Therapeutic cell protective role of histochrome under oxidative stress in human cardiac progenitor cells. *Mar. Drugs* **2019**, *17*, 6. [CrossRef]
8. Fedoreyev, S.A.; Krylova, N.V.; Mishchenko, N.P.; Vasileva, E.A.; Pislyagin, E.A.; Iunikhina, O.V.; Lavrov, V.F.; Svitich, O.A.; Ebralidze, L.K.; Leonova, G.N. Antiviral and Antioxidant Properties of Echinochrome A. *Mar. Drugs* **2018**, *16*, 12. [CrossRef]
9. Sayed, D.A.; Soliman, A.M.; Fahmy, S.R. Echinochrome pigment as novel therapeutic agent against experimentally-induced gastric ulcer in rats. *Biomed. Pharmacother.* **2018**, *107*, 90–95. [CrossRef]
10. Lennikov, A.; Kitaichi, N.; Noda, K.; Mizuuchi, K.; Ando, R.; Dong, Z.; Fukuhara, J.; Kinoshita, S.; Namba, K.; Ohno, S.; et al. Amelioration of endotoxin-induced uveitis treated with the sea urchin pigment echinochrome in rats. *Mol. Vis.* **2014**, *20*, 171–177.

11. Baumgart, D.C.; Carding, S.R. Inflammatory bowel disease: Cause and immunobiology. *Lancet* **2007**, *369*, 1627–1640. [CrossRef]
12. Zhang, Y.Z.; Li, Y.Y. Inflammatory bowel disease: Pathogenesis. *World J. Gastroenterol.* **2014**, *20*, 91–99. [CrossRef] [PubMed]
13. Neurath, M.F. Current and emerging therapeutic targets for IBD. *Nat. Rev. Gastroenterol. Hepatol.* **2017**, *14*, 269–278. [CrossRef] [PubMed]
14. Yarur, A.J.; Abreu, M.T.; Deshpande, A.R.; Kerman, D.H.; Sussman, D.A. Therapeutic drug monitoring in patients with inflammatory bowel disease. *World J. Gastroenterol.* **2014**, *20*, 3475–3484. [CrossRef]
15. Xu, X.R.; Liu, C.Q.; Feng, B.S.; Liu, Z.J. Dysregulation of mucosal immune response in pathogenesis of inflammatory bowel disease. *World J. Gastroenterol.* **2014**, *20*, 3255–3264. [CrossRef]
16. Wallace, K.L.; Zheng, L.B.; Kanazawa, Y.; Shih, D.Q. Immunopathology of inflammatory bowel disease. *World J. Gastroenterol.* **2014**, *20*, 6–21. [CrossRef]
17. Imam, T.; Park, S.; Kaplan, M.H.; Olson, M.R. Effector T Helper Cell Subsets in Inflammatory Bowel Diseases. *Front. Immunol.* **2018**, *9*, 1212. [CrossRef]
18. Chen, M.L.; Sundrud, M.S. Cytokine networks and T-cell subsets in inflammatory bowel diseases. *Inflamm. Bowel Dis.* **2016**, *22*, 1157–1167. [CrossRef]
19. Shapouri-Moghaddam, A.; Mohammadian, S.; Vazini, H.; Taghadosi, M.; Esmaeili, S.A.; Mardani, F.; Seifi, B.; Mohammadi, A.; Afshari, J.T.; Sahebkar, A. Macrophage plasticity, polarization, and function in health and disease. *J. Cell. Physiol.* **2018**, *233*, 6425–6440. [CrossRef]
20. Murray, P.J.; Wynn, T.A. Protective and pathogenic functions of macrophage subsets. *Nat. Rev. Immunol.* **2011**, *11*, 723–737. [CrossRef]
21. Zhou, X.; Li, W.; Wang, S.; Zhang, P.; Wang, Q.; Xiao, J.; Zhang, C.; Zheng, X.; Xu, X.; Xue, S.; et al. YAP aggravates inflammatory bowel disease by regulating M1/M2 macrophage polarization and gut microbial homeostasis. *Cell Rep.* **2019**, *27*, 1176–1189.e5. [CrossRef] [PubMed]
22. Zhu, W.; Yu, J.; Nie, Y.; Shi, X.; Liu, Y.; Li, F.; Zhang, X.L. Disequilibrium of M1 and M2 macrophages correlates with the development of experimental inflammatory bowel diseases. *Immunol. Investig.* **2014**, *43*, 638–652. [CrossRef] [PubMed]
23. Tsai, H.F.; Wu, C.S.; Chen, Y.L.; Liao, H.J.; Chyuan, I.T.; Hsu, P.N. Galectin-3 suppresses mucosal inflammation and reduces disease severity in experimental colitis. *J. Mol. Med. (Berl.)* **2016**, *94*, 545–556. [CrossRef] [PubMed]
24. Abron, J.D.; Singh, N.P.; Price, R.L.; Nagarkatti, M.; Nagarkatti, P.S.; Singh, U.P. Genistein induces macrophage polarization and systemic cytokine to ameliorate experimental colitis. *PLoS ONE* **2018**, *13*, e0199631. [CrossRef] [PubMed]
25. Song, W.J.; Li, Q.; Ryu, M.O.; Ahn, J.O.; Ha Bhang, D.; Chan Jung, Y.; Youn, H.Y. TSG-6 secreted by human adipose tissue-derived mesenchymal stem cells ameliorates DSS-induced colitis by inducing M2 macrophage polarization in mice. *Sci. Rep.* **2017**, *7*, 5187. [CrossRef]
26. Berns, M.; Hommes, D.W. Anti-TNF-alpha therapies for the treatment of Crohn's disease: The past, present and future. *Expert Opin. Investig. Drugs* **2016**, *25*, 129–143. [CrossRef]
27. Park, G.B.; Kim, M.J.; Vasileva, E.A.; Mishchenko, N.P.; Fedoreyev, S.A.; Stonik, V.A.; Han, J.; Lee, H.S.; Kim, D.; Jeong, J.Y. Echinochrome a promotes ex vivo expansion of peripheral blood-derived CD34(+) cells, potentially through downregulation of ROS production and activation of the Src-Lyn-p110delta pathway. *Mar. Drugs* **2019**, *17*, 9. [CrossRef]
28. Kim, H.K.; Cho, S.W.; Heo, H.J.; Jeong, S.H.; Kim, M.; Ko, K.S.; Rhee, B.D.; Mishchenko, N.P.; Vasileva, E.A.; Fedoreyev, S.A.; et al. A novel atypical PKC-iota inhibitor, echinochrome a, enhances cardiomyocyte differentiation from mouse embryonic stem cells. *Mar. Drugs* **2018**, *16*, 6. [CrossRef]
29. Brezar, V.; Tu, W.J.; Seddiki, N. PKC-theta in regulatory and effector T-cell functions. *Front. Immunol.* **2015**, *6*, 530. [CrossRef]

30. Genot, E.M.; Parker, P.J.; Cantrell, D.A. Analysis of the role of protein kinase C-alpha, -epsilon, and -zeta in T cell activation. *J. Biol. Chem.* **1995**, *270*, 9833–9839. [CrossRef]
31. Kim, H.S.; Shin, T.H.; Lee, B.C.; Yu, K.R.; Seo, Y.; Lee, S.; Seo, M.S.; Hong, I.S.; Choi, S.W.; Seo, K.W.; et al. Human umbilical cord blood mesenchymal stem cells reduce colitis in mice by activating NOD2 signaling to COX2. *Gastroenterology* **2013**, *145*, 1392–1403.e1-8. [CrossRef] [PubMed]

marine drugs

MDPI

Article

Antiviral and Antioxidant Properties of Echinochrome A

Sergey A. Fedoreyev [1,*], Natalia V. Krylova [2], Natalia P. Mishchenko [1], Elena A. Vasileva [1], Evgeny A. Pislyagin [1], Olga V. Iunikhina [2], Vyacheslav F. Lavrov [3], Oksana A. Svitich [3], Linna K. Ebralidze [3] and Galina N. Leonova [2]

1 G.B. Elyakov Pacific Institute of Bioorganic Chemistry, FEB RAS, Vladivostok 690022, Russia; mischenkonp@mail.ru (N.P.M.); vasilieva_el_an@mail.ru (E.A.V.); pislyagin@hotmail.com (E.A.P.)
2 G.P. Somov Institute of Epidemiology and Microbiology, FEB RAS, Vladivostok 690087, Russia; krylovanatalya@gmail.com (N.V.K.); olga_iun@inbox.ru (O.V.I.); galinaleon41@gmail.com (G.N.L.)
3 I.I. Mechnikov Research Institute of Vaccines and Sera, Moscow 105064, Russia; v.f.lavrov@inbox.ru (V.F.L.); svitichoa@yandex.ru (O.A.S.); lina.lidze@gmail.com (L.K.E.)
* Correspondence: fedoreev-s@mail.ru; Tel.: +7-914-651-2679

Received: 2 November 2018; Accepted: 12 December 2018; Published: 15 December 2018

Abstract: The aim of this study was to examine the in vitro antioxidant and antiviral activities of echinochrome A and echinochrome-based antioxidant composition against tick-borne encephalitis virus (TBEV) and herpes simplex virus type 1 (HSV-1). The antioxidant composition, which is a mixture of echinochrome A, ascorbic acid, and α-tocopherol (5:5:1), showed higher antioxidant and antiviral effects than echinochrome A. We suppose that echinochrome A and its composition can both directly affect virus particles and indirectly enhance antioxidant defense mechanisms in the hosting cell. The obtained results allow considering the echinochrome A and the composition of antioxidants on its basis as the promising agents with the both antioxidant and antiviral activities.

Keywords: echinochrome A; composition of antioxidants; antioxidant activity; antiviral activity

1. Introduction

Oxidative stress, arising through production of free radicals including reactive oxygen species (ROS), is usually defined as a disturbance in the balance between the level of ROS and antioxidant defenses [1]. Viral infections, along with other numerous human diseases, are accompanied by oxidative stress, which plays an important role in their pathogenesis [2,3]. Oxidative processes promote virus replication in infected cells, decrease cell proliferation, and induce cell apoptosis [4]. Intensification of the processes of free radical lipid oxidation and the sharp suppression of the antioxidant and antiradical protection system of the body are observed in patients with neurotropic virus infections such as tick-borne encephalitis [5] and herpes simplex [6,7]. Central nervous system tissues are especially sensitive to lipid peroxidation due to their high lipid content [8]. The lipid peroxides resulting from the ROS-induced peroxidation of membrane phospholipids, such as malondialdehyde, can transverse the circulation and cell membranes, with the resultant dysfunction of vital cellular processes such as membrane transport and mitochondrial respiration [9].

Antioxidants with different mechanisms of action are used to prevent or treat various diseases that are associated with oxidative stress and possess therapeutic effects in many cases [10–12]. Since the most important aspect of the treatment of viral diseases is the suppression of viral replication followed by cell survival, the search for drugs that have antiviral properties among antioxidants is promising. There are many examples showing that natural antioxidants such as vitamins C and E (ascorbic acid and α-tocopherol, respectively), curcumin, various polyphenols, and others are promising agents for antiviral therapy, since they decrease ROS levels in infected cells, the expression of pro-apoptotic signaling molecules, and modulate the cellular levels of stress-related proteins such as c-Jun N-terminal kinases (JNK), phospho-p38 mitogen-activated protein kinase (MAPK), extracellular signal-regulated kinases (ERK-1/2), and transcription factor NF-kB [13–18].

A well-known natural antioxidant echinochrome A (naphthoquinonoid pigment of sea urchins) is the active substance of the Russian drug Histochrome®, which is used in cardiology for the treatment of ischemic heart disease and myocardial infarction, and in ophthalmology for the treatment of degenerative diseases of the retina and cornea, macular degeneration, primary open-angle glaucoma, and others [19,20].

The aim of this research was to study the in vitro antioxidant and antiviral activities of echinochrome A (Ech) and the compositions based on Ech, including also other antioxidants, against RNA-containing tick-borne encephalitis virus (TBEV) and DNA-containing herpes simplex virus type 1 (HSV-1).

This paper was prepared for printing on the basis of materials presented as a lecture on the Third International Symposium on Life Science, Vladivostok, Russia, September 2018.

2. Results

2.1. Antioxidant Activity of Ech Formulations Alone or Combined with Other Antioxidants

We have compared antioxidant properties of Ech, α-tocopherol (Toc), and ascorbic acid (Asc), as well as their combinations, using the model of linetol peroxidation. The procedure that we applied relates to simple gravimetric methods via the measurement of weight increases following oxygen fixation on fatty acids [21]. Action of the studied substances on linetol was characterized as the induction time of the lipid auto-oxidation reaction ($\Delta\tau$, h-difference between times necessary for linetol oxidation in the presence and absence of an antioxidant). The determination of antioxidant activities made it possible not only to compare the antioxidant activities of the studied substances with each other, but also to find the optimal ratio of antioxidants in the most active compositions. It was established that Toc was the most effective antioxidant in this experiment ($\Delta\tau$ 125 h) (Table 1). Ech was some less effective ($\Delta\tau$ 100 h), while Asc showed no antioxidant effect on this model. The low efficiency of Asc may be explained by its high susceptibility to auto-oxidation in linetol solution. It is known that in experiments in vitro, Asc lacks antioxidant activity in the absence of Toc. This observation was confirmed by our experiments ($\Delta\tau$ of the mixture Asc + Toc (2:1) was 195 h, which is more than effect of Toc itself). A mixture of all three antioxidants (Ech + Asc + Toc) demonstrated a stronger effect on a model of linetol auto-oxidation as a result of the synergy of these compounds ($\Delta\tau$ 223 h) (Table 1). We calculated the effect of synergism (in %) according to Kancheva et al. by the formulas for binary and ternary mixtures of antioxidants [22].

Table 1. Antioxidant activity of the formulations on a model of linetol auto-oxidation. [1]

Antioxidants and their Compositions	$\Delta\tau$, h	The Efficiency of the Composition Compared to Ech
Ech	100 ± 5	-
Asc	24 ± 3	-
Toc	125 ± 7	-
Ech + Asc (1:1)	69 ± 4	No effect
Ech + Toc (1:1)	201 ± 8 *	Synergism 8%
Asc + Toc (2:1)	195 ± 7 *	Synergism 7%
Ech + Asc + Toc (5:5:1)	223 ± 10 **	Synergism 40%
Control-linetol	24 ± 2	

[1] The concentration of Ech, Asc, Toc and their compositions in test medium was of 0.05 mg/mL. * Statistically significant differences between Ech and antioxidant compositions ($p \leq 0.05$); ** statistically significant differences between three-component and two-component mixtures of antioxidants ($p \leq 0.05$). Asc: ascorbic acid, Ech: echinochrome A, Toc: α-tocopherol.

2.2. *Antioxidant Activity of the Formulations Against LPS-Induced ROS Formation in Vero Cells*

To determine whether Ech alone or combined with other antioxidants is able to decrease intracellular ROS level in Vero cells, we used the model of *E. coli* lipopolysaccharide (LPS)-induced ROS formation. The ROS levels in Vero cells treated with LPS increased by 20% in comparison to control–untreated cells (Figure 1). Ech, Ech + Asc + Toc, and Asc + Toc decreased the ROS formation by 61%, 68%, and 50% in Vero cells, correspondingly, in comparison to LPS-treated cells.

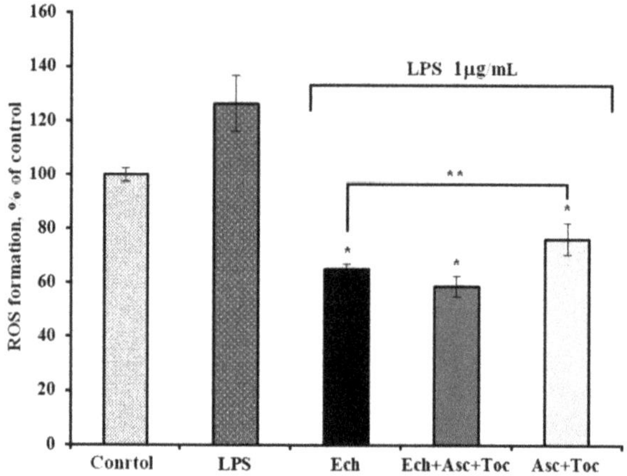

Figure 1. Influence of Ech and studied formulations on the lipopolysaccharide (LPS)-induced reactive oxygen species (ROS) formations in Vero cells. The formulations were tested at a concentration of five µg/mL. * $p < 0.05$; ** statistically significant differences between Asc + Toc and Ech ($p \leq 0.05$).

Ech and its composition with Asc and Toc showed significant antioxidant effects on both experimental models, which makes them promising agents for further investigations on TBEV and HSV-1 replications accompanied by oxidative stress.

2.3. *Cytotoxicity and Antiviral Activity of Formulations.*

Cytotoxicity assay was carried out to determine the concentration range of formulations for the subsequent study of its antiviral activity in the non-toxic range for pig embryo kidney (PK) and Vero cells. Acyclovir and ribavirin were used as standard antivirals for HSV-1 and TBEV, respectively. Based on the obtained methylthiazolyltetrazolium bromide (MTT) assay results, 50% cytotoxic concentrations (CC_{50}) against PK and Vero cells were determined for all of the studied formulations (Table 2). Further antiviral activity assay was performed at the concentrations of the formulations below 400 µg/mL.

Table 2. Cytotoxic and antiviral activities of formulations against tick-borne encephalitis virus (TBEV) and herpes simplex virus type 1 (HSV-1).

Formulation	TBEV			HSV-1		
	CC_{50} (µg/mL)	IC_{50} (µg/mL)	SI	CC_{50} (µg/mL)	IC_{50} (µg/mL)	SI
Ech + Asc + Toc (5:5:1)	57.9 ± 2.3 *	12.6 ± 1.5 **	4.8 ± 0.5 **	66.7 ± 3.2 *	11.2 ± 1.2 **	6.0 ± 0.6 **
Ech	54.4 ± 1.8 *	21.8 ± 2.6 *	2.5 ± 0.2 *	60.5 ± 3.1 *	18.8 ± 2.1 *	3.2 ± 0.3 *
Asc + Toc (5:1)	521.7 ± 5.3	1304 ± 145	0.4 ± 0.1	530.9 ± 9.4	885 ± 97	0.6 ± 0.1
Ribavirin	2010 ± 180	30.5 ± 4.6	66.0 ± 5.4			
Acyclovir				1470 ± 160	10.8 ± 1.2	133.6 ± 12.0

CC_{50}-50% cytotoxic concentration of a formulation, IC_{50}-50% virus-inhibiting concentration of a formulation, SI: selective index of the formulation. * Statistically significant differences between Asc + Toc and other formulation ($p \leq 0.05$), ** statistically significant differences between antioxidant composition and Ech ($p \leq 0.05$).

The anti-TBEV and anti-HSV-1 activity of tested formulations were assessed using cytopathic effect (CPE) inhibition assay. PK and Vero cells infected with the 10-fold dilutions of corresponding virus were simultaneously treated with different concentrations of the formulations. It was found that the formulations inhibited virus-induced CPE in a dose-dependent manner, and values of the 50% inhibitory concentrations (IC_{50}) and selective indices (SI) of the tested formulations for both viruses are presented in the Table 2. Ech and the Ech + Asc + Toc composition revealed moderate antiviral activities against TBEV and HSV-1 compared with Asc + Toc. Furthermore, based on IC_{50} and SI values, the Ech + Asc + Toc composition was more active toward TBEV and HSV-1 than Ech and Asc + Toc ($p \leq 0.05$) (Table 2). The obtained data revealed that the presence of Asc and Toc in composition with Ech enhances antiviral activity of this formulation up to two times compared with Ech alone.

2.4. Time-of-Formulation-Addition Assay

The inhibitory effects of tested formulations on different stages of TBEV and HSV-1 replication cycles were studied by time-of-addition experiments via MTT assay (Figure 2). Cells were pretreated with formulations before viral infection (pretreatment of cells), viruses were incubated with formulations before cell infection (pretreatment of virus), or infected cells were incubated with formulations after penetration of the virus into host cells (treatment of infected cells).

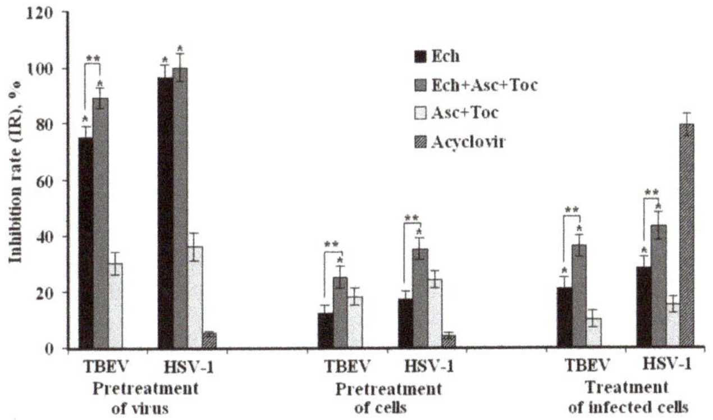

Figure 2. Antiviral action of the formulations on different stages of virus replication cycles. * Statistically significant differences between Asc + Toc and other formulation ($p \leq 0.05$), ** statistically significant differences between antioxidant composition and Ech ($p \leq 0.05$).

In the case of the pretreatment of viruses with the formulations (direct virucidal effect), Ech and the Ech + Asc + Toc composition considerably suppressed TBEV infection: inhibition rates (IR) were of 75 ± 4% and 89 ± 5%, respectively ($p < 0.05$). The corresponding pretreatment of HSV-1 by Ech and the Ech + Asc + Toc composition completely protected cells against this infection. However, only a minor effect on HSV-1 infection was detected when the virus was pretreated with acyclovir (Figure 2).

The treatment of PK and Vero cells with the tested formulations before infection (preventive effect) was much less effective. Ech, the Ech + Asc + Toc composition, and the Asc + Toc composition showed almost no preventive action against both virus infections. The same results were found when Vero cells were pretreated with acyclovir prior to infection.

When the formulations were added at an early stage of virus replication (one hour after infection), Ech and the Ech + Asc + Toc composition possessed moderate virus-inhibiting effects against TBEV infection with an IR of 21 ± 2% and 36 ± 3%, respectively, and against HSV-1 with an IR of 28 ± 3% and 43 ± 4%, respectively, compared to an inactive Asc + Toc formulation (~10%, $p < 0.05$). Meanwhile, acyclovir showed the highest antiviral activity, with an inhibition of the HSV-1 replication of 79 ± 4%.

3. Discussion

It was of interest that the Ech + Asc + Toc composition, which included three different antioxidants, demonstrated the most potent antioxidant action. Therefore, this composition showed a pronounced synergistic effect, which means that its antioxidant activity was much higher compared to each of the components added in the same amount to stabilize the lipid substrate due to the continuous regeneration of Toc from both the Ech and Asc. Moreover, the synergistic action of Ech in combination with other antioxidants was not so far reported. Ech and the Ech + Asc + Toc composition demonstrated high antioxidant activity on the model of LPS-induced ROS formation in Vero cells.

Since Ech and its composition with Asc and Toc showed significant antioxidant effects on both experimental models, and because of the ability of Ech to overcome the blood–brain barrier [23], further investigations of their effects on the replication cycles of neurotropic viruses such as TBEV and HSV-1 accompanied by oxidative stress were performed. Earlier combinations of antiviral agents with antioxidants have been used for the treatment of some other viral infections, for example, at influenza-associated complications [24]. In this study, we have shown the possibility of enhancing the antioxidant and antiviral effects of Ech due to combination with other antioxidants. We have found that the most effective method of application of Ech and the studied composition is the pretreatment of viruses with the formulations (virucidal action). The antioxidant composition Ech + Asc + Toc also demonstrated stronger antiviral activity against TBEV and HSV-1 compared to Ech. The inhibitory concentrations (IC_{50}) of the composition were half that of Ech, while the selective indices (SI) were twice as large as those of Ech (Table 2). It should be noted that regardless of the method of exposure of viruses and cells to the formulations, the virus inhibition rates of the composition of antioxidants was higher than that by Ech itself ($p < 0.05$, Figure 1).

It was shown that the main mechanism of the in vitro action of Ech and the composition of antioxidants at the stages of the life cycles of TBEV and HSV-1 is a direct inactivation of virus particles (Figure 2). Many authors have suggested that the virucidal activity of polyphenols (Ech is considered a polyphenol as well) might be caused by direct action on the viral particles inhibiting the adsorption of the virus to the host cell receptors [25–27]. At the same time, Li et al. reported that polyphenols can cause irreversible damage or the reversible blocking of certain regions of the viral capsid protein [28]. We suppose that Ech and its composition with antioxidants can bind with some envelope virus proteins that are necessary for the adsorption of the virus to cells. Since many polyphenols exhibit antioxidant and antiviral properties, we can assume that the activity of Ech and its composition in relation to TBEV and HSV-1 can also be caused by interfering with the redox imbalance caused by these viruses [16]. Thus, Ech, either alone or in varying compositions, can both directly affect virus particles and indirectly enhance the antioxidant defense mechanisms in the hosting cell.

Thus, the ability of Ech and its compositions to inactivate HSV-1 and TBEV virus particles makes it useful as an antiviral agent in preventing de novo viral infection, and thereby could help control viral spread and limit recurrent infections.

Our data on the antioxidant and antiviral activities of Ech—which earlier have been applied to the treatment of cardiovascular and eye diseases—and antioxidant composition based on Ech indicate the necessity of further studies of these formulations for the development of promising antiviral drugs.

4. Materials and Methods

4.1. Viruses and Cell Cultures

The RNA-containing tick-borne encephalitis virus (TBEV) strain Dal'negorsk that was isolated in 1973 from the brain of a patient with a fatal outcome of TBE, and characterized as a Far Eastern subtype, was used (Gene Bank Whole Genome Sequence Number: FJ402886) [29]. The DNA-containing herpes virus (HSV-1, strain VR3) was obtained from the National Collection of US Viruses (Rockville, MD, USA).

TBEV was grown on the pig embryo kidney (PK) cells using medium 199 supplemented with 10% fetal bovine serum (FBS) and 100 U/mL gentamicin. HSV-1 was grown in African green monkey kidney (Vero) cells using Dulbecco's Modified Eagle's Medium (DMEM) supplemented with 10% FBS, gentamicin, and glutamine.

Viral titers were determined by cytopathic effect (CPE) assay and expressed as the 50% tissue culture infectious dose ($TCID_{50}$/mL). The TBEV titer was $10^{8.8}$ $TCID_{50}$/mL, and the titer of HSV-1 was $10^{8.25}$ $TCID_{50}$/mL.

4.2. Studied Formulations

Echinochrome A (Ech, 2,3,5,7,8-pentahydroxy-6-ethyl-1,4-naphthoquinone) 98.0%, pharmaceutical, state registration number PN002362/01-2003, G.B. Elyakov Pacific Institute of Bioorganic Chemistry FEB RAS, Russia.

Ascorbic acid (Asc) 99.8%, pharmaceutical, AppliChem, Germany.
α-Tocopherol (Toc) ≥96%, pharmaceutical, Carl Roth, Germany.
The composition of antioxidants Ech + Asc + Toc at the weight ratio of 5:5:1.
The composition containing Asc and Toc at the weight ratio of 5:1.
Ribavirin®, pharmaceutical, Vertex, Russia.
Acyclovir®, pharmaceutical, Belmedpreparation, Republic of Belarus.

The tested formulations were dissolved in dimethylsulfoxide (DMSO, Sigma, Saint-Louis, MO, USA) and stored at −20 °C. The stock solutions (10 mg/mL) of formulations were diluted with a suitable cell culture medium so that the final concentration of DMSO was 0.5%.

4.3. Determination of Antioxidant Activity of the Formulations

Antioxidant activity of the formulations was determined on a model of linetol peroxidation containing a complex mixture of ethyl esters of polyunsaturated fatty acids (oleic, linoleic, and linolenic) of linseed oil at 37 °C [30]. Stock solutions of Ech, Asc, and Toc were prepared at a concentration of 10 mg/mL in ethanol. Two-component and three-component antioxidant compositions were obtained by mixing the volumes of stock solutions in the indicated proportions. First, 10 μL of each solution and 300 μL of linetol were placed in a glass vial. The reaction vessels were placed in an incubator (37 °C). The concentration of antioxidant in linetol in all cases was 0.05 mg/mL, or 0.005%. The mass of the reaction mixtures pre-cooled to room temperature was measured twice a day (accuracy 0.0005 g). When the mass of increased by 10 mg, the reaction was stopped. All of the experiments were repeated three times. The period of linetol oxidation inhibition ($\Delta\tau$) was calculated as the difference between times necessary for the weight of linetol to increase by 10 mg in experiments with and without the addition of antioxidants using the formula $\Delta\tau = \tau - \tau_0$, where τ is the time of linetol oxidation initiation in the presence of an antioxidant (h); and τ_0 is the time of linetol oxidation initiation without the addition of an antioxidant (h).

4.4. Antioxidant Activity of the Formulations Against LPS-Induced ROS Formation in Vero Cells

The Vero cells that were grown on 96-well plates (1×10^4 cells/well) were washed from the growth medium and treated with 100 μL/well of the tested compounds (five μg/mL) and 10 μL/well LPS from *E. coli* serotype 055:B5 (Sigma, 1.0 μg/mL), which were both dissolved in PBS and cultured at 37 °C in a CO_2-incubator for one hour. For the ROS levels measurement, 20 μL of 2,7-dichlorodihydrofluorescein diacetate (DCF-DA, Sigma, final concentration 10 μM) solution was added to each well, and the plates were incubated for 30 min at 37 °C. The intensity of DCF-DA fluorescence was measured at λ_{ex} 485 n/λ_{em} 518 nm using the plate reader PHERAstar FS (BMG Labtech, Offenburg, Germany) [31].

4.5. Cytotoxicity Assay of the Formulations

The cytotoxicity of the tested formulations was estimated by MTT assay in PK and Vero cell lines [32,33]. A monolayer of cells (1 × 10^4 cells/well) grown in 96-well plates was treated with different concentrations of tested formulations (from 0 to 2000 μg/mL) and cultured at 37 °C in a CO_2-incubator for six days; untreated cells were used as controls. Then 20 μL of MTT solution (5 mg/mL) (methylthiazolyltetrazolium bromide, Sigma, Saint-Louis, MO, USA) was added in each well followed by incubation at 37 °C for one hour. The MTT solution was removed, and 150 μL/well of isopropanol was added. Optical density (OD) was measured at 540 nm using an ELISA microplate reader (Labsystems Multiskan RC, Vantaa, Finland) with a reference absorbance at 620 nm. The viability of the cells was calculated as (ODt)/(ODc) × 100%, where ODt and ODc correspond to the absorbance of treated and control cells, respectively. Cytotoxicity was expressed as 50% cytotoxic concentration (CC_{50}) of the tested formulation that reduced the viability of treated cells by 50% compared with control cells. Experiments were performed in triplicate and repeated three times.

4.6. Antiviral Activity ASSAY of Formulations

The antiviral activity of formulations against TBEV and HSV-1 was evaluated using cytopathic effect (CPE) inhibition assay in PK and Vero cells, respectively. The overnight monolayer of cells grown on 96-well plates (1 × 10^4 cells/well) was infected with 100 μl/well of serial dilutions of virus suspension (10^{-1}–10^{-8}) and simultaneously treated by formulations (100 μL/well in triplicate) of different concentrations (from 0 to 400 μg/mL) for one hour at 37 °C. After virus absorption, the virus–formulations mixture was removed; the cells were washed, and a maintenance medium with 1% FBS was added. The plates were kept at 37 °C in CO_2-incubator for six days for TBEV or for three days for HSV-1 until CPE appeared. The antiviral activity was determined by the difference of the viral titers between treated infected cells and untreated infected cells and expressed as the inhibition rate (IR, %), using the formula [27]: IR = $(1 - T/C) \times 100$, where T is the antilog of the formulations-treated viral titers and C is the antilog of the control (without formulations) viral titers. The concentration of formulation that reduced the virus-induced CPE by 50% was determined as the 50% inhibitory concentration (IC_{50}). The selectivity index (SI) was calculated as the ratio of CC_{50} to IC_{50}. Experiments were repeated three times.

4.7. Time-of-Formulation-Addition assay

PK and Vero cells were grown in 96-well plates (1 × 10^4 cells/well). An infectious dose of both TBEV and HSV-1 was of 100 $TCID_{50}$/mL, tested formulations were used at a concentration of 20 μg/mL, and acyclovir was used at a concentration of 10 μg/mL. The plates were kept at 37 °C in CO_2-incubator for six days for TBEV or for three days for HSV-1 until 80–90% CPE was observed in viruses control compared with cells control.

- Pretreatment of cells with formulations. Monolayer of cells was pretreated with formulations in triplicate and incubated at 37 °C for one hour. Thereafter, the cells were washed and infected with virus at 37 °C for one hour. The cells were washed to remove unabsorbed virus and incubated with maintenance medium until CPE was observed.
- Pretreatment of virus with formulations. The virus was mixed with formulations at a ratio 1:1 (*v*/*v*), incubated for one hour at 37 °C, then applied to monolayer of cells in triplicate. After one hour adsorption at 37 °C, cells were washed, and maintenance medium was added, followed by incubation until CPE was observed.
- Treatment of infected cells. Monolayer of cells was infected with the virus at 37 °C for one hour, then washed, treated with tested formulations in triplicate, and incubated until CPE was appeared.

Antiviral activity of formulations was assessed by MTT test, and the viral inhibition rate (IR, %) was calculated according to the formula [34], IR = (ODtv − ODcv)/(ODcd − Odcv) × 100, where ODtv represents the OD of cells infected with virus and treated with the test formulation; ODcv corresponds to the OD of the untreated virus-infected cells, and ODcd is OD of control (untreated and noninfected) cells.

4.8. Statistical Analysis

CC_{50} and IC_{50} were calculated by regression analysis of the dose–response curve. Statistical processing of the data was performed using Statistica 10.0 software. The results are given as mean $\pm$ standard deviation (SD). The differences between parameters of control and experimental groups were estimated using the Wilcoxon test. Differences were considered significant at $p \leq 0.05$.

5. Conclusions

We have shown that the both Ech, an active substance of the permitted to clinical application in Russia drugs, belonging the Histochrome series, and an antioxidant composition, containing Ech, Asc, and Toc (5:5:1), possess in vitro antiviral activity against RNA-containing tick-borne encephalitis virus and DNA-containing herpes simplex virus type 1. The studied composition of antioxidants exhibits more potent antioxidant and antiviral properties than Ech itself, thus demonstrating the synergistic effects of its components.

Author Contributions: S.A.F. and N.V.K. planned, summarized the work and wrote the manuscript; N.P.M. prepared echinochrome A and antioxidant composition; E.A.V. examined the antioxidant activity; E.A.P. conducted the experiments with ROS measurement; V.F.L., O.V.I., O.A.S., L.K.E. investigated the HSV-1 antiviral activity; N.V.K. and G.N.L. examined the TBEV antiviral activity.

Funding: This work was supported by the Ministry of Science and Education of the Russian Federation (project RFMEF161317X0076).

Acknowledgments: Authors are grateful to V.A.S. for constructive comments for the results and discussion of the manuscript.

Conflicts of Interest: The authors declare no conflict of interest.

References

1. Betteridge, D.J. What is oxidative stress? *Metab. Clin. Exp.* **2000**, *49*, 3–8. [CrossRef]
2. Gullberg, R.C.; Steel, J.J.; Moon, S. Oxidative stress influences positive strand RNA virus genome. *Virology* **2015**, *475*, 219–229. [CrossRef]
3. Kumar, S.; Misra, U.K.; Kalita, J.; Khanna, V.K.; Khan, M.Y. Imbalance in oxidant/antioxidant system in different brain regions of rat after the infection of Japanese encephalitis virus. *Neurochem. Int.* **2009**, *55*, 648–654. [CrossRef] [PubMed]
4. Schreck, R.; Rieber, P.; Baeuerle, P.A. Reactive oxygen intermediates as apparently widely used messengers in the activation of the NF-kappa B transcription factor and HIV-1. *EMBO J.* **1991**, *10*, 2247–2258. [CrossRef] [PubMed]
5. Zaharicheva, T.A.; Koval'skij, Ju.G.; Lebed'ko, O.A.; Mzhel'skaja, T.V. Oxidative stress in patients with tick-borne encephalitis in the Far East of the Russian Federation. *Dal'nevost. Zhurn Infekc. Patol.* **2012**, *20*, 41–45. (In Russian)
6. Kavouras, J.H.; Prandovszky, E.; Valyi-Nagy, K.; Kovacs, S.K.; Tiwari, V.; Kovacs, M.; Shukla, D.; Valyi-Nagy, T. Herpes simplex virus type 1 infection induces oxidative stress and the release of bioactive lipid peroxidation by-products in mouse P19N neural cell cultures. *J. Neurovirol.* **2007**, *13*, 416–425. [CrossRef]
7. Sebastiano, M.; Chastel, O.; de Thoisy, B.; Eens, M.; Costantini, D. Oxidative stress favours herpes virus infection in vertebrates: A meta-analysis. *Curr. Zool.* **2016**, *62*, 325–332. [CrossRef]
8. Valyi-Nagy, T.; Dermody, T.S. Role of oxidative damage in the pathogenesis of viral infections of the nervous system. *Histol. Histopathol.* **2005**, *20*, 957–967. [CrossRef]
9. Schwarz, K.B. Oxidative stress during viral infection: A review. *Free Radic. Biol. Med.* **1996**, *21*, 641–649. [CrossRef]

10. Jin, H.; Kanthasamy, A.; Ghosh, A.; Anantharam, V.; Kalyanaraman, B.; Kanthasamy, A.G. Mitochondria-targeted antioxidants for treatment of Parkinson's disease: Preclinical and clinical outcomes. *Biochim. Biophys. Acta* **2014**, *1842*, 1282–1294. [CrossRef]
11. Kandhare, A.D.; Mukherjee, A.; Bodhankar, S.L. Antioxidant for treatment of diabetic nephropathy: A systematic review and meta-analysis. *Chem. Biol. Interact.* **2017**, *278*, 212–221. [CrossRef]
12. Krylova, N.V.; Popov, A.M.; Leonova, G.N. Antioxidants as Potential Antiviral Agents for Flavivirus Infections. *Antibiot Khimioter* **2016**, *61*, 25–31. [PubMed]
13. Malvy, D.J.M.; Richard, M.J.; Arnaud, J.; Favier, A.; Amedee-Manesme, O. Relationship of plasma malondialdehyde, vitamin E and antioxidant micronutrients to human immunodeficiency virus-1 seropositivity. *Clin. Chim. Acta* **1994**, *224*, 89–94. [CrossRef]
14. Allard, J.P.; Aghdassi, E.; Chau, J.; Tam, C.; Kovacs, C.M.; Salit, I.E.; Walmsley, S.L. Effects of vitamin E and C supplementation on oxidative stress and viral load in HIV-infected subjects. *Aids* **1998**, *12*, 1653–1659. [CrossRef] [PubMed]
15. Mathew, D.; Hsu, W.L. Antiviral potential of curcumin. *J. Funct. Foods* **2018**, *40*, 692–699. [CrossRef]
16. Di Sotto, A.; Checconi, P.; Celestino, I.; Locatelli, M.; Carissimi, S.; De Angelis, M.; Rossi, V.; Limongi, D.; Toniolo, C.; Martinoli, L.; et al. Antiviral and Antioxidant Activity of a Hydroalcoholic Extract from *Humulus lupulus* L. *Oxidative Med. Cell. Longev.* **2018**, *2018*, 5919237. [CrossRef] [PubMed]
17. El-Toumy, S.A.; Salib, J.Y.; El-Kashak, W.A.; Marty, C.; Bedoux, G.; Bourgougnon, N. Antiviral effect of polyphenol rich plant extracts on herpes simplex virus type 1. *Food Sci. Hum. Wellness* **2018**, *7*, 91–101. [CrossRef]
18. Di Sotto, A.; Di Giacomo, S.; Amatore, D.; Locatelli, M.; Vitalone, A.; Toniolo, C.; Rotino, G.L.; Lo Scalzo, R.; Palamara, A.T.; Marcocci, M.E.; et al. A Polyphenol Rich Extract from *Solanum melongena* L. DR2 Peel Exhibits Antioxidant Properties and Anti-Herpes Simplex Virus Type 1 Activity In Vitro. *Molecules* **2018**, *23*, 66. [CrossRef]
19. Elyakov, G.B.; Maximov, O.B.; Mischenko, N.P.; Koltsova, E.A.; Fedoreev, S.A.; Glebko, L.I.; Krasovskaya, N.P.; Artjukov, A.A. Composition Comprising di-and Trisodium Salts of Echinochrome for Treating Ocular Conditions. European Patent 1121929, 3 November 2004.
20. Elyakov, G.B.; Maximov, O.B.; Mischenko, N.P.; Koltsova, E.A.; Fedoreev, S.A.; Glebko, L.I.; Krasovskaya, N.P.; Artjukov, A.A. Drug preparation "Histochrome" for treating acute myocardial infarction and ischemic heart diseases. European Patent 1121930, 14 November 2007.
21. Olcott, H.S.; Einset, E. A weighing method for measuring the induction period of marine and other oils. *J. Am. Oil Chem. Soc.* **1958**, *35*, 161–162. [CrossRef]
22. Kancheva, V.D.; Slavova-Kazakova, A.K.; Angelova, S.E.; Kumar, P.; Malhotra, S.; Singh, B.K.; Saso, L.; Prasad, A.K.; Parmar, V.S. Protective effects of new antioxidant compositions of 4-methylcoumarins and related compounds with DL-α-tocopherol and L-ascorbic acid. *J. Sci. Food Agric.* **2018**, *98*, 3784–3794. [CrossRef]
23. Stonik, V.A.; Gusev, E.I.; Martynov, M.Yu.; Guseva, M.R.; Shchukin, I.A.; Agafonova, I.G.; Mishchenko, N.P.; Fedoreev, A.S. New medications for treatment of hemorrhagic stroke. High-resolution MRI in evaluation of histochrome in experimental hemorrhagic stroke. *Dokl. Boil. Sci.* **2005**, *405*, 421–423. [CrossRef]
24. Uchide, N.; Toyoda, H. Antioxidant therapy as a potential approach to severe influenza-associated complications. *Molecules* **2011**, *16*, 2032–2052. [CrossRef] [PubMed]
25. Torky, Z.A.; Hossain, M.M. Pharmacological evaluation of the hibiscus herbal extract against herpes simples virus-type 1 as an antiviral drug in vitro. *Int. J. Virol.* **2017**, *13*, 68–79. [CrossRef]
26. Garrett, R.; Romanos, M.T.V.; Borges, R.M.; Santos, M.G.; Rocha, L.; Silva, A.J.R.D. Antiherpetic activity of a flavonoid fraction from *Ocotea notata* leaves. *Rev. Bras. Farmacogn.* **2012**, *22*, 306–313. [CrossRef]
27. Astani, A.; Schnitzler, P. Antiviral activity of monoterpenes beta-pinene and limonene against herpes simplex virus in vitro. *Iran. J. Microbiol.* **2014**, *6*, 149–155. [PubMed]
28. Li, D.; Baert, L.; Xia, M.; Zhong, W.; Jiang, X.; Uyttendaele, M. Effects of a variety of food extracts and juices on the specific binding ability of norovirus GII.4 P particles. *J. Food Protect.* **2012**, *75*, 1350–1354. [CrossRef] [PubMed]
29. Leonova, G.N.; Maystrovskaya, O.S.; Kondratov, I.G.; Takashima, I.; Belikov, S. The nature of replication of tick-borne encephalitis virus strains isolated from residents of the Russian Far East with inapparent and clinical forms of infection. *Virus Res.* **2014**, *189*, 34–42. [CrossRef]

30. Veselova, M.V.; Fedoreev, S.A.; Vasilevskaya, N.A.; Denisenko, V.A.; Gerasimenko, A.V. Antioxidant activity of polyphenols from the Far East yew-sprouted plant. *Pharm. Chem. J.* **2007**, *41*, 29–34. [CrossRef]
31. Ivanchina, N.V.; Kicha, A.A.; Malyarenko, T.V.; Kalinovsky, A.I.; Menchinskaya, E.S.; Pislyagin, E.A.; Dmitrenok, P.S. The Influence on LPS-Induced ROS Formation in Macrophages of Capelloside A, a New Steroid Glycoside from the Starfish *Ogmaster Capella*. *Nat. Prod. Commun.* **2015**, *10*, 1937–1940.
32. Matsuda, M.; Shigeta, S.; Okutani, K. Antiviral activities of marine Pseudomonas polysaccharides and their oversulfated derivatives. *Mar. Biotechnol.* **1999**, *1*, 68–73. [CrossRef]
33. Mosmann, T. Rapid colorimetric assay for cellular growth and survival: Application to proliferation and cytotoxicity assays. *J. Immunol. Methods* **1983**, *65*, 55–63. [CrossRef]
34. Ngan, L.T.M.; Jang, M.J.; Kwon, M.J.; Ahn, Y.J. Antiviral activity and possible mechanism of action of constituents identified in *Paeonia lactiflora* root toward human rhinoviruses. *PLoS ONE* **2015**, *10*, e0121629. [CrossRef] [PubMed]

marine drugs

MDPI

Article

Spinochrome D Attenuates Doxorubicin-Induced Cardiomyocyte Death via Improving Glutathione Metabolism and Attenuating Oxidative Stress

Chang Shin Yoon [1], Hyoung Kyu Kim [1], Natalia P. Mishchenko [2], Elena A. Vasileva [2], Sergey A. Fedoreyev [2], Valentin A. Stonik [2] and Jin Han [1,*]

[1] National Research Laboratory for Mitochondrial Signaling, Department of Physiology, College of Medicine, Cardiovascular and Metabolic Disease Center (CMDC), Inje University, Busan 614-735, Korea; changshin73@gmail.com (C.S.Y.); estrus74@gmail.com (H.K.K.)

[2] G.B. Elyakov Pacific Institute of Bioorganic Chemistry, Far-Eastern Branch of the Russian Academy of Science, Vladivostok 690022, Russia; mischenkonp@mail.ru (N.P.M.); vasilieva_el_an@mail.ru (E.A.V.); fedoreev-s@mail.ru (S.A.F.); stonik@piboc.dvo.ru (V.A.S.)

* Correspondence: phyhanj@inje.ac.kr; Tel.: +82-51-890-6727; Fax: +82-51-894-5714

Received: 28 November 2018; Accepted: 15 December 2018; Published: 20 December 2018

Abstract: Doxorubicin, an anthracycline from *Streptomyces peucetius*, exhibits antitumor activity against various cancers. However, doxorubicin is cardiotoxic at cumulative doses, causing increases in intracellular reactive oxygen species in the heart. Spinochrome D (SpD) has a structure of 2,3,5,6,8-pentahydroxy-1,4-naphthoquinone and is a structural analogue of well-known sea urchin pigment echinochrome A. We previously reported that echinochrome A is cardioprotective against doxorubicin toxicity. In the present study, we assessed the cardioprotective effects of SpD against doxorubicin and determined the underlying mechanism. ^{1}H-NMR-based metabolomics and mass spectrometry-based proteomics were utilized to characterize the metabolites and proteins induced by SpD in a human cardiomyocyte cell line (AC16) and human breast cancer cell line (MCF-7). Multivariate analyses identified 12 discriminating metabolites (variable importance in projection > 1.0) and 1814 proteins from SpD-treated AC16 cells. Proteomics and metabolomics analyses showed that glutathione metabolism was significantly influenced by SpD treatment in AC16 cells. SpD treatment increased ATP production and the oxygen consumption rate in D-galactose-treated AC16 cells. SpD protected AC16 cells from doxorubicin cytotoxicity, but it did not affect the anticancer properties. With SpD treatment, the mitochondrial membrane potential and mitochondrial calcium localization were significantly different between cardiomyocytes and cancer cell lines. Our findings suggest that SpD could be cardioprotective against the cytotoxicity of doxorubicin.

Keywords: Spinochrome D; doxorubicin; cardioprotective effect

1. Introduction

Echinochrome A has a chemical structure of 6-ethyl-2,3,5,7,8-pentahydroxy-1,4-naphthoquinone, which exhibits cardioprotective activity and reduces the myocardial ischemia/reperfusion injury via its antioxidant effect and enhancement of mitochondria biogenesis [1–3]. Echinochrome A has a number of structural analogues and together they comprise the class of spinochrome pigments of sea urchins. Biological effects of spinochromes were investigated mainly on crude extracts [4] and there is not so much information on the activity of individual pigments, particularly regarding cardioprotective ability. Spinochrome D (SpD) is one of six main spinochromes and it is biosynthesized by many sea urchin species (Figure 1A) [5]. SpD is a side product of echinochrome A isolation from the flat sea urchin *Scaphechinus mirabilis*, which is utilized for the preparation of the active substance of the antioxidant and the cardioprotective drug *Histochrome*® [6]. Nevertheless, the content of SpD in sea urchins is usually pretty low (0.001–0.003% of dry weight), but recently by Balaneva et al. was developed a simple and effective synthesis scheme with the yield of SpD in 58% [7]. SpD might be assumed to inherit the cardioprotective ability of echinochrome A, but the detailed mechanism has been unknown.

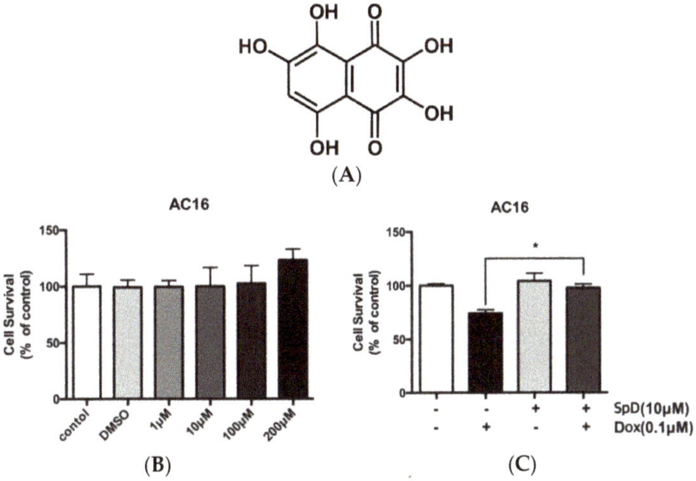

Figure 1. Spinochrome D (SpD) protected cardiac cells from the cytotoxicity of doxorubicin. (**A**) Chemical structure of SpD (MW, 238.15044); (**B**) AC16 human cardiomyocytes were treated with 0–200 μM SpD for 24 h and cell viability was measured using a Cell Counting Kit-8 reagent (CCK-8) assay. SpD did not affect the cell viability of cardiomyocytes. * $p < 0.05$ compared with control; (**C**) Treatment with SpD (10 μM, 24 h) attenuated the cardiotoxicity of doxorubicin (0.1 μM) in AC16 cells.

Doxorubicin is an anthracycline that was firstly extracted from *Streptomyces peucetius* and it has been routinely used for the treatment of several cancers, including breast, lung, gastric, ovarian, non-Hodgkin's, and Hodgkin's lymphoma [8,9]. There are several proposed anti-cancer mechanisms of doxorubicin, including intercalation into DNA and generation of reactive oxygen species (ROS). The inhibition of topoisomerase II has been known to induce apoptosis in cells [10–12].

Unfortunately, cumulative dose of doxorubicin over 550 mg/m^2 body surface area has been known to develop cardiomyopathy [13,14]. The exact mechanism of cardiomyopathy is still controversial but iron-related free radical formation and mitochondrial disruption have been considered to be the main causes [15]. There have been trials to overcome the doxorubicin's cardiac toxicity by reducing its oxygen radical formation to achieve important accomplishment [16–18].

In the present study, we demonstrated that SpD has a cardio-protective effect against the cardiac toxicity of doxorubicin without interfering the cytotoxicity to cancer cell lines. We used an integration of ^{1}H-NMR based metabolomics and mass-spectrometry based proteomics to specify molecular pathways that are affected by SpD treatment in human cardiomyocytes. We also measured changes of the mitochondrial membrane potential and mitochondrial calcium in SpD treated human cardiomyocytes.

2. Results

2.1. *SpD Protected AC16 Cells against Doxorubicin Cytotoxicity*

Human cardiomyocyte AC16 cells were treated with SpD at 1–200 μM (Figure 1B). We found no harmful effects on cell viability. Identical concentrations of SpD were tested on rat cardiomyocyte

H9c2 cells and also they showed no effect on cell viability (Figure S1). The cell viability of AC16 cells decreased after 0.1 μM doxorubicin treatment for 24 h, and an exposure duration of 48 h resulted in cell death for the majority of cells (data not shown). However, adding 10 μM SpD treatment in addition to doxorubicin for 24 h led to 80–90% AC16 cell survival (Figure 1C).

2.2. Liquid Chromatography–Mass Spectrometry-MS (LC-MS/MS)-Based Proteomics Analyses of SpD/Doxorubicin-Treated AC16 Cells

We performed LC-MS/MS analysis of cell lysates from SpD-treated and -untreated AC16 cells with or without doxorubicin for 24 h. The detected proteins are shown in Venn diagrams (Figure 2A,B) and full lists (Supplementary Information 2). We found networks of proteins forming clusters that are centered on "mitochondria" (Figure 2C and Figure S5). The affected pathways based on the Kyoto Encyclopedia of Genes and Genomes (KEGG) database listed proteins participating in gap junction, focal adhesion, aminoacyl-tRNA biosynthesis, and glutathione metabolism (Figure 2D).

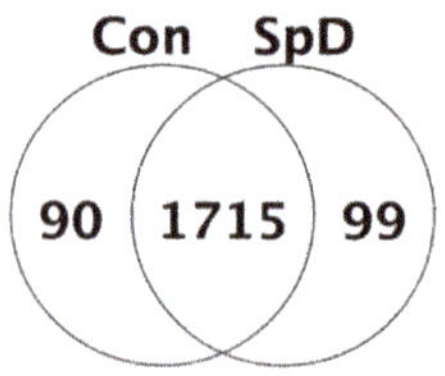

(A)

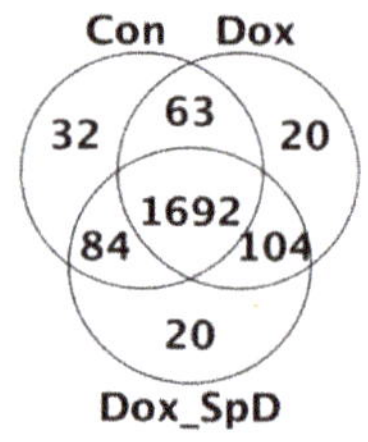

(B)

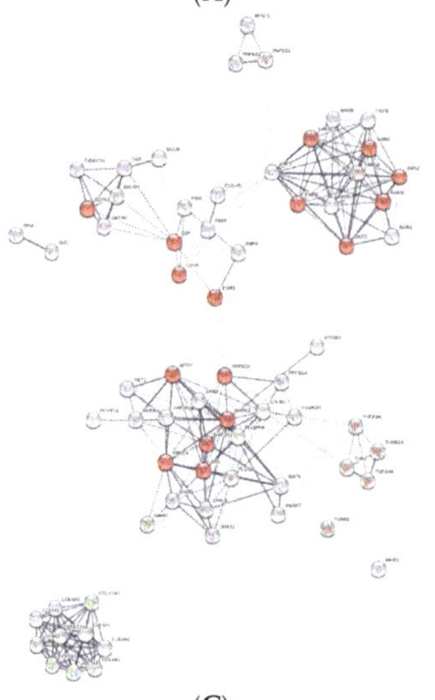

(C)

KEGG pathway from STRING analysis

pathway	Observed gene count	FDR
Gap junction	16	1.47×10^{-21}
Focal adhesion	18	1.81×10^{-18}
Aminoacyl-tRNA biosynthesis	12	2.22×10^{-18}
Glutathione metabolism	12	9.83×10^{-18}
PI3K-Akt signaling pathway	19	3.06×10^{-16}
Protein digestion and absorption	12	7.29×10^{-15}
GnRH signaling pathway	11	5.04×10^{-13}
Platelet activation	12	8.39×10^{-13}
Adrenergic signaling in cardiomyocytes	12	2.68×10^{-12}
Amoebiasis	11	2.68×10^{-12}

(D)

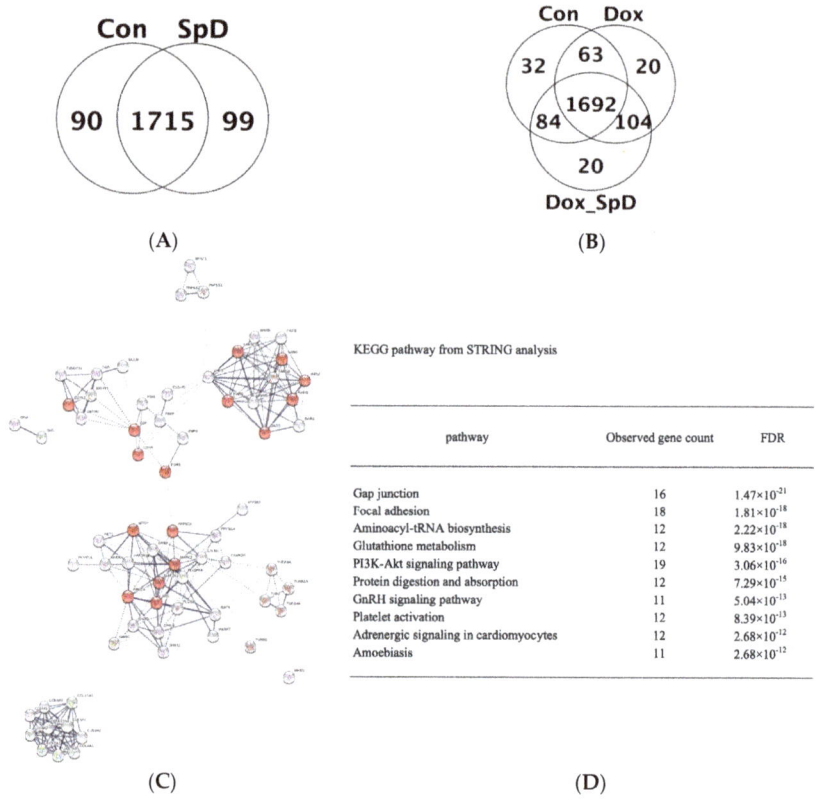

Figure 2. Mass spectrometry-based proteomics of SpD-treated AC16 cells. Liquid Chromatography–Mass Spectrometry-MS (LC-MS/MS) spectrometry-based proteomics detected proteins from SpD (10 μM, 24 h) (**A**) and SpD/doxorubicin (**B**) treated AC16 cells; (**C**) Search Tool for the Retrieval of Interacting Genes/Proteins (STRING) analysis showed that altered metabolic proteins clustered around "mitochondria" which are represented as red colored nodes. All filled nodes represent the 3D structures of proteins are known; and, (**D**) The top 10 influenced metabolic pathways are shown from the STRING analysis (Kyoto Encyclopedia of Genes and Genomes (KEGG) database).

2.3. ^{1}H-NMR Mediated Metabolomics Analysis of SpD-Treated AC16 Cells

To identify metabolite alterations that are induced by SpD, we used ^{1}H-NMR spectroscopy to characterize 30 mg of AC16 cells incubated with SpD (10 μM) for 24 h. Metabolic profiling (Chenomx, Edmonton, AB, Canada) was used to identify 32 metabolites in SpD-treated AC16 cells and untreated control cells (Table 1).

Table 1. Identified metabolites and their corresponding concentrations (mM; mean, standard deviation), as determined by Chenomx NMR Suit 7.1® peak fitting of individual ^{1}H-NMR spectra (600 MHz) for SpD (10 μM) treated AC16 cells (30 mg, n = 3).

Metabolite	Control		SpD	
	Mean (mM)	S.D.	Mean (mM)	S.D.
Acetate	8.218	5.815	4.820	1.541
Alanine	1.236	0.665	1.341	0.315
Asparagine	0.388	0.194	0.397	0.095
Aspartate	0.412	0.139	0.428	0.138
Choline	0.751	0.437	0.831	0.111
Creatine	0.463	0.190	0.557	0.051
Formate	0.230	0.034	0.197	0.048
Fumarate	0.143	0.047	0.164	0.043
Glutamate	2.877	1.640	3.622	0.791
Glutamine	0.129	0.048	0.101	0.006
Glutathione	0.383	0.158	0.572	0.081
Glycerol	0.912	0.405	0.788	0.088
Glycine	1.650	0.952	1.900	0.656
Hypoxanthine	0.285	0.222	0.349	0.089
Inosine	0.169	0.068	0.209	0.056
Isoleucine	0.169	0.080	0.235	0.031
Lactate	9.551	3.793	12.374	2.715
Leucine	0.829	0.536	0.824	0.073
Lysine	0.783	0.489	0.719	0.124
Methionine	0.064	0.017	0.090	0.029
O-Phosphocholine	0.274	0.124	0.392	0.066
O-Phosphoethanolamine	0.939	0.468	1.068	0.091
Phenylalanine	0.376	0.200	0.364	0.018
Proline	0.907	0.435	1.114	0.202
Serine	0.948	0.536	0.790	0.352
Taurine	0.505	0.270	0.723	0.198
Threonine	0.853	0.434	0.846	0.152
Tyrosine	0.323	0.168	0.329	0.004
Uracil	0.363	0.243	0.279	0.021
Valine	0.479	0.272	0.474	0.073
myo-Inositol	1.198	0.554	1.750	0.352
sn-Glycero-3-phosphocholine (GPC)	0.123	0.058	0.245	0.068

After normalization of the data (Figure 3), univariate and multivariate statistical analyses were used to comprehensively evaluate the effects of SpD on AC16 cells.

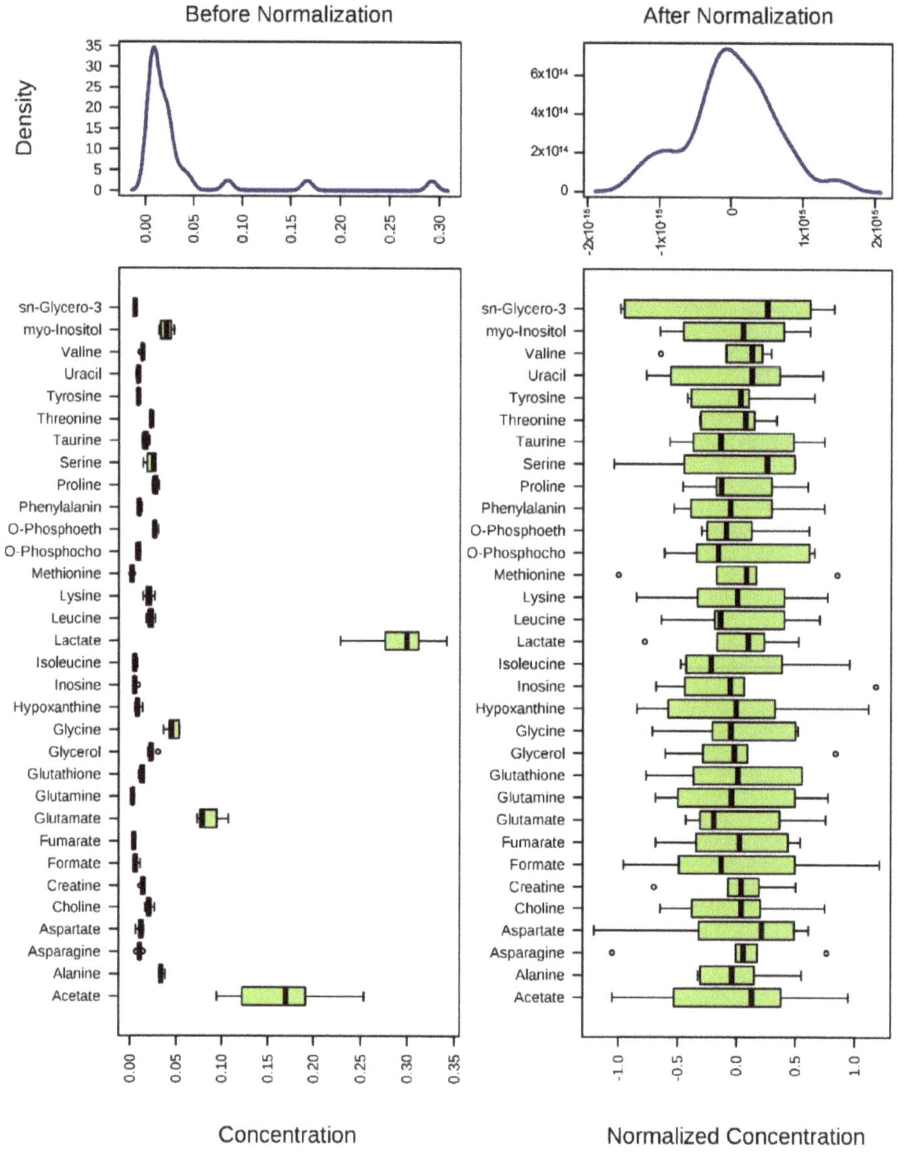

Figure 3. Normalization of ^{1}H-NMR aquired metabolite concentrations. The concentrations of metabolites were normalized by log-transformation followed by Pareto scaling (mean-centered and divided by the square root of the standard deviation of each variable). Changes of metabolites are represented as ratios of control metabolites.

Univariate volcano plots of log2(FC) > 1.2 ($p < 0.05$) metabolites showed that the levels of sn-glycero-3-phosphocholine (GPC), glutathione, myo-inositol, taurine, and O-phosphocholine were increased, while the levels of acetate and glutamine were decreased, by SpD (Figure 4).

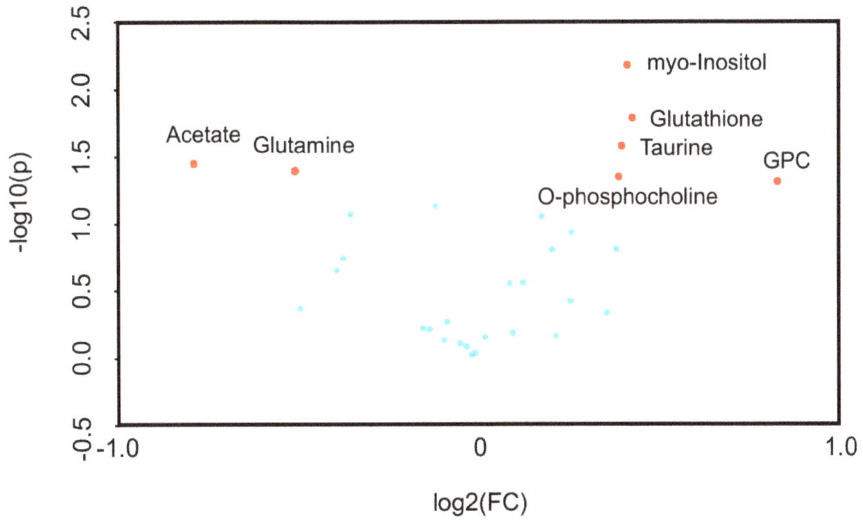

Figure 4. Volcano plots for SpD-induced metabolic changes compared with controls (n = 3). Metabolites are considered significant if log2(fold change) > 1.2. The p-value threshold was 0.05. The significantly changed metabolites included acetate, glutamine, myo-inositol, glutathione, taurine, O-phosphocholine, and sn-Glycero-3-phosphocholine (GPC).

Multivariate analysis is used to determine the relative differences in two or more systems that are large and complex. Therefore, as shown in Figure 5A, we performed principal component analysis (PCA) of metabolites from SpD-treated AC16 cells. The aim of PCA is to reduce the dimensionality of original data within the preservation of the variance.

To calculate variable importance in projection (VIP) scores of metabolites, we performed partial least-squares projections for latent structures-discriminant analysis (PLS-DA). Metabolites with VIP scores larger than 1.0 were considered as important (Figure S2). To confirm the "goodness" of the model and the predictive quality, we tested orthogonal partial least-squares projections to latent structures-discriminant analyses (OPLS-DA) on data from SpD-treated AC16 cells and control cells (Figure S3). In PCA, the SpD-treated group and control group revealed class differences showing 95% confidence regions separating each other. We extended the supervised PLS regression using orthogonal signal correction filters after selecting VIP > 1.0 metabolites. The metabolites from the SpD-treated AC16 cells significantly differed from the control cell group in the OPLS-DA model. The R^2Y model quality parameter was 0.937, demonstrating that the OPLS-DA model was robust (R^2Y value near 1.0), and the Q^2 parameter was 0.597, showing that the model was predictive ($Q^2 > 0.5$) (Figure S3). The loading plot of OPLS-DA is shown in Figure 5C. The heat-map analysis of VIP > 1.0 metabolites was represented with logarithmic fold changes (Figure 5B). In comparison with the control group, the most increased and decreased metabolites with SpD treatment were GPC and acetate, respectively.

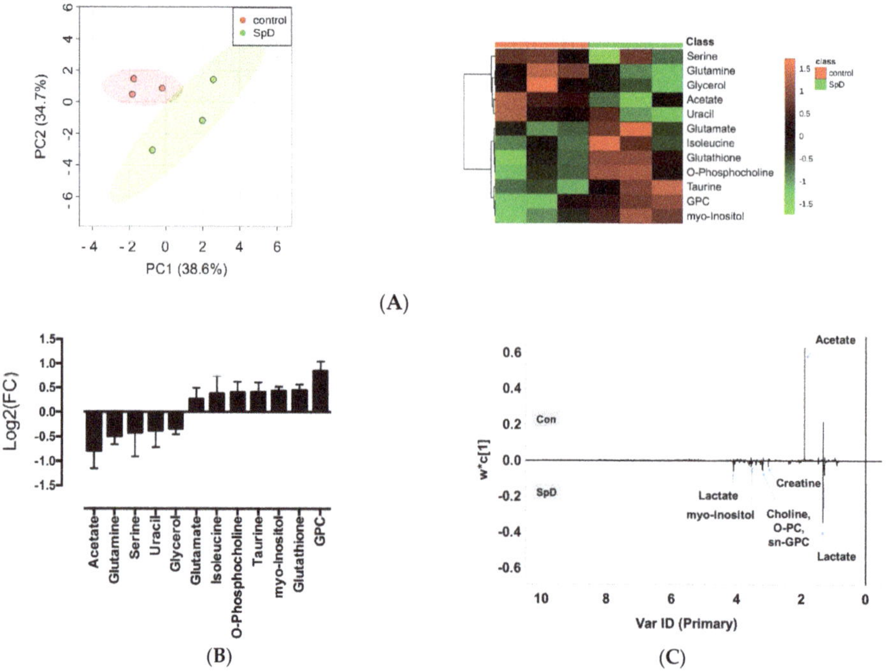

Figure 5. ^{1}H-NMR metabolomics for SpD-treated AC16 cells. (**A**) Principal component analysis (PCA) indicated that metabolites from the SpD-treated (10 μM, 24 h) group were significantly different from those in the control group; (**B**) Heat-map analysis of metabolites with variable importance in projection (VIP) score > 1.0. The logarithmic fold changes are shown below. GPC, sn-glycero-3-phosphocholine; (**C**) The loading plots from orthogonal partial least-squares discriminant analysis (OPLS-DA) for SpD metabolites compared with the control group.

To interpret metabolic changes, correlation networks were generated according to Pearson's correlation coefficients ($|r| > 0.9$) between metabolites, in a pair-wise fashion. In untreated controls, acetate shared 28 correlations and GPC shared one correlation with other metabolites. Upon SpD treatment, the number of correlations with acetate decreased to eight metabolites, while the number of metabolites correlating with GPC increased to 11 (Figure 6A,B). Pathway enrichment analyses showed that various metabolic processes, including inositol phosphate metabolism, glycerolipid metabolism, and glutathione metabolism, were involved in the SpD treatment effects (Figure 6C and Figure S4).

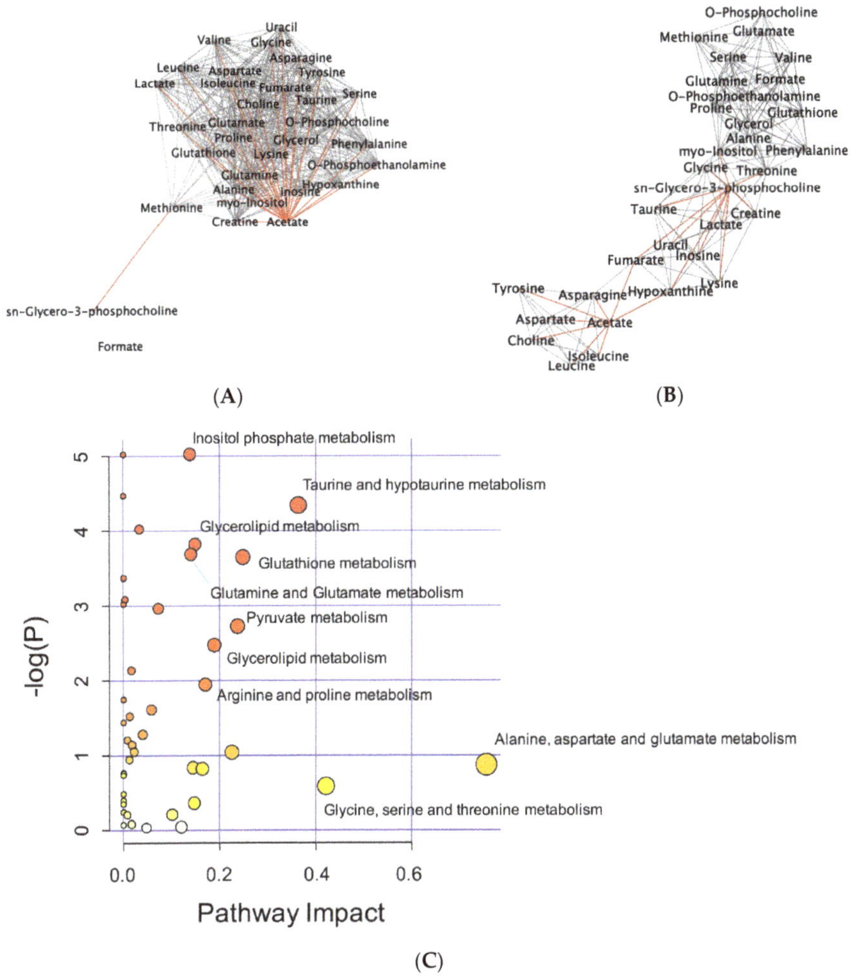

Figure 6. Network analysis of metabolites altered by SpD (10 μM, 24 h) treatment of AC16 cells. Networks of metabolites according to their Pearson's correlation coefficients were drawn using Cytoscape program. The networks with significantly increased GPC and decreased acetate are marked as red lines. (**A**) control and (**B**) SpD-treated cell metabolites; and, (**C**) Pathway impact analysis shows the most affected metabolic pathways affected by SpD. Varying colors from yellow to red represent metabolites' significance in the data.

2.4. Glutathione Metabolism in AC16 Cells Was Significantly Influenced by SpD Treatment

The integration of the metabolomic and proteomic data was carried out by Integrated Molecular Pathway Level Analysis (IMPaLa) to identify significantly influenced pathways from SpD-treated AC16 cells. The KEGG database showed that VIP > 1.0 metabolites were related to nine over-represented pathways, including glutathione metabolism, protein digestion and absorption, gap junction, and sulfur metabolism (Table 2). The related genes and metabolites are presented in Table S1. The directions of changes in the metabolite-specified proteins are listed in Table 3.

Table 2. Pathways determined from integration of metabolomic and proteomic data of SpD treated AC16 cells. Identified proteins and metabolites were analyzed using Integrated Molecular Pathway Level Analysis (IMPaLA) for pathway enrichment.

Pathway	No. of Overlapping Genes	No. of Genes in Pathway	No. of Overlapping Metabolites	No. of Metabolites in Pathway	*p*-Value	*q*-Value
Glutathione metabolism	12	54 (54)	2	38 (38)	8×10^{-6}	4×10^{-4}
Protein digestion and absorption	12	90 (90)	3	47 (47)	3×10^{-5}	9×10^{-4}
Gap junction	16	88 (88)	1	11 (11)	7×10^{-5}	0.002
Sulfur metabolism	4	10 (10)	2	33 (33)	8×10^{-5}	0.002
Aminoacyl-tRNA biosynthesis	12	66 (66)	2	52 (52)	9×10^{-5}	0.002
Choline metabolism in cancer	12	99 (99)	2	11 (11)	1×10^{-4}	0.002
Central carbon metabolism in cancer	11	65 (65)	2	37 (37)	1×10^{-4}	0.003
Long-term depression	9	60 (60)	1	9 (9)	0.003	0.033
Long-term potentiation	9	67 (67)	1	7 (7)	0.004	0.043

Table 3. Direction of log (FC) of metabolite-specified genes/proteins in SpD/Dox treated AC16.

Pathway	Gene	Direction of Log(FC) vs. Control			Protein
		SpD	Dox	Dox and SpD	
Glutathione metabolism	TXNDC12	DOWN	DOWN	UP	Thioredoxin domain-containing protein 12
Protein digestion and absorption	COL4A1	DOWN	DOWN	UP	Collagen alpha-1(IV) chain
	COL5A2	DOWN	DOWN	UP	Collagen alpha-2(V) chain
Gap junction	MAPK3	DOWN	UP	DOWN	Mitogen-activated protein kinase
	MAP2K1	UP	DOWN	UP	Dual specificity mitogen-activated protein kinase kinase 1
Sulfur metabolism	BPNT1	DOWN	DOWN	UP	3′(2′),5′-bisphosphate nucleotidase 1
Aminoacyl-tRNA biosynthesis	FARSB	DOWN	DOWN	UP	Phenylalanine–tRNA ligase beta subunit
	TARS	UP	UP	DOWN	Threonine–tRNA ligase, cytoplasmic
Choline metabolism in cancer	MAP2K1	UP	DOWN	UP	Dual specificity mitogen-activated protein kinase kinase 1
	AKT2	DOWN	UP	UP	RAC-beta serine/threonine-protein kinase
	RAC1	DOWN	DOWN	UP	Isoform B of Ras-related C3 botulinum toxin substrate 1
	RHEB	DOWN	UP	UP	GTP-binding protein Rheb
	MAPK3	DOWN	UP	DOWN	Mitogen-activated protein kinase
Central carbon metabolism in cancer	MAP2K1	UP	DOWN	UP	Dual specificity mitogen-activated protein kinase kinase 1
	PDHB	UP	DOWN	DOWN	Isoform 2 of Pyruvate dehydrogenase E1 component subunit beta, mitochondrial
	MTOR	UP	DOWN	UP	Serine/threonine-protein kinase mTOR
	AKT2	DOWN	UP	UP	RAC-beta serine/threonine-protein kinase
	MAPK3	DOWN	UP	DOWN	Mitogen-activated protein kinase
Long-term depression	MAP2K1	UP	DOWN	UP	Dual specificity mitogen-activated protein kinase kinase 1
	MAPK3	DOWN	UP	DOWN	Mitogen-activated protein kinase
Long-term potentiation	MAP2K1	UP	DOWN	UP	Dual specificity mitogen-activated protein kinase kinase 1
	CAMK2D	DOWN	UP	UP	

2.5. *SpD Functioned as an Antioxidant in AC16 Cells*

To test the antioxidant ability of SpD, oxidative stress was induced in AC16 cells using H_2O_2 or cobalt chloride with high glucose for 24 h. The DCF-DA fluorescence showed that SpD treatment reduced ROS in AC16 cells (Figure 7).

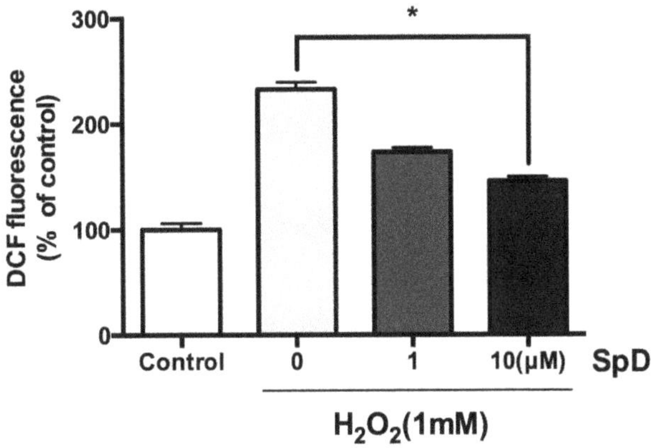

(**A**)

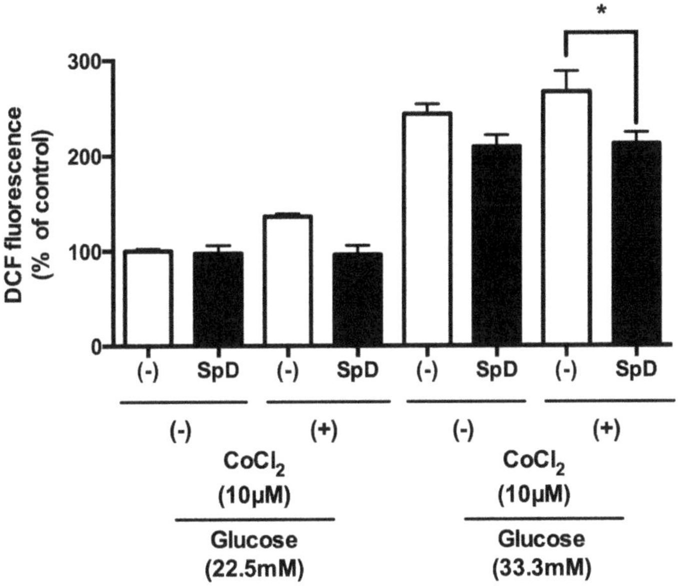

(**B**)

Figure 7. SpD showed antioxidant activity in AC16 cells treated with H_2O_2 or cobalt chloride and hyperglycemic stress. (**A**) Reactive oxygen species generation was induced in AC16 cells using 1 mM H_2O_2 and SpD (0–10 μM) was co-treated for 24 h. * $p < 0.05$ compared with 1mM H_2O_2 group without SpD; (**B**) Cobalt chloride (a hypoxia-mimetic agent) and hyperglycemia (33.3 mM glucose in media) were applied to AC16 cells. The cells were incubated with ′,7′-dichlorofluorescein diacetate (DCF-DA) (20 μM) for 20 min at 37 °C and the intensity of fluorescence was measured at 485 nm. * $p < 0.05$ compared with no SpD treated group.

2.6. SpD Increased Mitochondrial ATP Production and Oxygen Consumption

SpD treatment increased intracellular ATP production and the oxygen consumption rate (OCR) in AC16 cells (Figure 8A,B). In addition, SpD treatment increased ATP production in H_2O_2-treated cells (Figure 8C). Co-treatment with doxorubicin (0.1 μM) and SpD for 24 h increased ATP production as compared to doxorubicin treatment alone (Figure 8D). In our study, SpD showed enhanced antioxidant capacity when compared with equimolar echinochrome A (Figure S6).

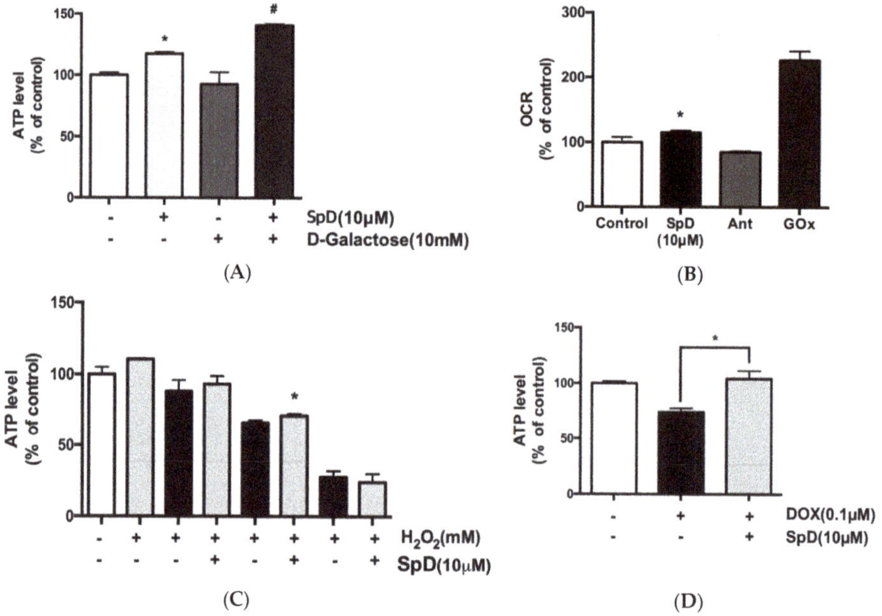

Figure 8. SpD caused increased ATP production and oxygen consumption rate (OCR) in AC16 cells. (**A**) SpD (10 μM) increased ATP production in AC16 cells. D-galactose (10 mM) was added to reduce cytosolic glycolytic ATP production. By changing energy metabolism in cardiomyocytes by replacing glucose with galactose, high concentrations of galactose could prevent ATP production except that of mitochondria by oxidative phosphorylation (OXPHOS); (**B**) SpD (10 μM) increased OCR. Antimycin A (Ant, 1 μM, a Complex III inhibitor) was used as a cell-based negative control and glucose oxidase (GOx, 1 mg/mL) was used as a cell-free positive control. (**C**) SpD increased ATP levels under H_2O_2 induced oxidative stress. (**D**) SpD increased ATP production in the presence of doxorubicin (0.1 μM). * $p < 0.05$ compared with untreated controls, # $p < 0.05$ compared with the D-galactose-treated group.

2.7. SpD Protected against Doxorubicin-Induced Mitochondrial Damage in AC16 Cells

Using tetramethylrhodamine (TMRE) and rhodamine-2 (rhod-2) staining, we compared mitochondrial membrane potential and mitochondrial Ca^{2+} in doxorubicin and SpD-treated AC16 cells (Figure 9). Doxorubicin treatment for 24 h decreased the TMRE intensity of AC16 cells in a dose-dependent manner. The doxorubicin-treated cells also showed increased cytosolic diffusion of rhod-2. We treated AC16 cells with 10 μM of SpD in the presence of 0.1–1.0 μM doxorubicin. SpD treatment attenuated the loss of mitochondrial membrane potential that is induced by doxorubicin (Figure 9A,B). SpD treatment reduced the cytosolic overload of mitochondrial Ca^{2+} in doxorubicin-treated cells (Figure 9C,D).

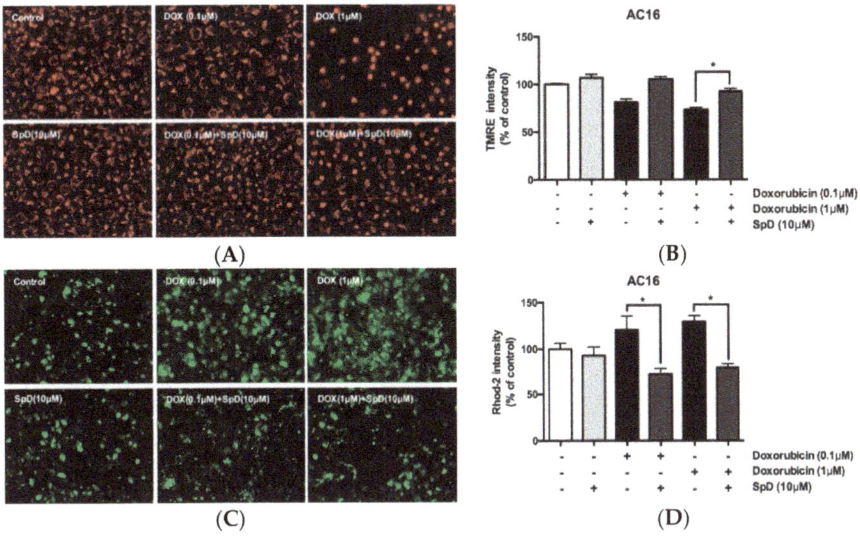

Figure 9. SpD attenuated doxorubicin-induced mitochondrial membrane potential and mitochondrial calcium changes in AC16 cells. (**A**) Mitochondrial membrane potential ($\Delta\psi_m$) in AC16 cells was indicated by TMRE fluorescence. The cells were treated with doxorubicin (0.1–1.0 μM) with/without SpD (10 μM); (**B**) The intensity of tetramethylrhodamine (TMRE) staining was measured using fluorometry at $550_{Ex}/590_{Em}$ nm. Doxorubicin decreased mitochondrial membrane potential in a dose-dependent manner. Co-treatment with SpD attenuated the membrane potential loss; (**C**) Mitochondrial calcium was localized using rhod-2, a selective indicator for mitochondrial Ca^{2+}; and, (**D**) The intensity of rhod-2 was measured at $552_{Ex}/581_{Em}$ nm. Doxorubicin induced diffusion of mitochondrial Ca^{2+} to the cytosolic space but SpD co-treatment attenuated the Ca^{2+} diffusion. * $p < 0.05$ compared with the doxorubicin-treated group.

2.8. SpD Did Not Interfere with the Anticancer Effects of Doxorubicin in MCF-7 Cells

SpD did not inhibit the cytotoxic activity of doxorubicin in MCF-7 cells (Figure 10). Human breast cancer MCF-7 cells and human cervical cancer HeLa cells showed reduced cell viability after treatment with SpD above 100 μM (Figure 10A and Figure S7A). When the SpD/doxorubicin co-treated cells were compared with the cells that were treated with doxorubicin alone, there were no significant differences in ROS level (Figure 10B), loss of mitochondrial membrane potential (Figure 10C,D), or Ca^{2+} overload (Figure 10E,F). Similar experiments using the HeLa human cervical cancer cell line showed the same lack of inhibition of cytotoxicity (Figure S7). Interestingly, SpD treatment inhibited cell migration in a wound healing test (Figure S8).

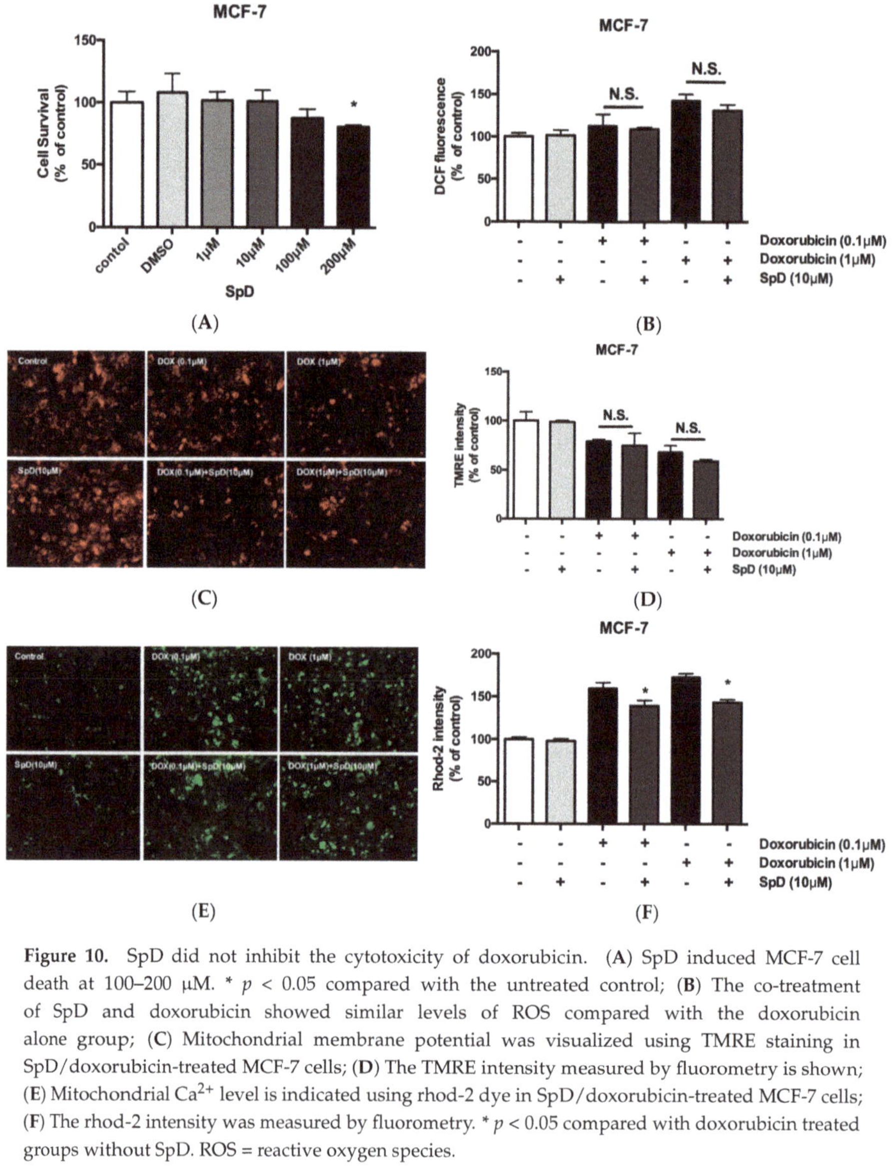

Figure 10. SpD did not inhibit the cytotoxicity of doxorubicin. (**A**) SpD induced MCF-7 cell death at 100–200 μM. * $p < 0.05$ compared with the untreated control; (**B**) The co-treatment of SpD and doxorubicin showed similar levels of ROS compared with the doxorubicin alone group; (**C**) Mitochondrial membrane potential was visualized using TMRE staining in SpD/doxorubicin-treated MCF-7 cells; (**D**) The TMRE intensity measured by fluorometry is shown; (**E**) Mitochondrial Ca^{2+} level is indicated using rhod-2 dye in SpD/doxorubicin-treated MCF-7 cells; (**F**) The rhod-2 intensity was measured by fluorometry. * $p < 0.05$ compared with doxorubicin treated groups without SpD. ROS = reactive oxygen species.

3. Discussion

There have been many efforts to overcome the cardiotoxicity of doxorubicin in cancer treatment. The IC_{50} (drug concentration required to inhibit cell growth by 50%) of doxorubicin for breast cancer cell lines has been reported to be between 1–4 μM after 24 h treatment (IC_{50} = 1 μM for MCF-10F; 4 μM for MCF-7; and, 1 μM for MDA-MB-231 cells) [19]. We used 10 μM of SpD, which induced no significant viability changes in either cardiomyocytes or cancer cells. From animal models using Histochrome® (echinochrome A), 1–10 mg/kg of doses have been reported to act as antioxidant in cardiomyocytes, which approximately correspond to 3–30 μM [20]. In our study, echinochrome A and SpD showed cardioprotective activity when treated with 0.1 μM doxorubicin. In equimolar treatment,

SpD showed better antioxidant activity and ATP production than echinochrome A. It might be reasonable to assume that cell viability decreases with increased doxorubicin incubation time. However, lower concentrations (<0.25 μM) of doxorubicin often show a low dose–time response relationship in cancer cells [21]. Cardiomyocytes and cancer cells have different mechanisms of doxorubicin-induced apoptosis. In cardiomyocytes, doxorubicin induces apoptosis by a H_2O_2-mediated mechanism, which is largely independent of p53 activation. In contrast, the p53 tumor suppressor plays an important role in doxorubicin-induced apoptosis in cancer cells [22–24].

Univariate analyses, such as fold change comparison, *t*-test, and volcano plot suggest overall shapes of measured data and multivariate analyses, including PCA, PLS-DA, and OPLS-DA, often reveal the latent structure of the data. When quantitatively analyzing multi-parametric metabolite responses, it is critical to specify all of the independent and dependent variables to be included [25]. In biological systems, metabolites are the end product of enzymatic and other protein activity, and therefore they are not independent from biological interactions. In our study, correlation network analysis and pathway enrichment analysis of VIP > 1.0 metabolites (e.g., GPC, acetate) showed that glycerolipid metabolism, glutathione metabolism, and pyruvate metabolism were significantly affected by SpD treatment in cardiomyocyte [26]. In addition to production during ethanol metabolism, acetate is transported into cells by proteins of the monocarboxylate transporter family or it is generated intracellularly by protein deacetylases and acetyl-CoA hydrolases [27,28]. In the cytosol, CoA is acetylated by acetyl-CoA synthetase to produce acetyl-CoA. In contrast, in mitochondria, acetyl-CoA is produced through the pyruvate dehydrogenase complex reactions. Acetyl-CoA participates in the citric acid cycle and β-oxidation of fatty acids to produce cellular energy (e.g., ATP). In addition to increased acetate consumption, SpD might increase cytosolic glycolysis and entrance of glutamate into the citric acid cycle, which could be shown by an increased lactate concentration and increased ratio of glutamate to glutamine (from 20.9 to 35.3; calculated as shown in Table 1). SpD treatment increased the accumulation of cytosolic osmolytes such as GPC, myo-inositol, and free amino acids (e.g., taurine and glycine), which are critical for the viability of cells. The integrated analysis with mass spectrometry based proteomics indicated that the glutathione metabolism of AC16 cells was most affected by SpD treatment. Since we measured the reduced form of glutathione (GSH) using Chenomx NMR Suit 7.1, the increased concentration of glutathione represents the increase of GSH $_{\text{reduced glutathione}}$/GSSG $_{\text{oxidized glutathione}}$ ratio. Using the luciferase mediated method, we confirmed the increase of GSH/GSSG ratio in a dose-dependent manner (Figure S9).

Based on the acquired results, we hypothesized that SpD mainly exerted its function as antioxidant in the process of protection of cardiomyocytes against the cytotoxicity of doxorubicin. Since the cytotoxicity of doxorubicin on cardiomyocytes is known to be based on ROS increase, we tested SpD activity in ROS generating environments. We tested 1 mM H_2O_2 concentration, which might be increased by constitutively active NADPH oxidase 4 (NOX4) [29]. In addition, we assessed the antioxidant ability of SpD in cobalt chloride and hyperglycemic condition. The hypoxia mimetic cobalt chloride and hyperglycemic concentrations of glucose (33.3 mM) are known to increase intracellular ROS [30–34]. Hyperglycemia induces hypoxia-induced cell death via the influx of calcium in diabetic cardiomyopathy [35–37]. Oxidative stress might cause cardiac mitochondrial dysfunction, leading to cell death [38,39].

Since the integrated analysis that is located the mitochondrial proteins clustered together at SpD treatment, we had to focus the mitochondrial ATP production by SpD treatment. To differentiate ATP production from the cytosol versus mitochondria, we added D-galactose (10 mM) to the culture media. By competing with glucose in the cytosol, D-galactose reduces cytosolic glycolysis, resulting in decreased cytosolic ATP production. Galactokinase produces galactose 1-phosphate from galactose, utilizing ATP. Uridine diphosphate (UDP)-galactose 4-epimerase converts UDP-glucose and galactose 1-phosphate into UDP-galactose and glucose 1-phosphate, respectively. Galactose participates in glycolysis by consuming ATP and reducing cytosolic glycolysis rates [40–42]. SpD treatment increased

ATP production, even in 10 mM galactose media, which suggested the enhancement of mitochondrial ATP production with increased OCR.

In cardiomyocytes, doxorubicin has been known to induce oxidized state in mitochondrial redox potential to trigger mitochondrial depolarization and elevated calcium levels, which suppresses ATP production via oxidative phosphorylation.

As the mitochondrial dysfunction occurs, the cells are subjected to ATP depletion and become more dependent on ADP metabolism to compensate the ATP/ADP ratio [43]. In our study, the SpD treatment did not inhibit the anticancer activity of doxorubicin while protecting cardiomyocytes at identical concentration via increasing ATP production. Our approaches might provide some clues for the potential cardioprotective mechanisms of SpD in a combination therapy with doxorubicin. Nevertheless, further studies are still needed for evaluation of the drug.

4. Materials and Methods

4.1. Cell Culture and Treatment

Human cardiomyocyte cell line AC16 were purchased from Merch Company (SCC 109). Rat cardiomyocyte cell line H9c2 (CRL-1466), human breast cancer cell line MCF-7 (HTB-22), and human cervical cancer cell line HeLa (CCL-2) were purchased from America Tissue Type Collection (ATCC, Bethesda, Rockville, MD, USA). Cells were routinely cultured in Dulbecco's modified Eagle's medium (DMEM) containing 25 mmol/L glucose and L-glutamine (Sigma, St. Louis, MO, USA) and 10% fetal bovine serum (FBS) (HyClone, Logan, UT, USA). Cells were maintained at 37 °C and 5% CO_2. For 10 mM galactose DMEM, D-galactose (Sigma, St. Louis, MO, USA) was added to the media. Spinochrome D (SpD, purity 98%) was isolated from the sea urchin *Scaphechinus mirabilis*, as described in [44], as the red powder with m.p. >320 °C and spectral characteristics, as in [45].

4.1.1. Cell Viability Assay

Cells were seeded in 96-well plates at 2×10^4 cells/well until adherent. Cells were treated with SpD for 24 h and then 10 µL of Cell Counting Kit-8 reagent (CCK-8, Dojindo Molecular Technologies, Kyushu, Japan) was added into each well for 20–30 min at 37 °C. The absorbance was read using a SpectraMax microplate reader (Molecular Devices, San Jose, CA, USA) at 450 nm.

4.1.2. Intracellular ATP Measurement

The ATP levels that are produced by cardiomyocytes were measured by the Luciferin-Luciferase reaction, according to the manufacturer's instructions (Cayman Chemicals, Ann Arbor, MI, USA). Cells were plated at 2×10^4 cells/well in 96-well plates and incubated with test compounds at 37 °C and 5% CO_2 for 24 h. Cells were lysed using 50 µL of lysis buffer (Triton X100; 0.1%), mixed with 50 µL of ATP measurement solution containing Luciferin-Luciferase, and then incubated at room temperature for 10–15 min. The luminescence was read using a luminometer (SpectraMax M2e; Molecular Devices, Sunnyvale, CA, USA) and expressed as relative light units. The ATP levels of the control and drug-treated samples were compared to ensure that the reading was exclusive to the ATP produced by drug-treated cardiomyocytes.

4.1.3. Oxygen Consumption Ratio (OCR) Measurement

The OCR in cardiomyocytes was measured using a MitoXpress® probe (Cayman Chemicals, Ann Arbor, MI, USA) according to the manufacturer's instructions. Cells were plated at 2×10^4 cells/well in 96-well plates and incubated with SpD at 37 °C and 5% CO_2 for 24 h. After replacing the spent media with 160 µL of 10% FBS-DMEM containing SpD, 10 µL of MitoXpress® Xtra Solution, and 100 µL of mineral oil were added to all wells. The plates were incubated at 37 °C and 5% CO_2 for 10–20 min and then the fluorescence was read at 380 nm excitation/650 nm emission on a fluorometer with a delay time of 100 µs (SpectraMax M2e).

4.1.4. Intracellular ROS Levels

The ROS levels were measured using 2′,7′-dichlorofluorescein diacetate (DCF-DA) (Sigma-Aldrich). Cells were plated at 2 × 10^4 cells/well in 96-well plates and incubated with test compounds at 37 °C and 5% CO_2 for 24 h. Subsequently, the cells were washed three times with phosphate-buffered saline (PBS) and incubated in the dark with 20 μM DCF-DA for 30 min at 37 °C. The cells were washed twice with PBS. The fluorescence was measured using a fluorometer at 485 nm excitation/535 nm emission.

4.1.5. Measurement of Mitochondrial Membrane Potential

Mitochondrial membrane potential was measured using tetramethylrhodamine (TMRE; Thermo Fisher Scientific, Scotts Valley, CA, USA). Cells were incubated with 200 nM TMRE in the dark for 30 min at 37 °C and 5% CO_2. After washing, the fluorescence was measured at 550 nm excitation/590 nm emission and cells were imaged using a fluorescence microscope (Olympus, IX71; Olympus, Tokyo, Japan).

4.1.6. Measurement of Mitochondrial Calcium

Mitochondrial calcium was measured using rhod-2/AM (TMRE; Thermo Fisher Scientific). Cells were incubated with 1 μM rhod-2 for 30 min. After PBS washing, the fluorescence was measured at 552 nm excitation/581 nm emission and cells were imaged using a fluorescence microscope.

4.1.7. Cell Migration Assay

Scratch wound assays were used for cancer cell mobility analyses. MCF-7 and HeLa cells were seeded into 25-well cell culture plates at a concentration of 2 × 10^4 cells and were maintained in 10% FBS-DMEM until 70–80% confluent. The scratch was carefully made using a 20P sterile pipette tip. The remaining cellular debris was gently removed with PBS. The wounded monolayer was incubated in 10% FBS-DMEM containing 10 μM SpD for 24 h. The cell migration was observed under 4× by using a phase contrast microscope.

4.2. LC-MS/MS Analysis and Database Searching

The trypsinized peptides from 50 μg of SpD-treated cell supernatant were analyzed using an LTQ-Orbitrap Velos^{TM} mass spectrometer coupled with an EASY-nLC II (Thermo Fisher Scientific, Waltham, MA, USA). The Uniprot human database was used for peptide searching. The protein identification was confirmed if the normalized fold change (FC) was higher than 1.30 (upregulated) or less than 0.77 (downregulated). The confidence level (CI) was 95% based on pair-wise analyses as compared with untreated controls. Relative peptide abundance was quantified with Scaffold using the Top 3 total ion chromatogram method. The differentially expressed proteins were categorized into Gene Ontology terms, i.e., biological process, cellular component, and molecular function.

4.3. ^{1}H-NMR Metabolomics

The high-resolution magic-angle spinning nuclear magnetic resonance (HR-MAS NMR) spectra were recorded using an Agilent 600 MHz spectrometer that was equipped with a 4 mm gHX NanoProbe (Agilent Technologies, Santa Clara, CA, USA). All spectra were acquired at 600.167 MHz. The acquisition time was 1.703 s, relaxation delay was 1 s, and a total of 128 scans was obtained. The Carr-Purcell-Meiboom-Gill (CPMG) pulse sequence was used for the suppression of water and compounds with high molecular mass. For data processing, Chenomx NMR Suit 7.1 professional with the Chenomx 600 MHz library database were used (Chenomx Inc., Edmonton, AB, Canada). The bin size for spectra was 0.001 ppm. The binning data were normalized to the total area. PCA, partial least-squares discriminant analysis (PLS-DA), and orthogonal partial least-squares discriminant analysis (OPLS-DA) were performed using SIMCA-P+ 12.0 (Umetrics, Malmö, Sweden).

For visualization of VIP scores of metabolites and Metabolic Set Enrichment Analysis, web-based software MetaboAnalyst 3.0 (http://www.metaboanalyst.ca) was used.

4.4. Pathway Enrichment Analysis

Integrated Molecular Pathway Level Analysis (IMPaLa, http://impala.molgen.mpg.de/) was used to specify the pathways that are affected by SpD. Only VIP > 1.0 metabolites and Log2(FC) > 1.2 proteins were considered. Search Tool for the Retrieval of Interacting Genes/Proteins (STRING, https://string-db.org) and Cytoscape (downloaded at https://cytoscape.org) were used for clustering molecular networks.

5. Conclusions

The present study investigated the effect of SpD on doxorubicin-treated cardiomyocytes through an integration of metabolic and proteomic analyses. Univariate and multivariate analyses of ^{1}H-NMR spectroscopy data identified the potentially affected metabolites and groups of proteins from SpD-treated cardiomyocytes. Based on the ^{1}H-NMR data, SpD increased glutathione, which regulates intracellular ROS stress. In addition, SpD treatment increased cytosolic and mitochondrial ATP production in cardiomyocytes, which was significantly correlated with increased lactate and decreased acetate levels. Co-treatment with SpD protected doxorubicin-treated cardiomyocytes, reducing the mitochondrial damage of doxorubicin. In contrast, SpD did not inhibit the cytotoxicity of doxorubicin in cancer cells. The integrated metabolomics and proteomics data suggest the involvement of the Akt/mTOR signaling pathway by which SpD might protect cardiomyocytes (Table 3). However, further study is still needed to verify these relationships.

Supplementary Materials: The following are available online at http://www.mdpi.com/1660-3397/17/1/2/s1, Figure S1. Spinochrome D (SpD) showed no harmful effect on H9c2 rat cardiac cells. H9c2 rat embryonic cardiomyocytes were treated with 0–200 μM of SpD for 24 h (2 × 104 cells/well, 96-well plates). The cell viability was measured using CCK-8 assay. SpD did not affect on the cell viability of cardiomyocytes. * mark indicates $p < 0.05$ compared with control. Figure S2. (A) PLS-DA from metabolites of SpD treated AC16 cells. (B) VIP > 0.1 metabolites from SpD treated AC16 cells from PLS-DA. Figure S3. OPLS-DA from metabolites of SpD treated AC16 cells ($R2X = 0.333$; $R2Y = 0.937$; $Q2 = 0.597$). Figure S4. Metabolite sets enrichment overview in SpD treated AC16 cells. Table S1. Genes and metabolites specified for the assigned pathways. Figure S5. STRING analysis revealed that metabolism associated proteins forms clusters around mitochondria (marked as red circles). Figure S6. Spinochrome D (SpD) showed enhanced antioxidant capacity compared with echinochrome A in AC16 and H9c2 cells. (A) SpD and echinochrome A showed no harmful effect on AC16 cells (2 × 104 cells/well, 96-well plate, 24 h). (B) SpD and echinochrome A protected AC16 cells against the cytotoxicity of doxorubicin. (C) SpD showed statistically enhanced antioxidant activity compared with echinochrome A. SpD produced enhanced ATP production in (D) AC16 cells and (E) H9c2 cells compared with echinochrome A. (F) SpD and echinochrome A showed enhanced OCR in AC16 cells. * mark indicates $p < 0.05$ compared with control. Figure S7. SpD did not inhibit the cytotoxicity of doxorubicin. (A) Mitochondrial membrane potential and mitochondrial calcium was visualized using TMRE and rhod-2 staining in MCF-7 cells. Doxorubicin decreased TMRE intensity and increased rhod-2 intensity in dose-dependent manner. The co-treatment of SpD (10 μM) did not affect doxorubicin-induced tendency of fluorescence intensity. (B) The fluorescence was measured using fluorescence spectrometer. SpD co-treatment did not affect the intensity of TMRE, rhod-2, and DCF-DA in MCF-7 cells. (C) TMRE and rhod-2 fluorescence images from HeLa cells with doxorubicin/SpD. (D) The fluorescence measures indicated that SpD did not affect the intensity of TMRE, rhod-2, and DCF-DA in HeLa cells. Figure S8. SpD inhibited cell migration of cancer cells. 2 × 104 cells of MCF-7 and HeLa were plated in 25-well cell culture plates and scratch wounds were made with 200 μL pipet tips. SpD was treated in 10–200 μM concentrations and incubated for 24 h. Figure S9. Total glutathione and ratio of reduced glutathione to oxidized glutathione (GSH/GSSG). (A) Total glutathione ratio (% of control) from SpD treated AC16 cells. (B) Ratio of reduced glutathione (GSH) to oxidized (GSSG) glutathione normalized by total glutathione concentration from control. The GSH/GSSG assay was measured using GSH/GSSG-Glo^{TM} Assay (Promega, WI, USA) according to the product's manual. * and ** mark indicates $p < 0.05$, $p < 0.01$ compared with control, respectively. Supplementary Information 2 lists all proteins detected by mass-spectrometry of SpD treated AC16 cells.

Author Contributions: C.S.Y. and H.K.K. conducted the experiments, tests, and data analyses. N.P.M., E.A.V., and S.A.F. isolated and purified the SpD and provided advice for the omics analysis. C.S.Y., H.K.K., V.A.S., and J.H. summarized the work and wrote the manuscript.

Funding: This research was funded by the Ministry of Education, Science, and Technology (2010-0020224, 2018R1D1A1A09081767, and 2017K1A3A1A49070056).

Acknowledgments: This study was supported by grants from the Priority Research Centers Program, Basic Science Research Program, and International Research & Development Program through the National Research Foundation of Korea (NRF). The study was carried out under support of the Ministry of Education and Science of the Russian Federation (RFMEFI61317X0076) using the equipment of the Collective Facilities Center (The Far Eastern Center for Structural Molecular Research (NMR/MS) PIBOC FEB RAS).

Conflicts of Interest: The authors declare no conflict of interest.

References

1. Lebedev, A.V.; Levitskaya, E.L.; Tikhonova, E.V.; Ivanova, M.V. Antioxidant properties, autooxidation, and mutagenic activity of echinochrome a compared with its etherified derivative. *Biochemistry* **2001**, *66*, 885–893. [PubMed]
2. Lebedev, A.V.; Ivanova, M.V.; Levitsky, D.O. Echinochrome, a naturally occurring iron chelator and free radical scavenger in artificial and natural membrane systems. *Life Sci.* **2005**, *76*, 863–875. [CrossRef] [PubMed]
3. Jeong, S.H.; Kim, H.K.; Song, I.S.; Lee, S.J.; Ko, K.S.; Rhee, B.D.; Kim, N.; Mishchenko, N.P.; Fedoryev, S.A.; Stonik, V.A.; et al. Echinochrome A protects mitochondrial function in cardiomyocytes against cardiotoxic drugs. *Mar. Drugs* **2014**, *12*, 2922–2936. [CrossRef]
4. Pozharitskaya, O.N.; Shikov, A.N.; Makarova, M.N.; Ivanova, S.A.; Kosman, V.M.; Makarov, V.G.; Bazgier, V.; Berka, K.; Otyepka, M.; Ulrichova, J. Antiallergic effects of pigments isolated from green sea urchin (*Strongylocentrotus droebachiensis*) shells. *Planta Med.* **2013**, *79*, 1698–1704. [CrossRef]
5. Anderson, H.A.; Mathieson, J.W.; Thomson, R.H. Distribution of spinochrome pigments in echinoids. *Comp. Biochem. Physiol.* **1969**, *28*, 333–345. [CrossRef]
6. Nagaoka, S.; Shiraishi, J.; Utsuyama, M.; Seki, S.; Takemura, T.; Kitagawa, M.; Sawabe, M.; Takubo, K.; Hirokawa, K. Poor prognosis of colorectal cancer in patients over 80 years old is associated with down-regulation of tumor suppressor genes. *J. Clin. Gastroenterol.* **2003**, *37*, 48–54. [CrossRef] [PubMed]
7. Balaneva, N.N.; Shestak, O.P.; Anufriev, V.F.; Novikov, V.L. Synthesis of Spinochrome D, A Metabolite of Various Sea-Urchin Species. *Chem. Nat. Compd.* **2016**, *52*, 213–217. [CrossRef]
8. Arcamone, F.; Cassinelli, G.; Fantini, G.; Grein, A.; Orezzi, P.; Pol, C.; Spalla, C. Adriamycin, 14-hydroxydaunomycin, a new antitumor antibiotic from S. peucetius var. caesius. *Biotechnol. Bioeng.* **1969**, *11*, 1101–1110. [CrossRef]
9. Cortes-Funes, H.; Coronado, C. Role of anthracyclines in the era of targeted therapy. *Cardiovasc. Toxicol.* **2007**, *7*, 56–60. [CrossRef]
10. Takemura, G.; Fujiwara, H. Doxorubicin-induced cardiomyopathy from the cardiotoxic mechanisms to management. *Prog. Cardiovasc. Dis.* **2007**, *49*, 330–352. [CrossRef]
11. Bachur, N.R.; Gee, M.V.; Friedman, R.D. Nuclear catalyzed antibiotic free radical formation. *Cancer Res.* **1982**, *42*, 1078–1081. [PubMed]
12. Sinha, B.K.; Katki, A.G.; Batist, G.; Cowan, K.H.; Myers, C.E. Adriamycin-stimulated hydroxyl radical formation in human breast tumor cells. *Biochem. Pharmacol.* **1987**, *36*, 793–796. [CrossRef]
13. Lefrak, E.A.; Pitha, J.; Rosenheim, S.; Gottlieb, J.A. A clinicopathologic analysis of adriamycin cardiotoxicity. *Cancer* **1973**, *32*, 302–314. [CrossRef]
14. Franco, Y.L.; Vaidya, T.R.; Ait-Oudhia, S. Anticancer and cardio-protective effects of liposomal doxorubicin in the treatment of breast cancer. *Breast Cancer* **2018**, *10*, 131–141. [CrossRef]
15. Thorn, C.F.; Oshiro, C.; Marsh, S.; Hernandez-Boussard, T.; McLeod, H.; Klein, T.E.; Altman, R.B. Doxorubicin pathways: Pharmacodynamics and adverse effects. *Pharmacogenet. Genom.* **2011**, *21*, 440–446. [CrossRef]
16. Siveski-Iliskovic, N.; Hill, M.; Chow, D.A.; Singal, P.K. Probucol protects against adriamycin cardiomyopathy without interfering with its antitumor effect. *Circulation* **1995**, *91*, 10–15. [CrossRef]
17. Mohamed, E.A.; Kassem, H.H. Protective effect of nebivolol on doxorubicin-induced cardiotoxicity in rats. *Arch. Med. Sci.* **2018**, *14*, 1450–1458. [CrossRef]
18. Studneva, I.; Palkeeva, M.; Veselova, O.; Molokoedov, A.; Ovchinnikov, M.; Sidorova, M.; Pisarenko, O. Protective Effects of a Novel Agonist of Galanin Receptors Against Doxorubicin-Induced Cardiotoxicity in Rats. *Cardiovasc. Toxicol.* **2018**, 1–11. [CrossRef] [PubMed]
19. Pilco-Ferreto, N.; Calaf, G.M. Influence of doxorubicin on apoptosis and oxidative stress in breast cancer cell lines. *Int. J. Oncol.* **2016**, *49*, 753–762. [CrossRef]

20. Agafonova, I.G.; Kotel'nikov, V.N.; Mischenko, N.P.; Kolosova, N.G. Evaluation of effects of histochrome and mexidol on structural and functional characteristics of the brain in senescence-accelerated OXYS rats by magnetic resonance imaging. *Bull. Exp. Biol. Med.* **2011**, *150*, 739–743. [CrossRef]
21. Al-Ghamdi, S.S. Time and dose dependent study of doxorubicin induced DU-145 cytotoxicity. *Drug Metab. Lett.* **2008**, *2*, 47–50. [CrossRef]
22. Wang, S.; Konorev, E.A.; Kotamraju, S.; Joseph, J.; Kalivendi, S.; Kalyanaraman, B. Doxorubicin induces apoptosis in normal and tumor cells via distinctly different mechanisms. intermediacy of H(2)O(2)- and p53-dependent pathways. *J. Biol. Chem.* **2004**, *279*, 25535–25543. [CrossRef]
23. Magnelli, L.; Cinelli, M.; Chiarugi, V. Phorbol esters attenuate the expression of p53 in cells treated with doxorubicin and protect TS-P53/K562 from apoptosis. *Biochem. Biophys. Res. Commun.* **1995**, *215*, 641–645. [CrossRef] [PubMed]
24. McCurrach, M.E.; Connor, T.M.; Knudson, C.M.; Korsmeyer, S.J.; Lowe, S.W. bax-deficiency promotes drug resistance and oncogenic transformation by attenuating p53-dependent apoptosis. *Proc. Natl. Acad. Sci. USA* **1997**, *94*, 2345–2349. [CrossRef] [PubMed]
25. Worley, B.; Powers, R. Multivariate Analysis in Metabolomics. *Curr. Metab.* **2013**, *1*, 92–107.
26. Kotze, H.L.; Armitage, E.G.; Sharkey, K.J.; Allwood, J.W.; Dunn, W.B.; Williams, K.J.; Goodacre, R. A novel untargeted metabolomics correlation-based network analysis incorporating human metabolic reconstructions. *BMC Syst. Biol.* **2013**, *7*, 107. [CrossRef]
27. Hosios, A.M.; Vander Heiden, M.G. Acetate metabolism in cancer cells. *Cancer Metab.* **2014**, *2*, 27. [CrossRef]
28. Knowles, S.E.; Jarrett, I.G.; Filsell, O.H.; Ballard, F.J. Production and utilization of acetate in mammals. *Biochem. J.* **1974**, *142*, 401–411. [CrossRef]
29. Rajaram, R.D.; Dissard, R.; Jaquet, V.; de Seigneux, S. Potential benefits and harms of NADPH oxidase type 4 in the kidneys and cardiovascular system. *Nephrol. Dial. Transpl.* **2018**. [CrossRef]
30. Wu, H.; Huang, S.; Chen, Z.; Liu, W.; Zhou, X.; Zhang, D. Hypoxia-induced autophagy contributes to the invasion of salivary adenoid cystic carcinoma through the HIF-1alpha/BNIP3 signaling pathway. *Mol. Med. Rep.* **2015**, *12*, 6467–6474. [CrossRef]
31. Kraskiewicz, H.; FitzGerald, U. Partial XBP1 knockdown does not affect viability of oligodendrocyte precursor cells exposed to new models of hypoxia and ischemia in vitro. *J. Neurosci. Res.* **2011**, *89*, 661–673. [CrossRef] [PubMed]
32. Chhunchha, B.; Fatma, N.; Kubo, E.; Rai, P.; Singh, S.P.; Singh, D.P. Curcumin abates hypoxia-induced oxidative stress based-ER stress-mediated cell death in mouse hippocampal cells (HT22) by controlling Prdx6 and NF-kappaB regulation. *Am. J. Physiol. Cell Physiol.* **2013**, *304*, C636–C655. [CrossRef] [PubMed]
33. Fakhruddin, S.; Alanazi, W.; Jackson, K.E. Diabetes-Induced Reactive Oxygen Species: Mechanism of Their Generation and Role in Renal Injury. *J. Diabetes Res.* **2017**, *2017*, 8379327. [CrossRef]
34. Volpe, C.M.O.; Villar-Delfino, P.H.; Dos Anjos, P.M.F.; Nogueira-Machado, J.A. Cellular death, reactive oxygen species (ROS) and diabetic complications. *Cell Death Dis.* **2018**, *9*, 119. [CrossRef]
35. Pang, Y.; Hunton, D.L.; Bounelis, P.; Marchase, R.B. Hyperglycemia inhibits capacitative calcium entry and hypertrophy in neonatal cardiomyocytes. *Diabetes* **2002**, *51*, 3461–3467. [CrossRef] [PubMed]
36. Feng, N.; Anderson, M.E. CaMKII is a nodal signal for multiple programmed cell death pathways in heart. *J. Mol. Cell Cardiol.* **2017**, *103*, 102–109. [CrossRef]
37. Singh, R.M.; Waqar, T.; Howarth, F.C.; Adeghate, E.; Bidasee, K.; Singh, J. Hyperglycemia-induced cardiac contractile dysfunction in the diabetic heart. *Heart Fail. Rev.* **2018**, *23*, 37–54. [CrossRef]
38. Adams, J.W.; Pagel, A.L.; Means, C.K.; Oksenberg, D.; Armstrong, R.C.; Brown, J.H. Cardiomyocyte apoptosis induced by Galphaq signaling is mediated by permeability transition pore formation and activation of the mitochondrial death pathway. *Circ. Res.* **2000**, *87*, 1180–1187. [CrossRef] [PubMed]

39. Diogo, C.V.; Suski, J.M.; Lebiedzinska, M.; Karkucinska-Wieckowska, A.; Wojtala, A.; Pronicki, M.; Duszynski, J.; Pinton, P.; Portincasa, P.; Oliveira, P.J.; et al. Cardiac mitochondrial dysfunction during hyperglycemia–the role of oxidative stress and p66Shc signaling. *Int. J. Biochem. Cell Biol.* **2013**, *45*, 114–122. [CrossRef]
40. Lane, R.S.; Fu, Y.; Matsuzaki, S.; Kinter, M.; Humphries, K.M.; Griffin, T.M. Mitochondrial respiration and redox coupling in articular chondrocytes. *Arthritis Res. Ther.* **2015**, *17*, 54. [CrossRef]
41. Aguer, C.; Gambarotta, D.; Mailloux, R.J.; Moffat, C.; Dent, R.; McPherson, R.; Harper, M.E. Galactose enhances oxidative metabolism and reveals mitochondrial dysfunction in human primary muscle cells. *PLoS ONE* **2011**, *6*, e28536. [CrossRef] [PubMed]
42. Kase, E.T.; Nikolic, N.; Bakke, S.S.; Bogen, K.K.; Aas, V.; Thoresen, G.H.; Rustan, A.C. Remodeling of oxidative energy metabolism by galactose improves glucose handling and metabolic switching in human skeletal muscle cells. *PLoS ONE* **2013**, *8*, e59972. [CrossRef]
43. Kuznetsov, A.V.; Margreiter, R.; Amberger, A.; Saks, V.; Grimm, M. Changes in mitochondrial redox state, membrane potential and calcium precede mitochondrial dysfunction in doxorubicin-induced cell death. *Biochim. Biophys. Acta* **2011**, *1813*, 1144–1152. [CrossRef] [PubMed]
44. Mishchenko, N.P.; Vasileva, E.A.; Fedoreev, S.A. Mirabiquinone, a new unsymmetrical binaphthoquinone from the sea urchin *Scaphechinus mirabilis*. *Tetrahedron Lett.* **2014**, *55*, 5967–5969. [CrossRef]
45. Vasileva, E.A.; Mishchenko, N.P.; Vo, H.M.; Bui, L.M.; Denisenko, V.A.; Fedoreyev, S.A. Quinoid pigments from the sea urchin *Astropyga radiata*. *Chem. Nat. Compd.* **2017**, *53*, 356–358. [CrossRef]

marine drugs

MDPI

Article

Effects of Carrageenans on Biological Properties of Echinochrome

Ekaterina V. Sokolova *, Natalia I. Menzorova, Victoria N. Davydova, Alexandra S. Kuz'mich, Anna O. Kravchenko, Natalya P. Mishchenko and Irina M. Yermak

G.B. Elyakov Pacific Institute of Bioorganic Chemistry, Far-East Branch of the Russian Academy of Sciences, Prospect 100-let Vladivostoku, 159, 690022 Vladivostok, Russia; menzor@piboc.dvo.ru (N.I.M.); vikdavidova@yandex.ru (V.N.D.); assavina@mail.ru (A.S.K.); Kravchenko_89@mail.ru (A.O.K.); mischenkonp@mail.ru (N.P.M.); imyer@mail.ru (I.M.Y.)

* Correspondence: eka9739@gmail.com; Tel.: +7-(423)2311430; Fax: +7-(423)2314050

Received: 9 October 2018; Accepted: 26 October 2018; Published: 1 November 2018

Abstract: Sea urchin pigment echinochrome A (Ech), a water-insoluble compound, is the active substance in the cardioprotective and antioxidant drug Histochrome® (PIBOC FEB RAS, Moscow, Russia). It has been established that Ech dissolves in aqueous solutions of carrageenans (CRGs). Herein, we describe the effects of different types of CRGs on some properties of Ech. Our results showed that CRGs significantly decreased the spermotoxicity of Ech, against the sea urchin *S. intermedius* sperm. Ech, as well as its complex with CRG, did not affect the division and development of early embryos of the sea urchin. Ech reduced reactive oxygen species production (ROS) in neutrophils, caused by CRG. The obtained complexes of these substances with pro- and anti-activating ROS formation properties illustrate the possibility of modulating the ROS induction, using these compounds. The CRGs stimulate the induction of anti-inflammatory IL-10 synthesis, whereas Ech inhibits this synthesis and increases the production of the pro-inflammatory cytokines IL-6 and TNFα. The inclusion of Ech, in the complex with the CRGs, decreases Ech's ability to induce the expression of pro-inflammatory cytokines, especially TNFα, and increases the induction of anti-inflammatory cytokine IL-10. Thus, CRGs modify the action of Ech, by decreasing its pro-inflammatory effect. Whereas, the Ech's protective action towards human epithelial HT-29 cells remains to be unaltered in the complex, with κ/β-CRG, under stress conditions.

Keywords: carrageenan; algae; echinochrome; reactive oxygen species; cytokines; HT-29

1. Introduction

With increasing awareness of functional properties of products from marine organisms, their attractiveness, both as a source of nutritious food items and stockpot of novel, biologically-active compounds, continuously expand [1]. The characteristic color of spines and armors of sea urchins are attributed to calcium salts of polyhydroxynaphthoquinone pigments derivatives—spinochromes and echinochromes—exhibiting a vast range of pharmacological activities. One of the most popular pigments is the echinochrome A (6-ethyl-2,3,5,7,8-pentahydroxy-1,4-naphthoquinone), which is known to be a biologically-active compound with antimicrobial, antialgal, and antioxidant activities [2]. Most of all, it has been ascertained that a treatment with echinochrome protected the mitochondrial functions in cardiomyocytes, against the acardiotoxic drugs (*tert*-Butyl hydroperoxide, sodium nitroprusside) [3]. There are controversial data in the literature, in terms of Ech's capacity to activate an immune response, some data suggest that Ech has an ability to activate inflammation, whereas others suggest that it can suppress inflammation [4,5]. Pharmacological studies in vitro and in vivo demonstrated that naphthoquinone pigments have a wide therapeutic latitude and are nontoxic, at therapeutic doses [6].

In Russia, echinochrome is produced from the sand dollar *Scaphechinus mirabilis*. It is the active substance in the cardioprotective and antioxidant drug Histochrome® (C (Ech) = 0.2 mg mL^{-1}) and is available in ampoules, permitted for subconjunctival, parabulbar, or intravenous administration [7,8]. One of the main setbacks to the wide use of Ech, is its insolubility in aqueous solutions and high susceptibility to oxidative destruction. Improvement of therapeutic efficacy of drugs can be achieved by modifying the formulation technique, for instance, by means of polymeric systems. Marine natural edible polymers have been widely used in hydrogels, drug encapsulation, and drug delivery because of their benefits, comprising such advantages as biocompatibility, biodegradability, and adhesiveness [9,10].

In order to provide a stable and biocompatible environment to the Ech, polymeric matrix systems, based on polysaccharides from red algae, have been proposed to be suitable candidates for oral delivery [11]. Polysaccharides of red algae, carrageenans (CRGs) are a class of linear galactans with alternating 1,3- and 1,4-linked galactose residues (D- and G-units). Several types of these polysaccharides were identified, based on the structure of their disaccharide repeating units, the pattern of sulfation, and the presence of 3,6-anhydrogalactose (DA-unit), as a 4-linked residue [12]. The three most industrially-exploited types, in the order of increasing sulfation degrees and decreasing gelation capabilities, respectively, are the κ-, ι- and λ- CRGs. Natural CRGs are often hybrids of more than one of these units and are composed of several carrabiose moieties, the proportions and structures of which vary with species, the life stages of seaweeds, and the ecophysiological and developmental conditions [13–15]. CRGs are widely utilized due to their excellent physical properties, such as thickening, gelling, and stabilizing effects in the food industry [16,17]. CRGs have successfully become appealing tools in immunotherapy and drug delivery, due to their immuno-active features and valuable physical properties as gelling [18,19].

Recently we have established that Ech is incorporated into the CRG supramolecular structure, which results in formation of complexes with altered Ech properties, such as decreased oxidative degradation and improved solubility. Along with the suitable physico-chemical properties, an Ech complex with CRG, in mice, revealed a high gastroprotective activity, surpassing the effect of either of the components used alone [11].

Unravelling the influence of CRGs–Ech complexes on some immunological parameters (ROS formation in phagocytic cells, the cytokine production in human whole blood model) and on human epithelial cell monolayers, will provide essential information for the rational design of CRG-based matrices for Ech delivery, for oral administration. It would also inspire the design of new approaches in assessing the modification of biological properties of biomaterials, used in delivery systems. The aim of this work was to investigate the biological properties of Ech that was included in a CRG matrix.

2. Results

CRGs were isolated by aqueous extraction from the non-fruited form of red algae *Chondrus armatus* (Gigartinaceae), *Tichocarpus crinitus* (Tichocarpaceae), and *Ahnfeltiopsis flabelliformis* (Phyllophoraceae), harvested along the Russian coast of the Japanese Sea and separated using 4% KCl into the KCl-insoluble and KCl-soluble fractions. The structures of polysaccharides were studied by ^{13}C-NMR and FT-IR-spectroscopy. The obtained spectra have been compared with the spectra of polysaccharides, which we had isolated earlier, from the above-mentioned species of algae [20–22]. The identity of the spectra indicates that the KCl-insoluble fraction form of *C. armatus*, *T. crinitus*, *A. flabelliformis*, were κ-, κ/β-, and ι/κ-types, respectively, and a KCl-soluble fraction from was *C. armatus*–λ-CRG.

The structures of disaccharide repeating units of the carrageenans and the sulfate content, as well as the average molecular weights of all the samples investigated, are summarized in Table 1. CRGs differ from each other in number and position of sulfated groups, and in the presence (κ, κ/β and ι/κ) or absence (λ) of 3,6-anhydrogalactose units (DA). The degree of sulfation decreased in the following row: $\lambda > \iota/\kappa > \kappa > \kappa/\beta$.

Table 1. The structures of disaccharides repeating units of carrageenans from algae of Gigartinaceae and Phyllophoraceae families.

Reference	Algal Species	CRG Sample	Structures of Disaccharide Repeating Units		SO_4^{2-} Contents
			3-Linked	4-Linked	
[20]	*C. armatus*	λ	G2S	D2S, 6S	26
[20]	*C. armatus*	κ	G4S	DA	22
[21]	*T. crinitus*	κ/β	G4S/G	DA/DA	19
[22]	*A. flabelliformis*	ι/κ	G4S/G4S	DA2S/DA	20

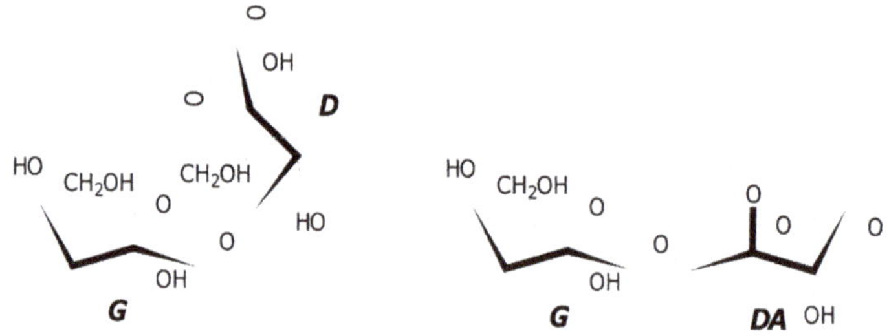

2.1. Toxicity

As a cellular model to study spermotoxic and embryotoxic properties, we used the spermatozoa and developing embryos of the sea urchin *S. intermedius*.

The spermotoxicities of Ech, CRGs, and the complexes Ech/CRGs were investigated by the Sea Urchins Sperm Cell Toxicity Test (SUSCT)-test [23,24]. These activities were determined by the degree of inhibition of the spermatozoa's ability to fertilize the sea urchin eggs. Previously, all types of CRGs (κ, λ, ι/κ) were investigated for spermotoxicity in seawater, at a concentration 50 to 200 μg mL^{-1}. The results showed that all of the studied CRGs had no toxic effect on the spermatozoa fertilization ability, at these concentrations. The current study with Ech in the concentration range from 1 to 10 μg mL^{-1} revealed that this substance exhibited spermotoxicity. The spermotoxicity of Ech was expressed in the 50% inhibition of the spermatozoa's ability to fertilize the egg-cells (IC_{50} values were of 3 μg mL^{-1}), at a sperm:egg ratio of 300:1. When the Ech was added to a solution of CRGs, with a concentration of the 100 μg mL^{-1}, the spermotoxicity of the Ech decreased significantly. The higher the concentration of the Ech, the greater was the protective effect of the CRG (Figure 1a). The protection of various CRGs types, against the spermotoxicity of the Ech (C = 3 μg mL^{-1}) was studied by the SUSCT-test, at the spermatozoa to eggs ratios of 300:1 and 150:1 (Figure 1b). From the data presented in Figure 1b, it can be seen that λ-CRG, with a higher degree of sulfation, showed a greater protective activity. This dependence of the protective effects of the CRGs on their structures, was particularly noticeable at the spermatozoa to eggs ratio of 150:1, when the sensitivity of the method was the highest.

To determine the embryotoxic effects of the Ech and its complex, with the CRG (100 μg mL^{-1}), fertilized eggs from the sea urchins were used. In a concentration range from 2–36 μg mL^{-1}, the Ech did not affect the division and development of early embryos of the sea urchin *Strongylocentrotus intermedius*, as well as its complex with the CRGs.

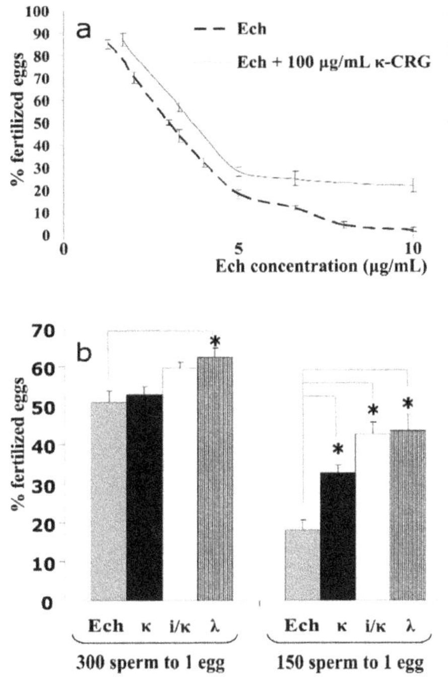

Figure 1. (**a**) The influence of Echinochrome (Ech) and its complex with the κ-carrageenans (CRGs) (100 µg mL^{-1}), on the sea urchin spermatozoa fertilizing ability (spermatozoa to eggs ratio 300:1). (**b**) The spermatozoa fertilizing ability of various types of CRGs (100 µg mL^{-1}), in the presence of Ech (3 mg mL^{-1}). * $p < 0.05$.

2.2. Reactive Oxygen Species (ROS)-Inducing Activity of the CRG and the Ech on the Human Blood Cells

The ROS induction in human neutrophils, in the presence of the Ech and its complexes with CRGs, was determined with the Ech concentration varying from 1 to 10 µg mL^{-1}. To assess the effect of the content of the polysaccharide in the complex with the Ech, on the formation of ROS, we used CRG concentrations in the range of 5 to 200 µg mL^{-1}. Thus, complexes with different CRGs/Ech ratios (5:1, 10:1, and 20:1) were prepared.

The corresponding effects were detected using a fluorescent probe and measured by means of flow cytometry (Figure 2). Lipopolysaccharide (LPS) from *E. coli* was used as a reference immunomodulator, in the current test, and the ROS production induced by the LPS, as a positive control, was approximately twice as much as the negative control (the vehicle). At low concentrations, the activity of Ech towards the ROS formation was comparable to the negative control, whereas at high concentrations its effect was lower than that of the control by 20%. The influence of the CRGs on the activation of ROS, at lower concentrations, was not significant except for the λ-CRG. In contrast, the CRGs at a concentration of 100 µg mL^{-1} intensified the induction of the ROS by up to 25–55%, relative to the negative control. The addition of the Ech to the CRGs, especially at high concentrations, resulted in significant diminishment of the ROS formation induced by the CRGs alone. The action of the complexes was compared to the negative control, where at higher concentrations, the effect of the samples was more noticeable.

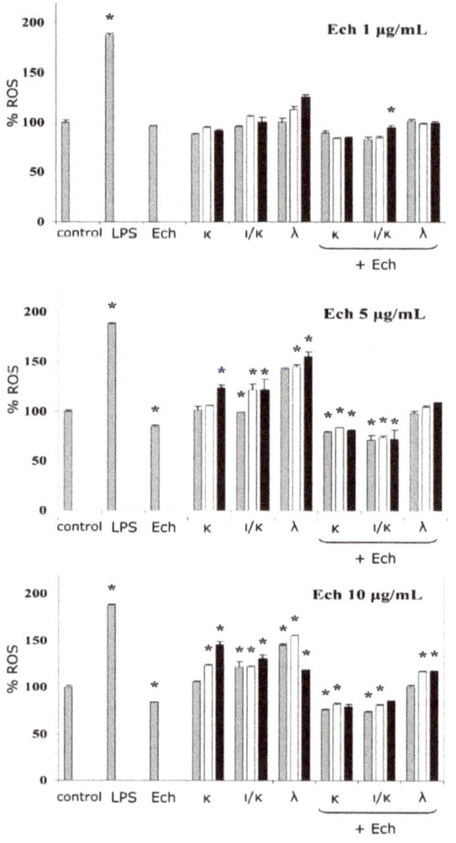

Figure 2. Neutrophils reactive oxygen species (ROS) formation in the presence of the Ech, CRGs, and their complexes. The concentration of the lipopolysaccharide (LPS) was 10 μg mL^{-1} and of the Ech was 1.0, 5.0, or 10.0 μg mL^{-1}, final value. The concentrations of the CRGs alone and in complexes with the Ech changed in the following ratios row: ■ = 5:1; □ = 10:1; ■ = 20:1. The results are expressed as % change in ROS, relative to the control (100%), * $p < 0.05$.

2.3. *IL-10-Inducing Action of the CRGs and the Ech on the Human Blood Cells*

The action of the carragenans, Ech, and their complexes on the pro-inflammatory (IL-6 and TNFα) and anti-inflammatory (IL-10) cytokines induction was conducted. In this experiment, Ech was used at one concentration, 1 μg mL^{-1} whereas, CRG concentrations individually and in complexes, varied in the following row 5.0, 10.0, and 20 μg mL^{-1}. As seen in Figure 3, κ- and λ-types (10 and 20 μg mL^{-1}) induced the expression of IL-10 in cells, by approximately 120 and 100 pg mL^{-1}, in comparison to the negative control, respectively. Ech significantly inhibited the synthesis of IL-10, reducing the induction of this anti-inflammatory cytokine by 50%, compared to the control. At the same time, the inclusion of Ech into the CRG complex increased the induction of IL-10 synthesis, compared to Ech. The greatest effect was shown by the complex of Ech with ι/κ-CRG (Figure 3). Regarding the pro-inflammatory cytokines, Ech (1 μg mL^{-1}) was a strong inductor, in comparison to the highest concentrations of the CRGs, but its action was decreased, especially in the complexes with the κ- or λ-types, by about 300 pg mL^{-1} for IL-6 and 350 pg mL^{-1} for TNFα. However, the combined action of the CRNs and the Ech complexes on the IL-6 still remained high, compared to the control. The ι/κ-CRG influenced the effect of Ech with less degree than the others, as complexes had formed. Thus, the CRGs modified the activity of Ech by decreasing its pro-inflammatory effect.

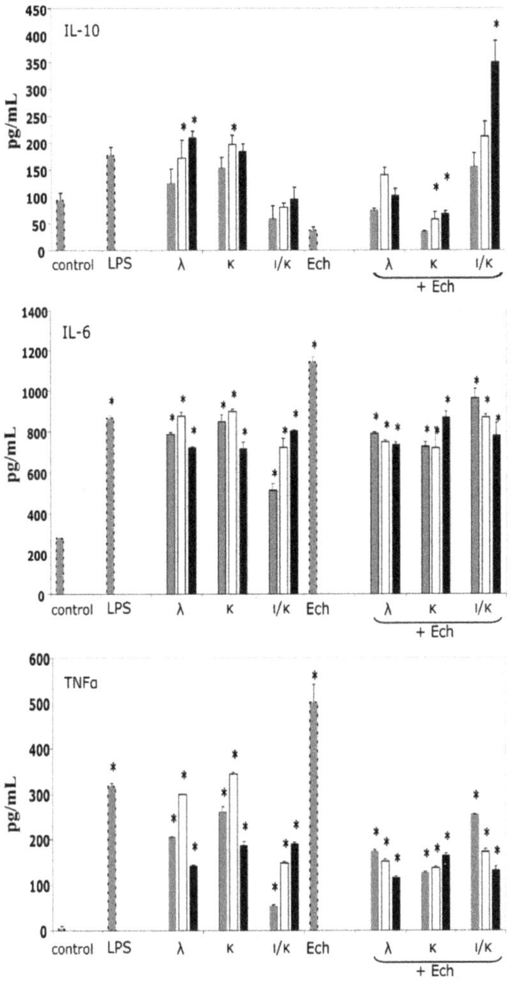

Figure 3. The induction of the necrosis factor-α, IL-6, and IL-10, in the presence of λ-, κ-, ι/κ-CRGs, Ech, and their complexes. The concentration of the LPS was 0.01 μg mL^{-1} and that of Ech was 1 μg mL^{-1}, which were the final value. The concentrations of the CRGs, alone and in complexes with the Ech (1 μg mL^{-1}), changed in the following rows: ▦ = control (saline/1 μg mL^{-1} of Ech); ▩ = 5 μg mL^{-1}, final value; □ = 10 μg mL^{-1}, final value; ■ = 20 μg mL^{-1}, final value. * $p < 0.05$.

2.4. Influence of the CRGs, the Ech and Their Complex, on the HT-29 Tumor Cells

The effect of the Ech, alone and in carrageenans complexes, on the HT-29 cells treated with ethanol was investigated. The exposure of cells to EtOH permits an assessment of the samples' ability to affect cell viability and, as a result, the permeability of the epithelial monolayer. All of the investigated samples were inert, in response to the intestinal epithelial HT-29 cells, under normal conditions. Under stress conditions, only the κ/β-CRG and the Ech, as well their complex, restored the cell viability after exposure to the EtOH. As to the CRG, the most prominent action was detected for the lowest concentrations, where protective effect preserved. The complex of κ/β-CRG with the Ech, also possessed an ability to restore the HT-29 cells after an exposure to ethanol (Figure 4).

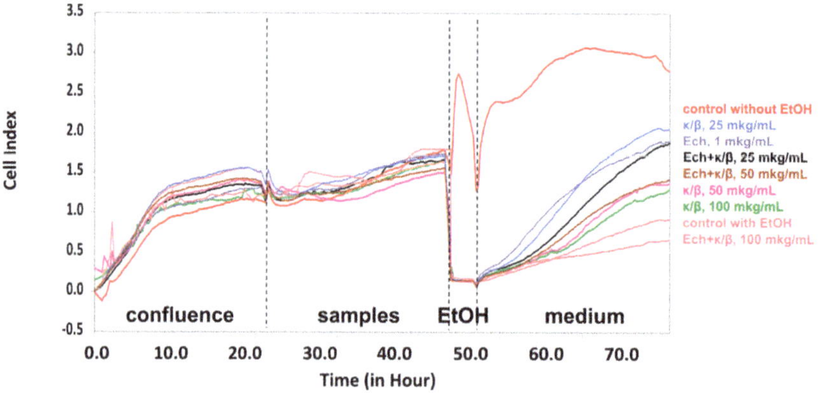

Figure 4. Time and dose-dependent cellular response profiling of HT-29 intestinal epithelial cells, in the presence of the κ/β-carrageenan, Ech, and their complex. Representative data are averaged from five wells. All experiments were repeated at least two times. Four stages of the experimental design are indicated with dashed lines: **1**—Growth of HT-29 cells to confluence; **2**—the stage of samples addition; **3**—incubation with ethanol; **4**—after the ethanol exposure. Concentration of the Ech (1 μg mL^{-1}, final value) was fixed. After each stage, the culture medium (McCoy's 5A Modified) was refreshed.

3. Discussion

Ech, a water-insoluble compound, is the active substance (P N002362/01) of the drug Histochrome®, registered in the Russian Federation. Earlier we have shown that Ech is soluble in aqueous solutions of CRGs, up to the concentration of 0.1 mg mL^{-1}. Moreover, the CRG environment protects the Ech from autooxidation [11]. In this work, we showed that carrageenans modified the biological activity of the Ech.

One of the manifestations of the biological effect of the drug is its ability to cause some disorders in the development and death of embryos (spermotoxic, embryotoxic, and cytostatic activities). The widespread use of the sea urchin embryos to test the toxicological and pharmacological effects of various drugs is due to the simplicity of the incubation of the synchronously developing embryos, under controlled conditions, and the ease of the intravital observation. The influence of the Ech and its complex with CRG, on sperm, was determined by the degree to which it inhibited the ability of spermatozoa to fertilize the sea urchin eggs and the further development of the early embryos of sea urchins, in comparison to the control. As the results showed, the CRGs significantly decreased the spermotoxicity of the Ech, towards the sea urchin *S. intermedius* sperm. Furthermore, neither the Ech, nor its complex with CRG, affected the division and development of the early embryos of the sea urchin.

Oxidative processes occurring during the neutrophils activation could be traced by the change in the ROS production [25]. In the case of the phagocytosis of the pathogens, the ROS were produced by the nicotinamide adenine dinucleotide phosphate oxidase (NOX) in a small volume of the phagosome [26]. During our study, we used an APF fluorescent probe (2-[6-(4-amino)phenoxy-3H-xanthen-3-on-9]benzoic acid), with a strong specificity towards the species of the reactive oxygen, localized predominantly in the phagosomes [27]. It should be noted that, in general, the activating effect of the CRGs was dependent on the polysaccharide concentration and the sulfation degree. In this study, a positive correlation between the impact on the ROS formation and the sulfation degree of the CRG (except for its highest concentration) was observed. Generally, the complex of the λ-CRG, with the Ech, was the most active out of all three types, their effect (complexes of the CRGs and the Ech with concentrations of 200:5 and 100:5 μg mL^{-1}) was about 15%, compared to control (Figure 2). The importance of the CRG sulfation degree, with regards to monocyte behaviour, have also been observed, previously [28].

In the complexes of the Ech with polysaccharides, containing 3,6-anhydrogalactose and the lower sulfate group contents (κ, ι/κ), the resultant action was closer to the level of the Ech alone. This was supported by results from the literature, which reported that the Ech significantly prevented an increase in the ROS levels in rat cardiac myoblast H9c2 cells and cardiomyocytes induced by some cardiotoxic agents [3], as well as in intraocular inflammation caused by endotoxin-induced uveitis [29]. Overall, this experiment indicated the modulation of the inductions of the ROS, in complexes with substances containing pro- (CRGs) and anti- (Ech) activating properties.

Depending on the ROS location in cells, the function of these molecules changes enormously. For example, mitochondrial ROS have a particularly interesting role in the immune response, since these ROS are currently considered essential for pathways initiating the production of pro-inflammatory cytokines [30]. The influence of the investigated samples on the synthesis of the immune mediators enabled the study of another facet of their immune activity, both separately and as complexes. Pro-inflammatory cytokines were exemplified by the IL-6, the most important inducer of the acute-phase proteins, and the TNFα, another pro-inflammatory molecule with cytotoxic effects in antitumor immunity, whereas the IL-10 is an important immunoregulatory cytokine with multiple biologic effects and strong tendencies of anti-inflammatory action [31]. The CRGs stimulated the induction of anti-inflammatory IL-10, whereas, the Ech inhibited the synthesis of this cytokine, and the addition of the CRGs to the Ech increased the induction of the expression of the anti-inflammatory IL-10 (Figure 3). Ech, at a concentration 1 μg mL^{-1}, increased the IL-6 and TNFα synthesis; however, the complexes with CRGs exhibited much less activity in the case of synthesizing the pro-inflammatory cytokine TNFα. The effect of the Ech on the cytokine balance towards the pro-inflammatory response corresponded to the literature data, which reported that spinochromes act as inductors of TNF-α production in LPS-stimulated macrophage cell cultures [5]. Another study underlined a pro-inflammatory action of the naphthoquinones, in mice [32].

Literature data suggest that the CRGs do not affect the epithelial cells of human gastrointestinal tract [33], but the influence of the Ech towards these cells, which is of special interest when one considers an oral administration of a drug, has not been investigated, to our knowledge.

HT-29 is a colorectal cancer cell line used as an in vitro model, for the intestinal epithelium, because it is a mucin secreting cell line which retains many features attributed to the lower small intestine [34]. Previously we have studied the influence of CRGs on these cells, under stress conditions and have found out that only the low-sulfated CRG had a protective action towards the HT-29 intestinal epithelial cells [35]. Our purpose in the study described in this report, was to determine the protective action of the Ech alone and in combination with the low-sulfated CRG on the survival of monolayers of these cells, treated with EtOH (Figure 4). The stress effect of ethanol on the state of the HT-29 cells provided an opportunity to assay the protective properties of polysaccharides from the red algae and the Ech. The Ech (1 μg mL^{-1}) also preserved the HT-29 cells, under stress conditions, to an extent similar to the κ/β-CRG (25 μg mL^{-1}). These results provide an opportunity to propose the CRGs as a possible matrix system, for oral delivery of Ech, which preserves the Ech-favorable qualities and mitigates its negative biological properties.

In general, the CRGs modified the Ech toxicity and the immunological properties. Our results showed that the CRGs significantly decreased the spermotoxicity of the Ech, against the sea urchin *S. intermedius* sperm. The Ech, as well as its complex with CRG, did not affect the division and development of the early embryos of the sea urchin. The influence of the investigated substances on the induction of the ROS, in the neutrophils, confirmed that Ech in a complex with a polysaccharide inhibited the induction of ROS induced by CRG.

The complexes obtained by us illustrated the modulation of the ROS induction, by these substances, with pro- (CRGs) and anti- (Ech) activating properties of the initial components. The CRG decreased the Ech's ability to induce the expression of pro-inflammatory cytokines and increased the expression of anti-inflammatory cytokines. Whereas, the Ech's protective action towards the intestinal cells exposed to EtOH, remained invariable in the complex with the κ/β-CRG.

4. Materials and Methods

The standardized echinochrome (pentahydroxyethylnaphthoquinone, Ech), registration number in the Russian Federation was P N002362/01 [Russian State Register of Drugs (as of 5 December 2016) Part 2]. It was obtained in powder form, from the G.B. Elyakov Pacific Institute of Bioorganic Chemistry, Vladivostok. The purity of the Ech (99.0%) was confirmed by liquid chromatography, coupled with mass spectrometry (LC-MS) data (Shimadzu LCMS-2020, Kyoto, Japan). The purified Ech that looked like red-brown needles, was soluble in ethanol, had a melting point of 219–221.5 °C, and a similar nuclear magnetic resonance (NMR) spectra to that reported previously in Reference [36]. We used an ethanolic solution of the Ech, at a concentration 10 mg mL^{-1}, as a stock solution.

The CRGs were isolated by aqueous extraction from the *Chondrus armatus* (Gigartinaceae), *Tichocarpus crinitus* (Tichocarpaceae), and *Anfeltiopsis flabelliformis* (Phyllophoraceae) red algae, harvested along the Russian coast of the Japanese Sea. The polysaccharides were separated into gelling KCl-insoluble and non-gelling KC1-soluble fractions and their structures were established according to the published protocols [20–22]. Viscosimetric molecular weights of the CRGs were calculated using the Mark-Houwink equation: $[\eta] = KM\alpha$, where $[\eta]$ is the intrinsic viscosity and K and α are empirical constants constituting 3×10^{-3} and 0.95 at 25 °C in 0.1 M NaCl, for the CRGs. The commercial LPS was from the bacterium *Escherichia coli* 055:B5 (Catalog No. L2880, Lot No. 102M4017V, Sigma, St. Louis, MO, USA). An APF probe (2-[6-(4-amino)phenoxy-3H-xanthen-3-on-9]benzoic acid) was purchased from Assay Designs (cat No 906-043).

4.1. Sea Urchin Models

The test samples in these experiments were polysaccharides of three CRG types. They were dissolved in sea water at 50 °C, to the level of the initial concentrations, from 0.5 to 1.0 mg mL^{-1}. Ech dissolved in 50% EtOH was used at the initial concentrations of 0.5 and 1 mg mL^{-1}. Adult sea urchins *Strongylocentrotus intermedius* (collected in the Troitsa Bay (Peter the Great Bay, the Sea of Japan) during August–September 2017, at a depth of 5–10 m) were stored in an aquarium with a closed-filter system, at a seawater temperature of 20 °C and salinity of 32 ± 0.5‰. Pooling male and female gametes and eggs, fertilizations were performed according to the standard procedures described in References [37,38]. The quality of the isolated sperms and eggs was checked with fertilization, prior to experiment. The fertilization membrane was formed within 1–2 min, after insemination, in at least 95–99% of the eggs, under normal conditions.

4.2. Sea Urchins Sperm Cell Toxicity Test (SUSCT Test)

We used the standard bioassay record of the SUSCT test for the analysis of the obtained preparations [23,24]. Sperm from sea urchins (15×10^6 cell mL^{-1}), prior to the experiment, were sustained in seawater for 30 min, with various concentrations of the substances. Next, the spermatozoa were added to the suspension of eggs (2.5×10^3 cell mL^{-1}). The final sperm:egg ratios were about 300 and 150:1. After 15 min, the percentage of fertilized eggs were counted on a Motic AE 21 inverted microscope (Xiamen, China). The experiments were carried out in triplicate using a 12-well plate. The effect of substance toxicity was assessed, visually, according to the number of unfertilized eggs in the four fields of view, in each experiment. The number of eggs fertilized by the sperms, after incubation in the seawater, without substances (control), was assumed to be 95–100%.

4.3. *Sea Urchin Embryos Development Test*

The preliminary fertilized eggs (2.5×10^3 cell mL^{-1}) were stored in seawater, with different concentrations of the tested Ech (10 to 40 μg mL^{-1}) and its complexes with CRGs, for 30 min, after which a suspension of native sperm was added. The number of embryos developed up to the stage of 2–4 blastomeres and of early blastula, in the presence of the test compounds, was evaluated using a microscope.

4.4. *Ethical Approval for Human Blood Samples*

The medical ethical committee of the local hospital (Vladivostok, Russian Federation) approved the study protocol. All subjects who participated in the experiments wrote an informed consent.

4.5. *Leukocytes*

Leukocytes were rapidly isolated from venous citrated blood by lyzing erythrocytes in a solution containing 0.15 M NH_4Cl, 10 mM $NaHCO_3$, and 0.1 mM EDTA [39].

4.6. *Detection of Reactive Oxygen Production*

Reactive oxygen production was detected by flow cytometry, with APF, as described elsewhere [40]. Cells (200,000 cells/well) were incubated for 1 hour, with the samples (12.5, 25, 50, and 100 μg mL^{-1}; final value). Free cells with (phosphate buffer saline) PBS, instead of the samples, were used as the negative control and were considered to be 100%. After 10 min on ice, the cells were analyzed, immediately, by a four color FACSCalibur (Becton Dickinson, San Jose, CA, USA) flow cytometer. Forward and side scatter light was used to identify the neutrophils cell populations.

4.7. *IL-6-, IL-10- and TNFα-Inducing Activity of CRGs and Ech on Human Blood Cells*

Blood processing was performed using the procedure described by De Groote et al. [41]. Heparinated peripheral blood was diluted 1:5 in sterile Medium 199 (Sigma, St. Louis, MO, USA) with glutamine (300 mg L^{-1}) (Gibco, Darmstadt, Germany) and gentamicin (50 μg ml^{-1}). Diluted blood (0.1 mL) was incubated with the investigated samples, in saline (37 °C, 5% CO_2). The CRGs were added to obtain the final concentrations of 5, 10, and 20 μg mL^{-1} Ech (to 1 μg mL^{-1}) and their complexes, to obtain final concentration values corresponding to the substances, separately. After 24 h, the supernatants were collected and frozen, followed by determining the cytokine content, using specific ELISA kits, according to the manufacture's protocol ("Cytokine", Saint-Petersburg, Russia).

4.8. *Cell culture*

The human cancer cell line HT-29 was obtained from the American Type Culture Collection (https://www.lgcstandards-atcc.org/). HT-29 cells were incubated at 37 °C in a 5% CO_2 humidified atmosphere, in McCoy's 5a Medium Modified, containing 10% *v*/*v* FBS (Lot RWH35894, HyClone, Logan, UT, USA), 2 mM L-glutamine, and 1% penicillin/streptomycin (Invitrogen, Paisley, UK).

4.9. *xCELLigence System*

Experiments on the xCELLigence system were conducted by means of the Real-Time Cell Analyzer Dual Plate (RTCA-DP) instrument (ACEA Bioscience, San Diego, CA, USA). The recommendations proposed by Ke et al. [42] and Sokolova et al. [35] were applied to study the effect of the samples on human intestinal epithelial cell monolayers.

Samples were added as follows:

Single samples. Carrageenans (20 μL, C = 250, 500, and 1000 μg mL^{-1}); Ech (20 μL, C = 10 μg mL^{-1}).

Complex samples. Carrageenan (10 μL, C = 500, 1000, and 2000 μg mL^{-1}) + Ech (10 μL, C = 20 μg mL^{-1}). (Concentrations are expressed as initial values.)

4.10. Statistical Analysis

All data are presented as means ± standard deviations. Statistical calculation was conducted by ANOVA one-way analysis of variance. Differences were suggested when statistically probable at $p < 0.01$.

5. Conclusions

The inclusion of Ech into the carrageenan matrix enables a decrease the spermotoxicity of the Ech (besides protection of the substance from oxidation and improvement its solubility [11]), preserving its protective properties against the ROS synthesis by neutrophils, and the protective action towards the HT-29 intestinal epithelial cells.

Author Contributions: E.V.S. conceived, designed, performed and described the experiment for cytokines and ROS on blood cells and epithelial HT-29 cells, V.N.D. performed the experiments on a flow cytometer and assisted in publishing the article, N.I.M. performed the experiments with sea urchins, A.S.K. performed maintenance of HT-29 cells and co-contributed to experiments with these cells, N.P.M. contributed Ech for the research, A.O.K. provided all carrageenans samples, I.M.Y. described the experiments on sea urchin models and management of the manuscript writing process.

Funding: This work was supported by the Russian Science Foundation (RScF grant, project 16-14-00051).

Acknowledgments: The authors enormously appreciated the support provided by the organizing committee of "The 3rd International Symposium on Life Science" and especially Valentin A. Stonik for his invaluable comments.

Conflicts of Interest: The authors declare no conflict of interest.

References

1. Sumich, J.L.; Pinkard-Meier, D.R. *Introduction to the Biology of Marine Life*, 1st ed.; Jones & Bartlett Learning: Burlington, MA, USA, 2016.
2. Pozharitskaya, O.N.; Shikov, A.N.; Laakso, I.; Seppänen-Laakso, T.; Makarenko, I.E.; Faustova, N.M.; Makarova, M.N.; Makarov, V.G. Bioactivity and chemical characterization of gonads of green sea urchin *Strongylocentrotus droebachiensis* from Barents Sea. *J. Funct. Foods* **2015**, *17*, 227–234. [CrossRef]
3. Jeong, S.H.; Kim, H.K.; Song, I.S.; Lee, S.J.; Ko, K.S.; Rhee, B.D.; Kim, N.; Mishchenko, N.P.; Fedoryev, S.A.; Stonik, V.A.; et al. Echinochrome A Protects Mitochondrial Function in Cardiomyocytes against Cardiotoxic Drugs. *Mar. Drugs* **2014**, *12*, 2922–2936. [CrossRef] [PubMed]
4. Pozharitskaya, O.N.; Ivanova, S.A.; Shikov, A.N.; Makarov, V.G. Evaluation of free radical-scavenging activity of sea urchin pigments using HPTLC with post-chromatographic derivatization. *Chromatographia* **2013**, *76*, 1353–1358. [CrossRef]
5. Brasseur, L.; Hennebert, E.; Fievez, L.; Caulier, G.; Bureau, F.; Tafforeau, L.; Flammang, P.; Gerbaux, P.; Eeckhaut, I. The Roles of Spinochromes in Four Shallow Water Tropical Sea Urchins and Their Potential as Bioactive Pharmacological Agents. *Mar. Drugs* **2017**, *15*, 179. [CrossRef] [PubMed]
6. Shikov, A.N.; Pozharitskaya, O.N.; Krishtopina, A.S.; Makarov, V.G. Naphthoquinone pigments from sea urchins: Chemistry and pharmacology. *Phytochem. Rev.* **2018**, *17*, 509–534.
7. Mishchenko, N.P.; Fedoreev, S.A.; Bagirova, V.L. Histochrome: A new original domestic drug. *Pharm. Chem. J.* **2003**, *37*, 48–52.
8. Elyakov, G.B.; Maximov, O.B.; Mischenko, N.P.; Koltsova, E.A.; Fedoreev, S.A.; Glebko, L.I.; Krasovskaya, N.P.; Artjukov, A.A. Drug Preparation "histochrome" for Treating Acute Myocardial Infarction and Ischaemic Heart Diseases. European Patent 1121930, 14 November 2007.
9. Santo, V.E.; Frias, A.M.; Carida, M.; Cancedda, R.; Gomes, M.E.; Mano, J.F.; Reis, R.L. Carrageenan-based hydrogels for the controlled delivery of PDGF-BB in bone tissue engineering applications. *Biomacromolecules* **2009**, *10*, 1392–1401. [CrossRef] [PubMed]
10. Shit, S.C.; Shah, P.M. Edible polymers: Challenges and opportunities. *J. Polym.* **2014**, *2014*, 13. [CrossRef]
11. Yermak, I.M.; Mischchenko, N.P.; Davydova, V.N.; Glazunov, V.P.; Tarbeeva, D.V.; Kravchenko, A.O.; Pimenova, E.A.; Sorokina, I.V. Carrageenans-Sulfated Polysaccharides from Red Seaweeds as Matrices for the Inclusion of Echinochrome. *Mar. Drugs* **2017**, *15*, 337. [CrossRef]

12. Knutsen, S.H.; Myslabodski, D.E.; Larsen, B.; Usov, A.I. A modified system of nomenclature for red algal galactans. *Bot. Mar.* **1994**, *37*, 163–170.
13. Falshaw, R.; Furneaux, R. Carragenan from the tetrasporic stage of *Gigartina decipiens* (Gigartinaceae, Rhodophyta). *Carbohydr. Res.* **1994**, *252*, 171–182. [PubMed]
14. Yermak, I.M.; Khotimchenko, Y.S. Chemical properties, biological activities and applications of carrageenan from red algae. In *Recent Advances in Marine Biotechnology*, 1st ed.; Fingerman, M., Nagabhushanam, R., Eds.; Science Publishing Inc.: New York, NY, USA, 2003; Volume 9, pp. 207–255.
15. Pereira, L.; Soares, F.; Freitas, A.C.; Duarte, A.C.; Ribeiro-Claro, P. Extraction, Characterization, and Use of Carrageenans. In *Industrial Applications of Marine Biopolymers*, 1st ed.; Sudha, P.N., Ed.; Taylor & Francis Group: Boca Raton, FL, USA, 2017; pp. 37–90.
16. Pereira, L. *Edible Seaweeds of the World*, 1st ed.; CRC Press. Taylor & Francis Group: Boca Raton, FL, USA, 2016.
17. Weiner, M.L. Food additive carrageenan: Part II: A critical review of carrageenan in vivo safety studies. *Crit. Rev. Toxicol.* **2014**, *44*, 244–269. [CrossRef] [PubMed]
18. Zia, K.M.; Tabasum, S.; Nasif, M.; Sultan, N.; Aslam, N.; Noreen, A.; Zuber, M. A review on synthesis, properties and applications of natural polymer based carrageenan blends and composites. *Int. J. Biol. Macromol.* **2017**, *96*, 282–301. [CrossRef] [PubMed]
19. Magnan, S.; Tota, J.E.; El-Zein, M.; Burchell, A.N.; Schiller, J.T.; Ferenczy, A.; Tellier, P.-P.; Coutlee, F.; Franco, E.L. Efficacy of a Carrageenan gel Against Transmission of Cervical HPV (CATCH): Interim analysis of a randomized, double-blind, placebo-controlled, phase 2B trial. *Clin. Microbiol. Infect.* **2018**, in press. [CrossRef] [PubMed]
20. Yermak, I.M.; Kim, Y.H.; Titlyanov, E.A.; Isakov, V.V.; Solov'eva, T.F. Chemical structure and gel properties of carrageenan from algae belonging to the Gigartinaceae and Tichocapaceae, collected from the Russian Pacific coast. *J. Appl. Phycol.* **1999**, *11*, 41–48. [CrossRef]
21. Barabanova, A.O.; Yermak, I.M.; Glazunov, V.P.; Isakov, V.V.; Titlyanov, E.A.; Solov'eva, T.F. Comparative study of carrageenans from reproductive and sterile forms of *Tichocarpus crinitus* (Gmel.) Rupr (Rhodophyta, Tichocarpaceae). *Biochem.* **2005**, *70*, 350–356. [CrossRef]
22. Kravchenko, A.O.; Anastyuk, S.D.; Sokolova, E.V.; Isakov, V.V.; Glazunov, V.P.; Helbert, W.; Yermak, I.M. Structural analysis and cytokine-induced activity of gelling sulfated polysaccharide from the cystocarpic plants of *Ahnfeltiopsis flabelliformis*. *Carbohydr. Pol.* **2016**, *151*, 523–534. [CrossRef] [PubMed]
23. Dinnel, P.A.; Link, J.M.; Sober, Q.J. Improved methodology for a sea urchin sperm cell bioassay for marine waters. *Arch. Environ. Contam. Toxicol.* **1987**, *16*, 23–32. [CrossRef] [PubMed]
24. Lera, S.; Macchia, S.; Pellegrini, D. Standardizing the methodology of sperm cell test with Paracentrotus lividus. *Environ. Monit. Assess.* **2006**, *122*, 101–109. [CrossRef] [PubMed]
25. Flannagan, R.S.; Jaumouillé, V.; Grinstein, S. The cell biology of phagocytosis. *Annu. Rev. Pathol. Mech. Dis.* **2012**, *7*, 61–98. [CrossRef] [PubMed]
26. Dupré-Crochet, S.; Erard, M.; N'uße, O. ROS production in phagocytes: Why, when, and where? *J. Leukoc. Biol.* **2013**, *94*, 657–670. [CrossRef] [PubMed]
27. Halliwell, B.; Whiteman, M. Measuring reactive species and oxidative damage in vivo and in cell culture: How should you do it and what do the results mean? *Br. J. Pharmacol.* **2004**, *142*, 231–255. [CrossRef] [PubMed]
28. Chan, W.I.; Zhang, G.; Li, X.; Leung, C.H.; Ma, D.L.; Dong, L.; Wang, C. Carrageenan activates monocytes via type-specific binding with interleukin-8: An implication for design of immuno-active biomaterials. *Biomater. Sci.* **2017**, *5*, 403–407. [CrossRef] [PubMed]
29. Lennikov, A.; Kitaichi, N.; Noda, K.; Mizuuchi, K.; Ando, R.; Dong, Z.; Fukuhara, J.; Kinoshita, S.; Namba, K.; Ohno, Sh.; Ishida, S. Amelioration of endotoxin-induced uveitis treated with the sea urchin pigment echinochrome in rats. *Mol. Vis.* **2014**, *20*, 171–177. [PubMed]
30. Schieber, M.; Chandel, N.S. ROS function in redox signaling and oxidative stress. *Cur. Biol.* **2014**, *24*, R453–R462. [CrossRef] [PubMed]
31. Commins, S.P.; Borish, L.; Steinke, J.W. Immunologic messenger molecules: Cytokines, interferons, and chemokines. *J. Allergy Clin. Immunol.* **2010**, *125*, S53–S72. [CrossRef] [PubMed]
32. Inoue, K.; Takano, H.; Hiyoshi, K.; Ichinose, T.; Sadakane, K.; Yanagisawa, R.; Tomura, S.; Kumaga, Y. Naphthoquinone enhances antigen-related airway inflammation in mice. *Eur. Respir. J.* **2006**, *29*, 259–267. [CrossRef] [PubMed]

33. McKim, J.M., Jr.; Baas, H.; Rice, G.P.; Willoughby, J.A., Sr.; Weiner, M.L.; Blakemore, W. Effects of carrageenan on cell permeability, cytotoxicity, and cytokine gene expression in human intestinal and hepatic cell lines. *Food Chem. Toxicol.* **2016**, *96*, 1–10. [CrossRef] [PubMed]
34. Langerholc, T.; Maragkoudakis, P.A.; Wollgast, J.; Gradisnik, L.; Cencic, A. Novel and established intestinal cell line models-an indispensable tool in food science and nutrition. *Trends Food Sci. Technol.* **2011**, *20*, S11–S20. [CrossRef]
35. Sokolova, E.V.; Kuz'mich, A.S.; Byankina, A.O.; Yermak, I.M. Effect of carrageenans alone and in combination with casein or lipopolysaccharide on human epithelial intestinal HT-29 cells. *J. Biomed. Mater. Res. Part A* **2017**, *105*, 2843–2850. [CrossRef] [PubMed]
36. Vasileva, E.A.; Mishchenko, N.P.; Tran, V.T.T.; Vo, H.M.N.; Bui, L.M.; Denisenko, V.A.; Fedoreyev, S.A. Quinoid pigments from the sea urchin *Astropyga radiata*. *Chem. Nat. Compd.* **2017**, *53*, 356–358. [CrossRef]
37. Buznikov, G.A.; Podmariov, V.K. Sea urchins *Strongylocentrotus drobachiensis*, *S. Nudus*, *S. intermedius*. In *Animal Species for Developmental Studies*, 1st ed.; Dettlaff, A., Vassetzky, S.G., Eds.; Springer: Boston, MA, USA, 1990; pp. 253–285, ISBN 0306110326.
38. Pinsino, A.; Mantranga, V.; Trinchella, F.; Roccheri, M.C. Sea urchin embryos as an in vivo model for the assessment of manganese toxicity: Developmental and stress response effects. *Ecotoxicology* **2010**, *19*, 555–562. [CrossRef] [PubMed]
39. Lehmann, A.K.; Sornes, S.; Halstensen, A. Phagocytosis: Measurement by flow cytometry. *J. Immunol. Methods* **2000**, *243*, 229–242. [CrossRef]
40. Setsukinai, K.I.; Urano, Y.; Kakinuma, K.; Majima, H.J.; Nagano, T. Development of novel fluorescence probes that can reliably detect reactive oxygen species and distinguish specific species. *J. Biol. Chem.* **2003**, *278*, 3170–3175. [CrossRef] [PubMed]
41. De Groote, D.; Zangerle, P.F.; Gevaert, Y.; Fassotte, M.F.; Beguin, Y.; Noizat-Pirenne, F.; Pirenne, J.; Gathy, R.; Lopez, I.M.; Dehart, I.; et al. Direct stimulation of cytokines (IL-1β, TNF-α, IL-6, IL-2, IFN-γ and GM-CSF) in whole blood. I. Comparison with isolated PBMC stimulation. *Cytokine* **1992**, *4*, 239–248. [CrossRef]
42. Ke, N.; Wang, X.; Xu, X.; Abassi, Y.A. The xCELLigence system for real-time and label-free monitoring of cell viability. *Methods Mol. Biol.* **2011**, *740*, 33–43. [PubMed]

marine drugs

MDPI

Article

Mutagenesis Studies and Structure-function Relationships for GalNAc/Gal-Specific Lectin from the Sea Mussel *Crenomytilus grayanus*

Svetlana N. Kovalchuk [1], Nina S. Buinovskaya [1], Galina N. Likhatskaya [2], Valery A. Rasskazov [1,†], Oksana M. Son [3], Liudmila A. Tekutyeva [3] and Larissa A. Balabanova [1,3,*]

1 Laboratory of Marine Biochemistry, G.B. Elyakov Pacific Institute of Bioorganic Chemistry, Far Eastern Branch, Russian Academy of Science, 159, Stoletya Vladivostoku str., Vladivostok 690022, Russia; s.n.kovalchuk@mail.ru (S.N.K.); ninok1993@mail.ru (N.S.B.)

2 Laboratory of Bioassays and Mechanism of Action of Biologically Active Substances, G.B. Elyakov Pacific Institute of Bioorganic Chemistry, Far Eastern Branch, Russian Academy of Science, 159, Stoletya Vladivostoku str., Vladivostok 690022, Russia; galinlik@piboc.dvo.ru

3 Innovative Technology Center, School of Economics and Management, Far Eastern Federal University, 8 Sukhanova St., Vladivostok 690090, Russia; oksana_son@bk.ru (O.M.S.); tekuteva.la@dvfu.ru (L.A.T.)

* Correspondence: balaban@piboc.dvo.ru; Tel.: +7-432-231-0703

† Deceased on 19 March 2018.

Received: 17 October 2018; Accepted: 21 November 2018; Published: 27 November 2018

Abstract: The GalNAc/Gal-specific lectin from the sea mussel *Crenomytilus grayanus* (CGL) with anticancer activity represents a novel lectin family with β-trefoil fold. Earlier, the crystal structures of CGL complexes with globotriose, galactose and galactosamine, and mutagenesis studies have revealed that the lectin contained three carbohydrate-binding sites. The ability of CGL to recognize globotriose (Gb3) on the surface of breast cancer cells and bind mucin-type glycoproteins, which are often associated with oncogenic transformation, makes this compound to be perspective as a biosensor for cancer diagnostics. In this study, we describe results on in silico analysis of binding mechanisms of CGL to ligands (galactose, globotriose and mucin) and evaluate the individual contribution of the amino acid residues from carbohydrate-binding sites to CGL activity by site-directed mutagenesis. The alanine substitutions of His37, His129, Glu75, Asp127, His85, Asn27 and Asn119 affect the CGL mucin-binding activity, indicating their importance in the manifestation of lectin activity. It has been found that CGL affinity to ligands depends on their structure, which is determined by the number of hydrogen bonds in the CGL-ligand complexes. The obtained results should be helpful for understanding molecular machinery of CGL functioning and designing a synthetic analog of CGL with enhanced carbohydrate-binding properties.

Keywords: galactose-specific lectin; *Crenomytilus grayanus*; carbohydrate-binding site; molecular docking; site-specific mutagenesis; carbohydrate-binding activity

1. Introduction

Lectins are specific carbohydrate-binding proteins, found in animals, plants and microorganisms, and involved in various biological processes including cell adhesion, innate immunity, fertilization, differentiation et al. [1–4]. First, classifications of lectins were based on the glycan structures, to which they exhibited high affinity [5]. Later, lectins were classified into families on the basis of similarity of amino acid sequences of their carbohydrate recognition domains (C-type lectins, L-, M-, P-, R-, F-type lectins, galectins et al.) [1,2,6]. To date, the amino acid sequences of several hundreds of lectins have been determined, and a number of their three-dimensional structures have been elucidated. Recently, a new lectin classification based on their three-dimensional structures was proposed and 48 lectin families were characterized [7].

In the last two decades, many lectins from marine invertebrates were identified, and their functions in various immune events were demonstrated [3]. Earlier, we reported on a novel GalNAc/Gal-specific lectin from the mussel *Crenomytilus grayanus* (CGL), which did not share sequence homology with known lectins and consisted of three tandem-repeat subdomains with high (up to 73%) sequence identity to each other [8,9]. Three-dimensional structure prediction revealed that CGL adopted a ß-trefoil fold and contained three binding sites including conserved HPY(K)G motifs [9,10], which was later confirmed by X-ray analysis [11,12].

CGL was shown to possess anti-cancer activity through binding globotriose Gb3 [12]. The ability of CGL to recognize Gb3 on the surface of breast cancer cells [12] and bind mucin-type glycoproteins [8,9], which are often associated with oncogenic transformation, makes structural studies highly valuable to discern mechanistic details of its function. In our previous study the role of three conserved HPK(Y)G motifs in hemagglutinating and carbohydrate binding activities of CGL was experimentally shown by site-specific mutagenesis studies [10]. To investigate CGL functions and peculiarities of its molecular organization in more detail, in this study we evaluated the contribution of individual amino acid residues from CGL binding sites into the lectin activity using analysis of recombinant CGL mutants and in silico evaluation of mono- and oligosaccharide structures impacts on CGL binding properties.

2. Results

2.1. Analysis of CGL Contacts with Galactose/Galactosamine for Mutagenesis

The theoretical model of the spatial structure of lectin CGL was previously constructed by us [10] based on the crystal structure of the lectin MytiLec determined at 1.05 Å resolution (Protein Data Bank accession: PDB 3WMV) [13]. Superimposition of all Cα atoms of obtained CGL model and CGL crystal structure (PDB 5F8S) [12] showed that they were almost completely superimposable (values of the root-mean-square deviation (RMSD) were 0.4 Å). Thus, the predicted structure of the lectin CGL was in good agreement with the experimentally established CGL structure and suitable for in silico mutagenesis and molecular docking studies.

The analysis of CGL contacts with α-galactose (Protein Data Bank accession: PDB 5F8W) and galactosamine (PDB 5F8Y) showed that CGL amino acid residues His37 and Asn119 from Site 1; His85 and Asn27 from Site 2; Asp127, His129, and Glu75 from Site 3 formed hydrogen bonds with these monosaccharides (Figure 1). These residues were selected for mutagenesis experiments.

2.2. Mutagenesis Studies

To obtain the recombinant CGL of the wild type and Asn27Ala, His37Ala, Glu75Ala, His85Ala, Asn119Ala, Asp127Ala and His129Ala mutants, expression plasmids were constructed on the basis of pET40/CmAP plasmid described earlier [10,14]. The alkaline phosphatase CmAP in the hybrid CGL-CmAP protein allowed for monitoring recombinant lectins during expression and purification steps [10,14].

CGL was shown to exhibit high affinity to porcine stomach mucin [15]. The mucin-binding activity of the recombinant CGL of the wild and mutant types was evaluated by measuring the alkaline phosphatase activity provided by CmAP domain [10] (Figure 2).

The mucin-binding activity of the obtained mutants varied in a wide range and was from 9% to 73% of the wild lectin (Figure 2). CGL mutants with the alanine substitutions of His37, His129, Glu75, Asp127 and His85, Asn27, Asn119 showed decreased mucin-binding activities in 1.4, 2.3, 3.2, 4.5, 5.0, 5.9 and 11.1 times, respectively.

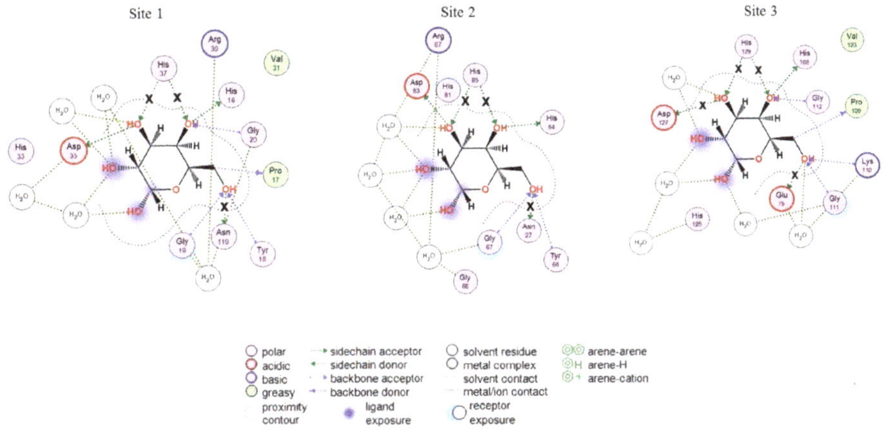

Figure 1. 2D-diagrams of the galactose-binding sites (Site 1, 2, 3) in the wild type CGL. Hydrogen bonds lost in the corresponding mutant are indicated with a cross (**x**).

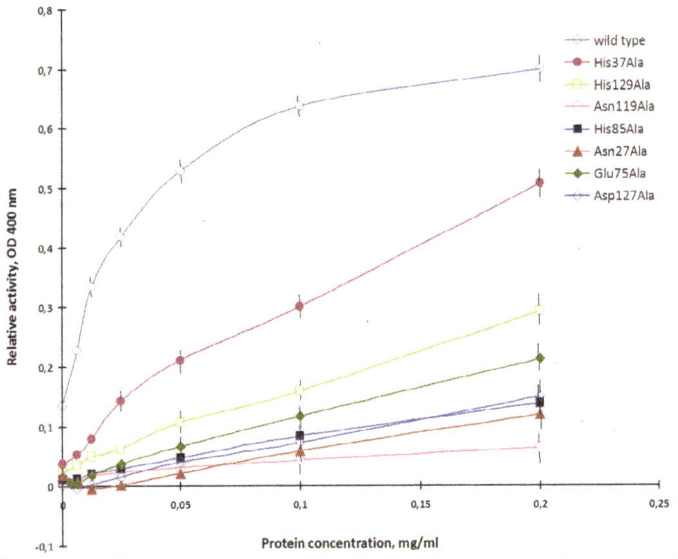

Figure 2. Mucin-binding activity of the wild and mutant types of CGL. The lectin-mucin complexes (axis *X*—mucin concentration) were monitored by measuring the phosphatase activity of CGL/CmAP hybrid (axis *Y*).

2.3. Analysis of Contacts in Complexes of CGL and Its Mutants with Oligosaccharides

It was found that the mucin-binding activities of the obtained mutants did not correlate with changes in the calculated binding energy of galactose with CGL mutants that can be explained by the fact that CGL affinity to different ligands depends on their structure (Table 1). To clarify the impact of the ligand structure on CGL binding activity and binding mechanisms of the attachment of CGL to ligands, in silico analysis of contacts of CGL mutants in complexes with globotriose Gb3 was carried out with MOE 2018.01 program. The obtained results showed that the alanine substitution of His37,

His129, Glu75, Asp127, His85, Asn27 and Asn119 residues changed CGL contacts with Gb3 (Figure 3) and the total binding energy of CGL with ligands (Table 1).

Table 1. The mucin-binding activity of the recombinant CGL of wild and mutant types and the change in the binding energy (ΔE = Emut-Ewt) of the CGL mutants with galactose and globotriose.

Lectin	Gal Binding ΔE^{a}, kcal/mol	Globotriose Binding ΔE^{b}, kcal/mol	Mucin-Binding Activity [c], %
Asn119Ala *	1.9	4.9	9
Asn27Ala **	2.0	5.2	17
Asp127Ala ***	4.0	4.3	22
His85Ala **	3.6	3.4	20
Glu75Ala ***	3.4	4.7	31
His129Ala ***	3.5	3.6	43
His37Ala *	3.5	3.1	73

[a/b]—change in the binding energy of the CGL mutants with galactose (ΔE^{a}) or globotriose (ΔE^{b}); [c]—mucin-binding activity of the wild type CGL was 100%; *—amino acid residues (aa) from Site 1, **—aa from Site 2, ***—aa from Site 3.

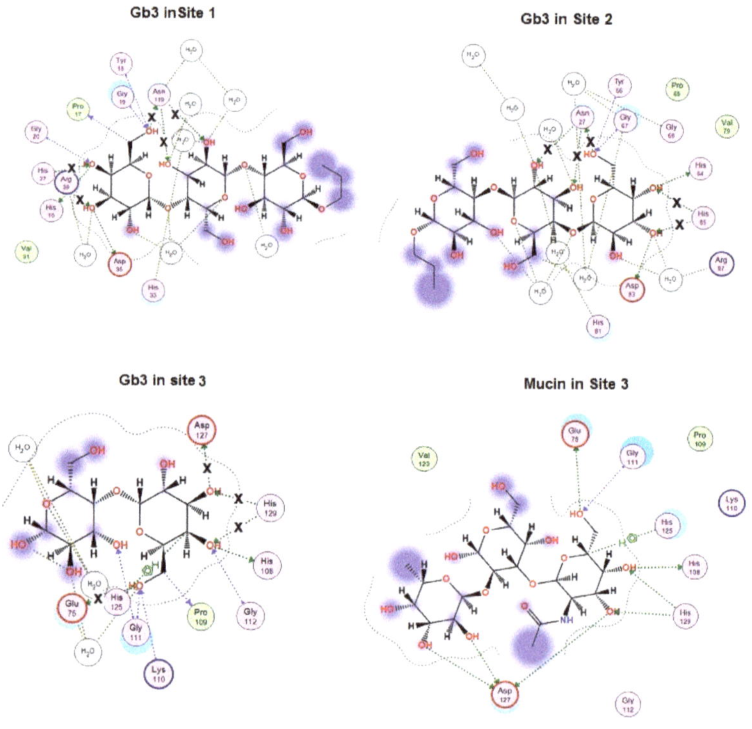

Figure 3. 2D-diagram of Gb3-binding sites (Site 1, 2, 3) and mucin binding in Site 3 of the wild type CGL. Hydrogen bonds lost in the corresponding mutant are indicated with a cross (**x**).

The analysis of contacts between CGL and Gb3 has shown that Asn27 and Asn119 residues formed the hydrogen bond not only with C6-OH group of Gb3 terminal galactose residue, but also with the neighboring galactose residue (Figure 3).

It was found that Asn27Ala and Asn119Ala mutants lost three hydrogen bonds with Gb3 in Sites 1 and 2 in comparison with the wild type CGL (Figure 3), what correlates with a drastic decrease in their affinity towards mucin that has two terminal galactose as Gb3 (Table 1, Figure 2).

The residue Glu75 in CGL Site 3 is located in the same position as Asn27 and Asn119 from Sites 1 and 2 and forms the hydrogen bond with C6-OH group of terminal monosaccharide residue similarly to Asn27 and Asn119. According to the modeling results, the mutant Glu75Ala lost only one hydrogen bond (Figure 3) and therefore retained a higher percentage (31%) of the lectin activity than Asn27Ala and Asn119Ala mutants (Table 1).

The His37, His85 and His129 residues form two hydrogen bonds only with the terminal Gb3 monosaccharide residue and the binding energy of His37Ala, His85Ala and His129Ala mutants with both galactose and globotriose are similar (Table 1, Figure 3). However, the lectin activities of the mutants His37Ala, His85Ala and His129Ala were different (Table 1, Figure 2). Apparently, the activities of these CGL mutants depend also on the structural rearrangement of the sites after alanine substitutions of His37, His85 and His129. Distinctive affinities of Sites 1–3 of CGL toward galactose were also shown by NMR titrations [12].

According to the modeling data, Asp127 forms only one hydrogen bond with the terminal monosaccharide of Gb3 (Figure 3). These results fully coincided with crystallographic data from Protein Data Bank (PDB accession numbers: 5F8W, 5F8Y and 5F90). However, the mutant Asp127Ala activity with the use of porcine stomach mucin (PSM) as ligand was only 22% compared to the wild lectin although only one hydrogen bond disappeared in the complexes with galactose and globotriose (Table 1, Figure 3).

To explain the drastic change in the activity of this mutant, a model of the mutant Asp127Ala complex with the PSM oligosaccharide was constructed using molecular docking of CGL with the PSM-like trisaccharide of the blood group A epitope GalNAcα1-3Gal [Fucα1-2] since data concerning crystal structure of PSM itself were not available in literature (Figures 3 and 4).

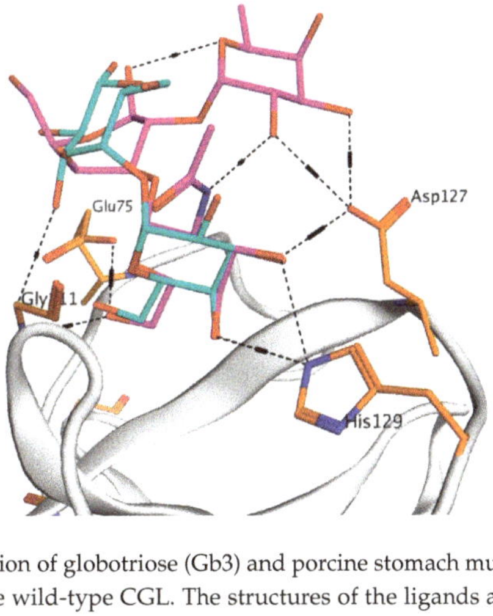

Figure 4. 3D-superimposition of globotriose (Gb3) and porcine stomach mucine (PSM) trisaccharides in the binding Site 3 of the wild-type CGL. The structures of the ligands are shown as stick in blue (Gb3) and in pink (PSM).

The analysis of contacts between Site 3 of CGL and the PSM-trisaccharide GalNAcα1-3Gal [Fucα1-2] has shown that Asp127 forms a hydrogen bond with C3-OH group of the terminal monosaccharide galactose and two additional hydrogen bonds with OH groups at C2 and C3 of the third residue fucose (Figures 3 and 4). Asp127Ala mutant lost all three hydrogen bonds with the PSM trisaccharide, which can explain a sharp decrease (down to 22% of the wild type CGL) in the mucin-binding activity of Asp127Ala mutant (Table 1, Figure 2).

Asp35 and Asp83 residues in the binding Sites 1 and 2 are located in the same positions as Asp127 in Site 3 and can form three hydrogen bonds with the PSM trisaccharide. The activities of Asp35Ala and Asp83Ala mutants have not been yet studied experimentally, but it may be assumed those will decreased like the case of Asp127Ala mutant.

3. Discussion

CGL is the GalNAc/Gal- and mucin-specific lectin with an amino acid sequence that distinguishes it from lectins of known families [9]. To date, this new lectin family which was proposed to name mytilectin [13] includes, besides CGL, five lectins from the sea mussels *Mytilus trossulus* (MTL), *Mytilus galloprovincialis* (MytiLecs 1–3) and *Mytilus californianus* (MCL) [15–19]. These lectins share common ß-trefoil fold and contain three carbohydrate-binding sites [9–13,19]. A β-trefoil fold was proposed for the first time for the crystal structure of Kunitz soybean tripsin inhibitor [20]. Now, it is known that β-trefoil fold is shared by proteins from several subfamilies, including cytokines, ricin B-like lectins, agglutinins, actin-cross-linking proteins etc. [21], which have no sequence similarity and have distinctive ligands, modes of ligand binding and functions.

According to the crystal data, CGL exhibits a characteristic pseudo three-fold symmetry and contains three structurally conserved subdomains [11,12]. Each of these subdomains is composed of four β-strands. Two strands from each subdomain collectively form a six-stranded β-barrel and the remaining two β-strands from each subdomain together form a β-hairpin triplet that caps one end of the barrel [11]. The putative glycan-binding pocket in the first CGL subdomain is formed by the side chains of His16, Tyr18, Val31, His33, Asp35, His37 and Arg39, and the backbone of Gly19 and Gly20 (HYGGVHDHR). The second binding pocket of CGL is formed by the same amino acid residues (HYGGVHDHR). Whereas in the third pocket of CGL, tyrosine is substituted by lysine, and arginine is replaced by alanine (HKGGVHDHA) [11]. The structure of the CGL-galactosamine complex obtained by Liao et al. [12] also revealed in CGL three carbohydrate-binding sites: Site 1 consisted of His16, Gly19, Asp35, His37 and Asn119; Site 2 included His64, Gly67, Asp83, His85, and Asn27; Site 3 comprised His108, Gly111, Asp127, His129, and Glu75. Superimposition of the three carbohydrate binding sites indicates that all three sites contain the same amino acid compositions except for the replacement of Asn for Glu in Site 3. These data confirmed our predications based on homology modeling [10].

In our previous study, we evaluated the contribution of three conserved HPK(Y)G motifs in hemagglutinating and carbohydrate binding activities of CGL by site-specific mutagenesis [10]. According to the obtained data, alanine substitutions of His16, Pro17, Gly19 of Site 1 and His64, Pro65 and Gly67 in Site 2 resulted in complete loss of the CGL hemagglutinating and mucin-binding activities, whereas the mutant CGL with His108Ala, Pro109Ala and Gly111Ala mutations in the Site 3 kept the binding activity against mucin [10].

In this study, we applied the same approach to elucidate the individual contribution of the amino acid residues from CGL binding Sites 1–3 to the carbohydrate binding activity. It was found that the alanine substitution of none of the studied amino acid residues (His37 and Asn119 from Site 1; His85 and Asn27 from Site 2; Asp127, His129, and Glu75 from Site 3) did not lead to the complete loss of the mucin-binding activity of CGL due to the presence of two other normal Sites. But the contribution of these amino acid residues to the mucin-binding activity of CGL was not the same. The replacements of Asn119Ala in Site 1 and Asn27Ala in Site 2 were found to lead to the greater decreasing of the mucin-binding activity of CGL (up to 9% and 17%, respectively) in comparison with the alanine substitution of Glu75 located in Site 3 in the same position as Asn119 and Asn27 from Sites 1 and 2, respectively (Table 1). This confirmed the suggestion of Jakób with co-authors [11] about differences in the affinity (or specificity) for glycan moieties between binding sites and with our previous experimental data [10].

Moreover, in silico analysis of the CGL binding to galactose, globotriose and mucin have shown that the affinity of CGL to these ligands depends on their structures, which determine the number of hydrogen bonds in the CGL-ligand complex and, consequently, its binding energy in total. The maximal decrease in the mucin-binding activity observed for the mutants Asn119Ala in Site 1 and Asn27Ala in

Site 2 could be explained by the loss of all three hydrogen bonds with two terminal galactose residues of oligosaccharides in comparison with the wild-type CGL (Table 1, Figure 3). The amino acid residue Asp127 in Site 3 (and similar residues Asp35 and Asp83 in Sites 1 and 2) was found to play a decisive role in the higher lectin specificity to mucin than globotriose (Figure 4). Thus, the efficiency of CGL binding depends on the composition of terminal monosaccharide units in oligosaccharides due to the different capability of CGL amino acid residues from Site 1–3 to bond with OH-groups of the second galactose and third fucose in the addition to the binding with the terminal galactose.

4. Materials and Methods

4.1. In Silico Analysis of Contacts between CGL and Ligands and Mutagenesis

The model of CGL spatial structure was constructed as described previously [10] on the basis of the crystal structure of the lectin MytiLec established with a resolution of 1.05 Å (PDB code 3WMV) [13]. The analysis of contacts between CGL and ligands, in silico mutagenesis, molecular docking and visualization of the results were carried out with the Ligand interaction and Dock modules of MOE 2018.01 program [22]. The crystal structure of CGL complexes with galactose (PDB 5F8W), galactosamine (PDB 5F8Y), globotriose Gb3 (PDB 5F90) and trisaccharide motif GalNAcα1-3Gal [Fucα1-2] from porcine stomach mucin (PSM-trisaccharide), which is identical with terminal trisaccharide of the blood group A human histo-blood group antigen (HBGA A-trisaccharide) (PDB 2WMI) [23], were used in docking analysis. Molecular docking of PSM-trisaccharide GalNAcα1-3Gal [Fucα1-2] with CGL was carried out using complex with galactosamine (PDB 5F8Y) as a template. The ligand binding energy (the molecular mechanics generalized Born interaction energy) was the non-bonded interaction energy between the receptor and the ligand and comprised van der Waals, Coulomb and generalized Born implicit solvent interaction energies [24]. The change in the binding energy of the CGL mutants with galactose or globotriose was calculated as ΔE = Emut-Ewt. The results were obtained with the use of IACP FEB RAS Shared Resource Center "Far Eastern Computing Resource" equipment (https://cc.dvo.ru).

4.2. Construction of Recombinant Plasmids, Protein Expression and Purification

Expression plasmid encoding CGL mutants was constructed as described earlier [10] on the basis of pET40/CmAP plasmid which carried the gene of alkaline phosphatase CmAP as a reporter gene. CGL mutants were genetically engineered by oligonucleotide-specific mutagenesis approach. The amino acid substitutions were introduced into the forward and reverse gene-specific primers (Table 2).

Table 2. Primers for construction of the recombinant plasmids.

Mutation	Sense Primer	Antisense Primer
Asn27Ala	5′–AGTAGCAACCCTGCTAACGCCACTAAGTTG–3′	5′–GCAGGACCAACTTAGTGGCGTTAGCAGGGT–3′
His37Ala	5′–GTCCTGCATAGCGATATCGCTGAAAGAATG–3′	5′–GGAAGTACATTCTTTCAGCGATATCGCTAT–3′
Glu 75Ala	5′–AGCTAATCCACCAAATGCCACCAATATGGTTC–3′	5′–TGATGCAGAACCATATTGGTGGCATTTGGTG–3′
His85Ala	5′–GTTCTGCATCAAGATCGTGCTGATCGGGCA–3′	5′–GAATAGTGCCCGATCAGCACGATCTTGAT–3′
Asn119Ala	5′–ATCCCCGAATCCACCGAATGCTACCGAAACAG–3′	5′–GTATAACTGTTTCGGTAGCATTCGGTGGAT–3′
Asp127Ala	5′–CAGTTATACATGGAGCTAAACATGCAGCCA–3′	5′–GAATTCCATGGCTGCATGTTTAGCTCCATGTA–3′
His129Ala	5′–ATACATGGAGATAAAGCTGCAGCCATGGAA–3′	5′–CAAAAATGAATTCCATGGCTGCAGCTTTATCT–3′

The resultant mutant genes were amplified with the primers CGL-dir: 5′-AGCTGAGCTCGATG ACGATGACAAGATGACAACGTTTCTTATCAAACACAAGGCCAGTG-3′ and CGL-rev: 5′-AGC TGTCGACTTAGGCATAAACTAAAACGCGCTTGTCTTT-3′, and ligated with the vector of pET-40b(+)/CmAP linearized by endonucleases SacI and SalI. The correct CGL cDNA sequence was verified by sequencing with ABI Prism Big Dye Terminator 3.1 Cycle Sequencing Kit and ABIPrism 310 Genetic Analyzer (Applied Biosystems, Foster City, CA, USA).

Recombinant lectins were expressed in *E. coli* Rosetta (DE3) and purified as described previously [10].

4.3. Lectin Activity Assay

The lectin activity assay was performed as described earlier (10). Briefly, 150 of porcine stomach mucin (PSM) with concentration of 0.1 mg/mL (0.1 M carbonate buffer, pH 9.5, containing 0.15 M NaCl) was added to each well of a polystyrene 96-well ELISA microtiter plate Maxisorp (Thermo Fisher Scientific, Waltham, MA, USA), incubated at 4 °C overnight, washed three times with the buffer containing 0.01 M Tris-HCl, pH 7.5, 0.15 M NaCl, 0.05% Triton X-100 (TBS-T) and three times with water. Bovine serum albumin (1 mg/mL) in TBS-T was added as described above. Samples containing recombinant CGL (0.2 mg/mL) were two-fold serially diluted in TBS-T and added in 150 mL aliquots to each well. The plate was incubated at room temperature for 1 h and then washed three times as described above. TBS-T was used as a negative control. Standard assay for alkaline phosphatase activity was carried out as described earlier [10]. One unit of AP activity was defined as the quantity of the enzyme required to release 1.0 µmol of p-nitrophenol from pNPP in 1 min. The specific activity was calculated as units per 1 mg of protein. All lectin activity assays were performed in three independent parallels for three to five times. Data were analyzed using the Student's t-test of the SigmaPlot 2000 version 6.0 program (SPSS Inc.). Differences from controls were considered significant at $p \leq 0.05$.

5. Conclusions

In this report we presented new details of structure-function relationships for a novel lectin from the mussel *C. grayanus*. In silico analysis of CGL complexes with galactose, globotriose and PSM-trisaccharide helped us to suggest the binding mechanisms of CGL. For the first time, it was shown that point mutation of residues that form hydrogen bonds with a terminal monosaccharide and not included in the conservative motif HPY(K)G, led to a change in the mucin-binding activity of mutants. The maximal decrease in the mucin-binding activity of the mutants Asn119Ala in Site 1 and Asn27Ala in Site 2 was due to the loss of all three hydrogen bonds with two terminal galactose residues of oligosaccharides in comparison with the wild type CGL. However, the efficiency of CGL binding depends on the composition of at least three terminal monosaccharide units in oligosaccharides. The amino acid residue Asp127 in Site 3 (and similar residues Asp35 and Asp83 in Sites 1 and 2) was found to play a decisive role in the higher lectin affinity to mucin due to forming an additional bond with the third fucose.

The ability of CGL to recognize Gb3 on the surface of breast cancer cells and bind mucin-type glycoproteins, which are often associated with oncogenic transformation, make it prospect in construction of a biosensor for cancer diagnostics. In this regard, the results elicited the individual contribution of His37, His129, Glu75, Asp127, His85, Asn27 and Asn119 amino acid residues from carbohydrate-binding sites to CGL activity could be helpful for designing an artificial analog of CGL with enhanced Gb3- and mucin-binding properties for applying in cancer diagnostics or anticancer therapy.

Author Contributions: S.N.K., N.S.B., G.N.L. and L.A.B. contributed equally to this work; V.A.R., O.M.S. and L.A.T. improved the manuscript through careful review and helpful suggestions.

Funding: This research was funded by Ministry of Education and Science of Russia (Agreement 02.G25.31.0172, 01.12.2015), and the APC was partially funded by the program "Far East" grant number 18-4-051.

Conflicts of Interest: The authors declare no conflict of interest.

References

1. Sharon, N.; Lis, H. History of lectins: From hemagglutinins to biological recognition molecules. *Glycobiology* **2004**, *14*, 53–62. [CrossRef] [PubMed]
2. Kilpatrick, D.C. Animal lectins: A historical introduction and overview. *Biochim. Biophys. Acta* **2002**, *1572*, 187–197. [CrossRef]
3. Iwanaga, S.; Lee, B.L. Recent advances in the innate immunity of invertebrate animals. *J. Biochem. Mol. Biol.* **2005**, *38*, 128–150. [CrossRef] [PubMed]
4. Vasta, G.R.; Ahmed, H. *Animal Lectins: A Functional View*; CRC Press: Boca Raton, FL, USA, 2008; ISBN 9780849372698.
5. Varki, A.; Cummings, R.D.; Esko, J.D.; Stanley, P.; Hart, G.W.; Aebi, M.; Darvill, A.G.; Kinoshita, T.; Packer, N.H. (Eds.) *Essentials of Glycobiology*, 3rd ed.; Cold Spring Harbor Laboratory Press: Cold Spring Harbor, NY, USA, 2015–2017. Available online: https://www.ncbi.nlm.nih.gov/books/NBK310274 (accessed on 5 September 2017).
6. Classification of Animal Lectins. Part I: Structures and Functions of Animal Lectins. Available online: http://www.imperial.ac.uk/research/animallectins/ctld/lectins.html (accessed on 1 January 2014).
7. Fujimoto, Z.; Tateno, H.; Hirabayashi, J. Lectin Structures: classification based on the 3-D structures. In *Lectins*; Hirabayashi, J., Ed.; Methods in Molecular Biology (Methods and Protocols); Humana Press: New York, NY, USA, 2014; Volume 1200.
8. Belogortseva, N.I.; Molchanova, V.I.; Kurika, A.V.; Skobun, A.S.; Glazkova, V.E. Isolation and characterization of new GalNAc/Gal-specific lectin from the sea mussel *Crenomytilus grayanus*. *Comp. Biochem. Physiol. C Pharmacol. Toxicol. Endocrinol.* **1998**, *119*, 45–50. [CrossRef]
9. Kovalchuk, S.N.; Chikalovets, I.V.; Chernikov, O.V.; Molchanova, V.I.; Li, W.; Rasskazov, V.A.; Lukyanov, P.A. cDNA cloning and structural characterization of a lectin from the mussel *Crenomytilus grayanus* with a unique amino acid sequence and antibacterial activity. *Fish. Shellfish Immunol.* **2013**, *35*, 1320–1324. [CrossRef] [PubMed]
10. Kovalchuk, S.N.; Golotin, V.A.; Balabanova, L.A.; Buinovskaya, N.S.; Likhatskaya, G.N.; Rasskazov, V.A. Carbohydrate-binding motifs in a novel type lectin from the sea mussel *Crenomytilus grayanus*: Homology modeling study and site-specific mutagenesis. *Fish. Shellfish Immunol.* **2015**, *47*, 565–571. [CrossRef] [PubMed]
11. Jakób, M.; Lubkowski, J.; O'Keefe, B.R.; Wlodawer, A. Structure of a lectin from the sea mussel *Crenomytilus grayanus* (CGL). *Acta Crystallogr. F Struct. Biol. Commun.* **2015**, *71*, 1429–1436. [CrossRef] [PubMed]
12. Liao, J.H.; Chien, C.T.; Wu, H.Y.; Huang, K.F.; Wang, I.; Ho, M.R.; Tu, I.F.; Lee, I.M.; Li, W.; Shih, Y.L.; et al. Multivalent marine lectin from *Crenomytilus grayanus* possesses anti-cancer activity through recognizing globotriose Gb3. *J. Am. Chem. Soc.* **2016**, *138*, 4787–4795. [CrossRef] [PubMed]
13. Terada, D.; Kawai, F.; Noguchi, H.; Unzai, S.; Hasan, I.; Fujii, Y.; Tame, J.R.H. Crystal structure of MytiLec, a galactose-binding lectin from the mussel *Mytilus galloprovincialis* with cytotoxicity against certain cancer cell types. *Sci. Rep.* **2016**, *6*, 28344. [CrossRef] [PubMed]
14. Balabanova, L.; Golotin, V.; Kovalchuk, S.; Bulgakov, A.; Likhatskaya, G.; Son, O.; Rasskazov, V.A. A novel bifunctional hybrid with marine bacterium alkaline phosphatase and Far Eastern holothurian mannan-binding lectin activities. *PLoS ONE* **2014**, *9*, e112729. [CrossRef] [PubMed]
15. Fujii, Y.; Dohmae, N.; Takio, K.; Kawsar, S.M.; Matsumoto, R.; Hasan, I.; Koide, Y.; Kanaly, R.A.; Yasumitsu, H.; Ogawa, Y.; et al. A lectin from the mussel *Mytilus galloprovincialis* has a highly novel primary structure and induces glycan-mediated cytotoxicity of globotriaosyl ceramide expressing lymphoma cells. *J. Biol. Chem.* **2012**, *287*, 44772–44783. [CrossRef] [PubMed]
16. Chikalovets, I.V.; Kovalchuk, S.N.; Litovchenko, A.P.; Molchanova, V.I.; Pivkin, M.V.; Chernikov, O.V. A new Gal/GalNAc-specific lectin from the mussel *Mytilus trossulus*: Structure, tissue specificity, antimicrobial and antifungal activity. *Fish. Shellfish Immunol.* **2016**, 27–33. [CrossRef] [PubMed]
17. Gerdol, M.; Venier, P. An updated molecular basis for mussel immunity. *Fish. Shellfish Immunol.* **2015**, *1*, 17–38. [CrossRef] [PubMed]
18. Hasan, I.; Gerdol, M.; Fujii, Y.; Rajia, S.; Koide, Y.; Yamamoto, D.; Kawsar, S.M.; Ozeki, Y. cDNA and gene structure of MytiLec-1, a bacteriostatic R-type lectin from the Mediterranean mussel (*Mytilus galloprovincialis*). *Mar. Drugs* **2016**, *14*, 92. [CrossRef] [PubMed]

19. García-Maldonado, E.; Cano-Sánchez, P.; Hernández-Santoyo, A. Molecular and functional characterization of a glycosylated galactose-binding lectin from *Mytilus californianus*. *Fish. Shellfish Immunol.* **2017**, *66*, 564–574. [CrossRef] [PubMed]
20. Murzin, A.G.; Lesk, A.M.; Chothia, C. Beta-trefoil fold. Patterns of structure and sequence in the Kunitz inhibitors interleukins—1 beta and 1 alpha and fibroblast growth factors. *J. Mol. Biol.* **1992**, *223*, 531–543. [CrossRef]
21. SCOPe 2.06. Available online: http://scop.berkeley.edu/sunid=50352 (accessed on 2 March 2018).
22. *Molecular Operating Environment (MOE), 2018.01*; Chemical Computing Group ULC: Montreal, QC, Canada, 2018.
23. Tian, P.; Engelbrektson, A.; Mandrell, R. Two-log increase in sensitivity for detection of norovirus in complex samples by concentration with porcine gastric mucin conjugated to magnetic beads. *Appl. Environ. Microbiol.* **2008**, *74*, 4271–4276. [CrossRef] [PubMed]
24. Labute, P. The generalized born/volume integral (GB/VI) implicit solvent model: Estimation of the free energy of hydration using london dispersion instead of atomic surface area. *J. Comput. Chem.* **2008**, *29*, 1693–1698. [CrossRef] [PubMed]

marine drugs

Review

Metabolites of Seaweeds as Potential Agents for the Prevention and Therapy of Influenza Infection

Natalia Besednova [1], Tatiana Zaporozhets [1], Tatiana Kuznetsova [1], Ilona Makarenkova [1], Lydmila Fedyanina [2], Sergey Kryzhanovsky [2], Olesya Malyarenko [3] and Svetlana Ermakova [3,*]

1 Federal State Budgetary Scientific Institution, Somov Research Institute of Epidemiology and Microbiology, Sel'skaya street, 1, Vladivostok 690087, Russia; besednoff_lev@mail.ru (N.B.); niiem_vl@mail.ru (T.Z.); takuznets@mail.ru (T.K.); ilona_m@mail.ru (I.M.)
2 Far Eastern Federal University, School of Biomedicine, bldg. M25 FEFU Campus, Ajax Bay, Russky Isl., Vladivostok 690922, Russia; fedyanina.ln@dvfu.ru (L.F.); kryzhanovskii.sp@dvfu.ru (S.K.)
3 G.B. Elyakov Pacific Institute of Bioorganic Chemistry, Far Eastern Branch of the Russian Academy of Sciences, Pr. 100-letiya Vladivostoka, 159, Vladivostok 690022, Russia; malyarenko.os@gmail.com
* Correspondence: ermakova@piboc.dvo.ru; Tel.: +7-914-725-2424

Received: 15 May 2019; Accepted: 20 June 2019; Published: 22 June 2019

Abstract: Context: Seaweed metabolites (fucoidans, carrageenans, ulvans, lectins, and polyphenols) are biologically active compounds that target proteins or genes of the influenza virus and host components that are necessary for replication and reproduction of the virus. Objective: This review gathers the information available in the literature regarding to the useful properties of seaweeds metabolites as potential agents for the prevention and therapy of influenza infection. Materials and methods: The sources of scientific literature were found in various electronic databases (i.e., PubMed, Web of Science, and ScienceDirect) and library search. The retrospective search depth is 25 years. Results: Influenza is a serious medical and social problem for humanity. Recently developed drugs are quite effective against currently circulating influenza virus strains, but their use can lead to the selection of resistant viral strains. In this regard, new therapeutic approaches and drugs with a broad spectrum of activity are needed. Metabolites of seaweeds fulfill these requirements. This review presents the results of in vitro and in vivo experimental and clinical studies about the effectiveness of these compounds in combating influenza infection and explains the necessity of their use as a potential basis for the creation of new drugs with a broad spectrum of activity.

Keywords: Flu; alga; sulphated polysaccharides; alginates; lectins; polyphenols; anti-viral activity

1. Introduction

The socioeconomic losses associated with viral infections of the respiratory tract are enormous at present. In Russia, acute respiratory infections (ARIs), including influenza, occupy a leading position for infectious diseases [1]. According to the Russian Federal Service for Surveillance on Consumer Rights Protection and Human Wellbeing (Rospotrebnadzor), 27.3–41.2 million cases of these diseases are registered in Russia each year. The total economic damage from ARIs in Russia ranges from 40 to 100 billion rubles annually [2]. In the United States, more than 400,000 people per year are hospitalized with respiratory viral infections [3].

Influenza is a serious medical and social problem for humanity. This acute infectious disease is caused by an enveloped ribonucleic acid (RNA) containing virus belonging to the family Orthomyxoviridae. Every year, more than 500 million people in the world get the flu; about 2 million of them die [4]. In Russia, every seventh person is involved in the influenza virus' annual epidemic [5]. When a new antigenic variant of the virus appears, a new pandemic covers all regions of the Earth. It is characterized by high morbidity with a large number of patients requiring hospitalization and mortality among all age groups of the population [6]. The 2009 pandemic of influenza A (H1N1)pdm09 was accompanied by wide coverage of the population of many countries of the world, including the Russian Federation, with serious clinical complications and high mortality [7,8]. Adverse outcomes were observed not only among immunocompromised individuals in high risk groups but also in healthy young people with no significant previous pathology, including pregnant women. The influenza virus can cause disease not only in humans but also in various animals (e.g., birds, pigs, horses) [9]. In recent years, cases of human infection with avian influenza viruses of the H5N1, H7N7, and H7N9 subtypes have been reported [10].

Despite the presence of a significant number of anti-influenza drugs, this infection is still dangerous, as annual flu epidemics remain insufficiently controlled. Recently developed drugs are quite effective against currently circulating influenza virus strains, but their use can lead to the selection of resistant viral strains [11]. In this regard, there is a need for new therapeutic approaches and drugs with a broad spectrum of activity. Sulphated polysaccharides of algae (red and brown), such as carrageenans and fucoidans fulfill these requirements. This review presents the in vitro and in vivo results of experimental and clinical studies demonstrating the excellent effectiveness of these compounds in combating influenza infection and explain the need to use them as a potential basis for the creation of new drugs with a broad spectrum of activity. Despite their pronounced antiviral properties, they have not been entered the category of drugs yet, because of the difficulties of these compounds' standardization [12].

The purpose of this review is to draw the attention of researchers working on the problem of prevention and therapy of influenza to coordinate their efforts for the creation of standard samples of these highly active biopolymers.

2. Influenza Virion

Influenza virions are particles with a diameter of 80–100 nm, coated with a lipid membrane with an integrated surface of three types of glycoproteins: hemagglutinin (HA), neuraminidase (NA), and the viral ion channel (M2) [13]. On one side, this membrane is in contact with the cytoplasmic domains of HA and NA, and on another, with the core of the virion. The ribonucleoprotein (RNP) is represented by eight segments of the genome: single-stranded negative-polarity RNA in a complex with the nucleoprotein protein and three subunits of the polymerase complex [14,15]. After the virus enters the cell, the ribonucleoprotein gets to the nucleus, where transcription, translation, and replication of segments of the viral genome occur (Figure 1).

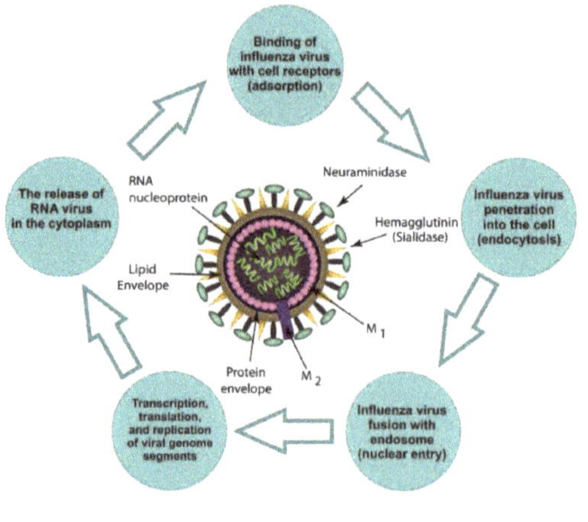

Figure 1. The life cycle of influenza virus.

The binding of the influenza virus with cell sial-containing receptors creates surface glycoproteins, i.e., hemagglutinin (HA), neuraminidase (NA), and viral ion channel (M2). Influenza virus penetration into the cell and fusion with endosome: HA contributes to the release of free nucleocapsid in the cytoplasm (the so-called fusion sites). M2 is involved process of "disassembly" of the virus in endosomes and the Golgi apparatus. Transcription and replication of the viral genome creates transcription and replication of virus-specific RNAs carried out by a viral polymerase complex. Ribonucleoprotein (RNP) enters the cytoplasm and then into the nucleus. The release of the RNA virus in the cytoplasm allows for NA to end the replication and helps to separate matured virion from epithelial cells. Further, the matrix protein (M1) comes into contact with the cytoplasmic domains of HA, NA, and the core of virion. M1 plays an important role in the assembly and disassembly processes of new virus particle.

Transcription and replication of virus-specific RNAs are carried out by a viral polymerase complex. Unlike the polymerases of eukaryotic cells, viral polymerase has no error correction mechanism. Therefore, the frequency of mutations of the viral genome is, according to various estimates, from 10^{-4} to 10^{-6} nucleotides per replication cycle [16,17]. This is several orders of magnitude higher than the rate of mutation in bacteria and eukaryotes [18]. Due to a short life cycle, the evolution of the influenza virus is fast. As a result, the rapid appearance of mutations allows the virus to escape the host's immune response [19,20]. Thus, it can cause annual epidemics, despite the formation of an immune layer in the population due to vaccination and natural incidence. In addition, as result of the use of antiviral drugs, drug-resistant strains of the virus have developed, leading in a decrease in the effectiveness of antiviral chemotherapy [21].

Influenza virus, like all complex viruses, has a supercapsid, i.e., an additional envelope or peplos, the structural elements of which are peplomer, including HA and NA [22]. The capsid encloses the genome of the virus. Three types of influenza virus (genera) have been described: A, B, and C [23]. Type B and C viruses cause disease only in humans. Hemagglutinin and neuraminidase carry antigenic determinants of the influenza virus and determine its subtype (H5N1, H3N2, H1N1, etc.). Influenza hemagglutinin is a highly variable surface glycoprotein, with 17 known antigenic subtypes [24]. The main function of hemagglutinin is receptory, i.e., it mediates the attachment of virions to target cells by binding to sial-containing receptors [25]. Hemagglutinin is the main specific antigen of the virus, causing the formation of antibodies that neutralize the infectivity of the virus. The presence of antibodies against HA is the main criterion for assessing the post-infectious or post-vaccination humoral immune response to the influenza virus [21].

However, the value of HA is not limited to physical contacts between the virus and the cell. It continues to act in the subsequent stages of infection, contributing to the release of free nucleocapsid into the cytoplasm. This occurs in the acidic environment of endosomes (phagolysosomes), due to the special structures of HA (its so-called fusion sites) that promote the unification of viral and cellular membranes.

The NA of influenza destroys sialic acid-based cell receptors on infected cell surfaces and on virions after generation, and thereby prevents virion self-aggregation, facilitating the passage of the virus through mucin during a natural infection. In influenza A viruses, there are nine subtypes of NA, but there is only one NA in B and C viruses. The NA separates the virions from sialylated mucins that cover the mucosa, promoting virus attachment to the surface of epithelial cells. At the end of the replication cycle, it helps to separate mature virions from epithelial cells. In both cases, NA acts as a spreading factor, expanding the area of infection. That is why antibodies to NA show a protective effect, but weaker than antibodies against HA [26].

The nucleoprotein of influenza virus (NP) is the main antigen recognized by cytotoxic T lymphocytes. Amino acid sequences 260–283 of the nucleoprotein of influenza A virus induce the T cell response. The NP of influenza virus is a major factor in the cycle of viral infection when switching the synthesis of influenza virus RNA from transcription mode to replication mode [25].

Protein M1 is the matrix protein of the influenza virus; it covers the lipid membrane. It is in contact with the cytoplasmic tails of HA and NA, and it is bound to the ribonucleoprotein complex of the virus [27]. This protein plays an important role in the assembly and disassembly processes of new virus particles [28]. Membrane protein M2 is an influenza virus surface protein that participates in the creation of an ion channel that regulates pH while disassembling the virus in endosomes and the Golgi apparatus. An acidic pH is a prerequisite for disassembly the virus and stabilizing it during intracellular transport. Viruses with a defect in the activity of this ion channel have poor reproduction efficiency [29].

3. Pathogenic Targets of Influenza Viruses in Humans

Cells of the single-layer multi-row cylindrical ciliated epithelium of the respiratory tract are main targets of the influenza virus. For infection, the virus must overcome the factors of non-specific resistance of the organism such as the viscous properties of mucus, the movement of the cilia of the cylindrical epithelium, action of non-specific inhibitors of viral replication in mucus, the macrophagal barrier and IgA [30]. With the help of HA, the virus attaches to the receptors of target cells and penetrates them, where the replication cycle takes place [5]. After 4–6 h, a batch of new viruses appears in the cell and then they are pushed out through the cell membrane to the outside. After 24 h, the number of viruses whose "parent" entered the cell can reach several hundred million. The released virions infect neighboring cells and some of them enter in the blood. The subsequent death of epithelial cells is caused not only by the cytopathogenic effect of the virus but also by the inability of the cell to fully recover after the replication of the pathogen. In the early stages of infection, Toll-like receptors (TLR) are involved in the recognition of conservative molecules characteristic of pathogenic microorganisms. The influenza virus stimulates the TLR responses of innate and adaptive immunity [31]. On the cell membrane, TLR4 and C-type lectin receptors (MMR-mannose and MGL-galactose) interact with the glycoproteins of the viral membrane, HA, and NA [32]. Inside cells, the endosomal receptors TLR3, TLR7, TLR10, and cytoplasmic RIG1 respond to viral RNA and RNP [33,34].

Since this article summarizes obtaining experimental data on potential next generation of anti-viral agents: biopolymers from brown, red, and green algae, the above-discussed information concerning virus action is important for understanding of mechanisms of the action of marine sulphated polysaccharides on the influenza virus and its targets in the body.

4. Recent Anti-Influenza Drugs

Despite the use of a significant number of anti-influenza drugs in medicine of different countries, the search for and development of new, effective and whenever possible harmless drugs continue [35,36]. Currently, for the prevention and treatment of influenza infection, a number of drugs are available with different mechanisms of action, such as limiting the infection at the early stages, stimulating innate immunity, and manipulating the effect of interferons (Table 1).

For a long time, rimantadine and amantadine were very actively used to treat the flu. Leibbrand et al. [37] reported that these anti-influenza drugs act on two stages of the life cycle of the influenza virus: stripping the virus and releasing virus particles from the cell after replication. Rimantadine is able to increase the acidity inside vacuoles surrounding viral particles after they penetrate into the cell. As a result, the fusion of the influenza virus with the vacuole membrane is prevented, which makes it impossible to transfer viral genetic material from the virus particle to the cytoplasm of the cell. Thus, rimantadine becomes an obstacle between the influenza virus and the genome of the host. Along with clinical efficacy, these drugs caused side effects in the gastrointestinal tract and the nervous system [38]. In addition, many influenza A viruses (for example, H3N2, H1N1) quickly became resistant to these agents [39].

Table 1. Anti-influenza drugs.

Direct Acting Antiviral Drugs	Mechanism of Action of Antiviral Drugs	Side Effects
Oseltamivir (Tamiflu)	Competitive and selective inhibitor of neuraminidase of influenza viruses A and B	The gastrointestinal tract can be involved (nausea and vomiting; diarrhea, abdominal bloating, and fecal incontinence); central nervous system (dizziness, migraine, sleep disturbance, weakness); respiratory tract system (bronchitis, cough, infections of the upper respiratory tract); generalized pain
Zanamivir (Relenza)	Selective inhibitor of neuraminidase of influenza viruses A, inhibitor of replication and release of new virus particles	Allergies, breathing problems, dermatological disorders
Umifenovir (Arbidol)	A specific inhibitor of the fusion of a viral lipid membrane with cell membranes. Interacts with NA, prevents its conformation, which is necessary for the fusion of NA with endosome membranes. Interferon inductor. Stimulator of humoral and cellular immunity	Pruritus, rash, angioedema, urticaria, anaphylaxis
Riamylovir (Triazavirin)	Inhibitor of viral RNA synthesis and replication of genomic fragments	Allergies; the gastrointestinal tract can be involved (nausea and vomiting; diarrhea, abdominal bloating, and fecal incontinence)
Rimantadine, amantadine	M2 channel blockers. An inhibitor of the early stage of virus reproduction from the moment it enters the cell until the beginning of the transcription process. RNA inhibitor	The gastrointestinal tract can be involved (diarrhea); central nervous system (dizziness, migraine, sleep disturbance, weakness); respiratory tract system (cough); generalized pain; allergies

At present, adamantane group of drugs are recommended in case all other measures fail. In the last decade, a number of drugs with direct action on the influenza virus (direct-acting antivirals, DAA) have appeared [39]. These include NA inhibitors (oseltamivir/Tamiflu^{TM} and undecivir/Relenza^{TM}), M2 channel blockers, and fusion inhibitors (umifenovir/Arbidol^{TM}). Zanamivir and oseltamivir have shown lower than expected efficacy in clinical trials. At the same time, these drugs are more effective in children, in whom the drugs reduce the duration of the disease if they are applied within 48 h after the onset of the first symptoms; they also reduce the number of serious complications. Moreover, these drugs are successfully used to prevent and reduce the intensity of symptoms of seasonal flu. The disadvantages of these chemotherapy drugs are a decrease in their effectiveness during the later stages of infection [40]. In cases of prolonged, complicated flu, pathogenic therapy preparations are used to eliminate the effects of the cytokine storm, reducing the severity of reactive processes [15]. Such processes are induced by the virus, but are carried out by the host mechanisms. These include toxic shock syndrome, hyperproduction of proinflammatory cytokines, cellular tissue infiltration, haemorrhagic syndrome, etc. Although modern drugs are quite effective against currently circulating influenza virus strains, their use often leads to the selection of resistant viruses and resistant strains [11].

In this regard, we need new therapeutic approaches and broad-spectrum drugs. Drugs aimed at various viruses or impairing different stages of influenza virus replication will represent a serious means of fighting infections and minimizing the development of resistant viruses. The sulphated polysaccharides of algae (red, brown and green), such as carrageenans, fucoidans, and ulvans, have been studied as anti-influenza drugs and met these requirements. At the same time, there are other compounds from algae that also have antiviral effects, including anti-influenza action, which should be subjected to further experimental and clinical study.

5. Polysaccharides

These compounds represent a class of biopolymers, the content and structure of which vary depending on the type of algae, its place of growth, climatic conditions, harvest season, method of extraction and many other factors [41]. According to the literature, sulphated polysaccharides (fucoidans, galactofucans, dextran sulphates, carrageenans, sulphated chitosans, synthetic polyvinyl, and polyethylene sulphates) have antiviral activity not only against the influenza virus but also against many other viruses, such as those that cause hepatitis C, tick-borne encephalitis, haemorrhagic fever with renal syndrome, dengue fever, and AIDS. It is known that, in the human body, the most prevalent heteropolysaccharides are glycosaminoglycans, negatively charged long unbranched polysaccharides consisting of disaccharides repeating units [42]. The binding of glycosamines with different ligands leads to post-translational modifications that facilitate cell migration, proliferation, and differentiation. The glycosaminoglycans, a class of heparan/heparan sulphates present in the basement membrane, in the extracellular matrix, and on the cell surface that are able to specifically interact with macromolecules of the extracellular matrix (fibronectin and laminin), enzymes, and an extensive class of heparan-binding molecules (growth factors and chemokines) [42]. Mimetics of glycosaminoglycan, including heparan/heparan sulphates provide a wide range of biological effects and modulate the effect of many signaling molecules in cells [43]. Sulphated polysaccharides of algae are natural mimics of heparan sulphates. Fucoidans and carrageenans can mimic the action of endogenous factors and regulate the functions of microorganism systems through key cell and enzyme receptors. Due to this, sulphated polysaccharides have the ability to bind to various receptors on the surface of the host cell and compete with viruses for glycoprotein receptors [44].

One of the characteristic features of algal polysaccharides is the presence of sulphate groups and uronic acid residues in their structures, which distinguishes them from the polysaccharides of land plants [45]. In the last decade, quite a lot of scientific articles have appeared that presents the effectiveness of fucoidans and carrageenans in influenza infection, as well as acute viral "colds".

5.1. Carrageenans

Carrageenans are sulphated polysaccharides of red algae whose chemical structure is based on a disaccharide repeating unit consisting of two D-galactose residues joined with each other by β-1,4 glycosidic bonds. These units are bound in polysaccharides by α-1,3 bonds [46]. The structural diversity of carrageenans is due to the presence of β-(l,4)-linked residues in the form of 3,6-anhydrogalactose, as well as the number and position of sulphate groups in monosaccharide residues [47]. Regular polysaccharides, the polymer chain of which is built from repeating disaccharide units of the same type, represent a different class of carrageenans. Natural carrageenans are rarely regular, as more often they contain repeating units of several types and have an irregular or hybrid structure (Figure 1), structures of which are explained by the multi-stage biosynthesis of polysaccharides in the algal cell wall.

The variability of the primary structure of carrageenans determines the diversity of their macromolecular organisation and defines a wide range of their biological activity [46]. The uniqueness of these hydrocolloids is in the alternating galactose and 3,6-anhydrogalactose residues, which are linked by α-1,3 and β-1,4 glycosidic bonds. A characteristic feature of carrageenan molecules is the large number of sulphate groups [48].

The quantity and location of sulphuric acid residues determine the type, form, and functions of carrageenans, which are actively used in food industry for the production of meat, dairy, and confectionery to improve the microtexture of nutritive products, i.e., as gelling agents, emulsifiers, and thickeners. Among the polysaccharides of algae, carrageenans are the most studied regarding their toxicity, pyrogenicity, and allergenicity [49]. The safety of their use in food and medical purposes has been confirmed by numerous studies [50]. Among the diverse biological properties of these sulphated polysaccharides, their antiviral, anticoagulant, immunomodulatory, antitumor, and anti-ulcer activity are currently attracting the greatest interest [46,51,52]. Sulphated polysaccharides interact with a variety of eukaryotic cell proteins and have a multidirectional effect on the body's immune response, both inhibitory and stimulatory, which makes it possible to consider carrageenans as possible immunomodulators. It is assumed that the immunomodulatory effect of carrageenans is initiated by α-Gal-(1,3)-Gal epitopes [53]. Recently, new data have appeared on the antioxidant activity of algae polysaccharides [46,54].

Carrageenans have attracted the attention of researchers investigating the problem of influenza and other acute respiratory viral infections, particularly in terms of the possibility of creating a physical barrier in the nasal cavity against respiratory viruses, including the flu virus [55]. For this purpose, kappa (k), iota (ι), and lambda (λ) carrageenans were used. It is known that carrageenans block the interaction of viruses with cells and also inhibit the formation of a syncytium, induced by influenza A viruses. A. Leibbrand et al. [37] carried out an investigation showing the effectiveness of carrageenan against human influenza A viruses. The authors determined the sensitivity of the H1N1 influenza virus strains, as well as the pandemic H3N2 strain, to carrageenan subtypes ι and k using the plaque formation method in canine kidney epithelial cells (MDCK). The most active in this test was ι-carrageenan (IC_{50} or 50% inhibitory concentration = 0.04 μg/mL); k-carrageenan was less active (IC_{50} = 0.3 μg/mL). The purity of the ι- and k-carrageenans used in these studies was above 95%, and the molecular weight of both polymers was more than 100,000 Da. At the concentrations of 40 and 4 μg/mL, ι-carrageenan effectively reduced viral replication by 2–4 log units within 96 h after infection. Thus, it was found that ι-carrageenan contributes to the survival of cells infected with the virus by direct exposure to the virus. In another series of experiments, the same authors investigated the effect of carrageenans on an influenza virus-infected primary cell culture of the human epithelium from the nasal cavity. Under these conditions, ι-carrageenan inhibited the formation of plaques by the pandemic strain H1N1/2009 (IC_{50} about 0.04 μg/mL). At the same time, an interesting fact was established: to obtain an effect when cells were infected with another virus (A/PR8/34 H1N1), a higher concentration of polysaccharide was required, i.e., the sensitivity of different strains to carrageenan was different.

Carrageenans are high molecular weight compounds and therefore it is unlikely that they can pass through the barriers of the body. However, local administration has a pronounced effect, for example, with influenza infection and other viral diseases of the respiratory system. In this case, carrageenans reduce the spread of the virus in the surface epithelium of the respiratory organs of infected animals and contribute to survival.

Unfortunately, the solubility of carrageenans is limited, especially in aqueous solutions containing potassium and calcium ions [52], since in their presence carrageenans form viscous gels. Another disadvantage of carrageenans is their anticoagulant properties. Despite this, ι-carrageenan has passed clinical trials and a nasal spray based on it has already been successfully sold in Europe for use in viral infections of the respiratory tract in humans. The effectiveness of the spray for ARIs was also reported by Eccles et al. [56]. The authors showed that, compared with persons receiving placebo, patients in the experimental group noted such significantly reduced symptoms of the disease as nasal congestion, runny nose, cough, and sneezing. Moreover, nasal congestion at the end of the observation period was noted by 63.6% of persons in the placebo group and 28.6% of the group receiving carrageenan. Viral capacity in the nasal mucosa in patients treated with the spray was significantly decreased (92%), while placebo treatment did not affect viral replication. The nasal spray was effective when used during the first 48 h after the onset of symptoms. Similar results were obtained by Ludvig et al. [57].

Spray application reduced the expression of pro-inflammatory cytokines and increased the level of IL-1 and IL-12p40 receptor antagonists, which are known to have anti-inflammatory action in the nasal lavage of patients with respiratory viral infections [56]. It is known that IL-12p40 is necessary for inhibiting the hyperactivity of airway and peribronchial fibrosis [58]. The expression of inflammatory mediators during viral infection may complicate underlying diseases in the form of asthma [59,60]. In this regard, a decrease in the intensity of the immune response due to a lower viral load seems to be an attractive property of treatment of ι-carrageenan. To increase their efficiency, oligosaccharides and their sulphated derivatives having a lower molecular weight were obtained from the high molecular weight

ATP carrageenan [61]. So, the oligosaccharide CO-1 with a molecular weight of 1–3 kDa effectively dose-dependently inhibited the replication of influenza A (H1N1) virus in MDCK cells (selectivity index >25.0). CO-1 did not bind to the cell surface, but it was bound to viral particles during the pre-treatment process. Unlike high molecular weight native carrageenan, this oligosaccharide can penetrate into MDCK cells and inhibit the expression of viral proteins and mRNA after its internalization into the cell, but before it leaves the cell, i.e. in one replication cycle. The main factors affecting the antiviral activity of oligosaccharides are the degree of sulphation and Mw. The most active oligosaccharide CO-1 contained 0.8–1.0 mol/mol sulphate, and its molecular weight was 1–3 kDa. The preparation CO-1 and its full sulphated derivative (COS) significantly increased the survival rate of mice infected with a lethal dose of influenza virus and reduced the viral load in the lungs of these animals [62]. Taking into account these findings, the authors proposed using low molecular weight oligosaccharides of carrageenan in the treatment of influenza as an alternative strategy to combat this infection.

Shao et al. [63] investigated the molecular mechanisms of cell protection using k-carrageenan against SW731 influenza virus penetration. The authors showed that the polysaccharide specifically and effectively inhibited the reproduction of the influenza virus. The MDCK cells were infected with various strains of the influenza virus, after which they were treated with carrageenan at different doses. After 24 h, a dose-dependent decrease in the titer of SW731 and CA04 viruses (homologous MDCK) was recorded. The remaining experimental strains of influenza virus (PR8, WSN, ZB07, and H1N1) were insensitive to carrageenan. Thus, k-carrageenan prevented the development of the extra- and intracellular stages of influenza virus replication. To determine the stage of reproduction of the virus affected by carrageenan, the authors added polysaccharide to infected cells during the period of adsorption (0 h), internalization (1 h), early replication (2–6 h), and release (8 h). Then, after 24 h, the inhibitory effect was evaluated, in response to treatment at the time points of 0, 1, 2, 4, and 6 h. After 8 h, there was no inhibition. Thus, it was shown that not only extracellular, but also some intracellular stages of influenza virus replication were affected by k-carrageenan. The titer of influenza virus SW731 was decreased in cases where the virus was treated with the polysaccharide before or during infection of the cells. When treating cells with carrageenan, there was no such effect, i.e. the best results were obtained by the action of the polysaccharide at the adsorption stage. The same authors showed that carrageenan does not inactivate the influenza virus, since no differences were found between the pre-treatment group and the adsorption group. Carrageenan specifically inhibited the binding of the HA virus to its receptor, sialic acid. The effect of polysaccharides on the exit stage was insignificant. The authors have proposed the use of carrageenan against the H1N1/2009 influenza virus and other viruses containing HA/H1N1/2009. The carrageenan used in these experiments contained both high- and low-molecular components, and therefore it acted on the extracellular and intracellular stages of reproduction.

Other authors [64], investigating the polysaccharides of the red alga *Gyrodinium impudicum*, obtained sulphated galactan conjugated with uronic acid and studied its activity as an anti-influenza agent. As in the studies by Wang W. [61,62] it was shown that the antiviral activity (IC_{50} against the influenza virus at doses 0.19–0.48 μg/mL) of the galactan is related to its ability to interact with viral particles, which preventing virus adsorption and internalization.

Yu et al. [65] suggested using hybrid carrageenan (ι/κ/ν-carrageenan) as a potential inhibitor of influenza A virus. In this study, the authors obtained three polysaccharides from the red alga *Eucheuma denticulatum* by successive extraction with cold and hot water and an aqueous solution of NaOH: hybrid polysaccharide (EW), preparation EH, containing only ι-carrageenan, and α-1,4α-D-glucan (EA), which consisted of 88% of glucan and 12% carrageenan as an impurity. The molecular weights of the compounds were 480, 580, and 510 kDa, respectively. Antiviral activity against the H1N1 influenza virus was highest when used the hybrid polysaccharide (276.5 μg/mL), and the H1N1 virus suppression index was 52% using a polysaccharide dose of 250 μg/mL. The IC_{50} for ι-carrageenan EH was 366.4 μg/mL. The polysaccharide EA showed the lowest antiviral activity (IC_{50} > 430 μg/mL).

The study of Fazekas T. et al. [66] was very important, because it was conducted in a clinical setting with the participation of patients (children and adults aged from 1 to 18 years) with respiratory viral infections, including influenza B. Intranasal spray was used three times a day in for seven days. Symptom dynamics was monitored and viral load was determined. In this study iota-carrageenan did not alleviate symptoms in children with acute symptoms of common cold, but significantly reduced viral load in nasal secretions that may have important implications for future studies. In this study, ν-carrageenan as part of the spray did not reduce the severity of symptoms in children with acute cold symptoms, but significantly reduced the viral load in the nasal lavage of patients who received the spray compared with the control group (27% versus 13%, respectively).

A positive evaluation of the effectiveness of nasal sprays in patients with acute respiratory viral infections was provided in two randomized double-blind, placebo-controlled trials by Koenighofer et al. [67]. In patients treated with carrageenan, the duration of the disease decreased by two days, there were fewer relapses, and the body was cleared of viruses more rapidly. The spray was effective in both children and adults. The treatment of patients with influenza by carrageenan gel was shown to significantly facilitate respiratory tract, reduces the duration of illness, and the severity of symptoms of intoxication. Carrageenans were found to provide a more pronounced synergistic effect with anti-influenza drugs with a different mechanism of action.

A number of authors have proposed increasing the effectiveness of the treatment by combining carrageenan with other drugs. Thus, a combined intranasal spray, including carrageenan and zanamivir (an NA inhibitor) was proposed by Morokutti-Kurz et al. [68]. Previously, the authors investigated the efficacy of in vivo and in vitro intranasal administration of zanamivir in different doses for the prevention and treatment of influenza. Their study showed that treatment of animals before infection and 36 h after infection with a virus was not accompanied by adverse events.

Zanamivir and carrageenan separately exhibited different antiviral activity against different strains of the influenza virus. Since the mechanism of action of these agents is quite different, one could expect protection against a wider spectrum of viruses than with their individual use. Both compounds and the complex preparation were non-toxic at the highest concentration (400 μg/mL zanamivir and 533 μg/mL carrageenan). The effectiveness of the suppression of the replication by both substances depended on the virus strain. The IC_{50} value for zanamivir ranged from 0.18 μg/mL for H5N1 and 22.97 μg/mL for H7N7. The IC_{50} values for carrageenan ranged from 0.39 μg/mL to 118.40 μg/mL for H1N1 and H7N7, respectively. Thus, zanamivir and carrageenan target different strains of influenza virus to varying degrees and, therefore, they can provide broader anti-influenza activity by acting synergistically. At the same time, the physical interaction of carrageenan with the virus did not violate the inhibition of NA by zanamivir. The effectiveness of the spray increased when ι-and k-carrageenans were used simultaneously. Mice infected with a lethal dose of the influenza virus that received the placebo dies, as did the animals in all groups receiving monotherapy; however, the combined spray statistically significantly increased the survival of animals. The authors believed that if a vaccine does not keep up with a virus that has changed its composition, such a spray will to some extent protect the population from the impending epidemic.

In addition, an interesting combination of two drugs was suggested [69]. For more than 50 years, xylometazoline has been used to relieve vasoconstriction and oedema of the nasal mucosa in acute respiratory viral infections caused by a wide variety of respiratory viruses, including the influenza virus. The authors combined this vasoconstrictor and ι-carrageenan in one preparation, which had an antiviral effect. It was found that the polysaccharide did not reduce the efficacy and safety of xylometazoline, and the antiviral efficacy of ι-carrageenan remained unchanged.

Thus, carrageenan is currently widely used as a therapeutic and prophylactic agent and was also proposed as an integral part of various antiviral drugs. On the other hand, there is evidence in the literature that oral administration of carrageenan by laboratory animals can lead to the development of inflammation of the gastrointestinal tract [52,70]. However, carrageenan compounds are considered safe and approved for use [48,71]. The Joint Expert Committee on Food Additives (JECFA) concluded that the use of carrageenan is acceptable, even in childhood: "The use of carrageenan in a formula for children or for special medical purposes at concentrations up to 1000 mg/mL does not cause concern" [72]. This confusion, it seems, may be due to imperfect terminology. Some authors combine low molecular weight products of carrageenan hydrolysis, such as polyginan and degraded carrageenan, which are clearly toxic, and native non-degraded food carrageenan, which is considered safe, under the general term "carrageenan" [71]. However there have already been reports of the ability of dietary λ-carrageenan to cause enteritis in rats with prolonged oral ingestion [70].

Among the many study associated with influenza infection, we did not find reports of adverse side effects of carrageenans at intranasal use. Moreover, in Europe, as already mentioned above, the use of the spray for intranasal administration as a preventive and therapeutic agent for influenza and ARIs is permitted. Apparently, attention should be paid to reports of negative phenomena associated with the use of carrageenans and to study this issue separately with respect to these infections.

Thus, it was reported that carrageenans created a physical barrier in the nasal cavity against respiratory viruses, including various strains of influenza virus. At an early stage of viral infection carrageenans are directly associated with the influenza virus, preventing its adsorption, penetration, and replication. At the same time, the antiviral effect of carrageenans is specific and is due to the screening of the cellular structures involved in the binding of the virus to its receptors.

5.2. Fucoidans

Fucoidans are highly sulphated, usually branched polysaccharides, often containing, in addition to fucose residues, glucose, galactose, xylose, mannose, and uronic acids, as well as acetyl groups [45]. The structures of polysaccharides from brown algae are very diverse and depends on the type of alga, its reproductive status, and other abiotic factors. In fact, each new polysaccharide isolated from algae is a new substance, and its molecule contain unique structural elements. This is why the determination of the structure of fucoidans, as well as the clarification of the structure/function relationship of these polysaccharides, is extremely difficult.

It should be noted that the effectiveness of fucoidans of brown algae as potential anti-influenza agents has been studied quite actively in recent years due to the polyvalence of their effects (antiviral, antibacterial, anti-inflammatory, immunomodulatory effects, etc.), as well as the fact that fucoidans penetrate biological membranes. Efficiency of oral administration of fucoidan is confirmed by data of its transformation in macroorganism, which are presented in articles [73,74]. The possibility of the appearance of fucoidan derivatives in the peripheral blood was confirmed by Irhimeh M.R. et al. [73]. Authors using monoclonal antibodies to highly sulfated fucoidan found its derivatives in plasma of healthy participants who took orally for 12 days at 3 g/d Undaria algae powder, containing 10% of fucoidan derivatives and purified galactofucane sulfate. The average concentration of fucoidan detected in plasma was 4.002 mg/L and 12.989 mg/L, respectively. Tokita Y. et al. [74] also found fucoidan from Cladosiphon okamuranus in the serum and urine of healthy participants 6 and 9 h after ingestion of the polysaccharide orally. These facts indicate the possibility of degradation of fucoidan molecules in the human body and the participation of its derived structures in the implementation of antiviral properties.

After administration, these polysaccharides can be detected in the urine and serum [74,75]. Histological studies using monoclonal antibodies against fucoidan made it possible to detect it in the small intestine, the epithelial cells of the jejunum, in mononuclear cells, and in sinusoidal non-parenchymal cells of the liver [76]. The same authors established the active transport of fucoidan through a monolayer of Caco2 cells in vitro and the excretion of fucoidan in the urine of a patient after oral administration. The level of fucoidan increased from 3 to 9 h after administration [77]. To prevent the destruction of fucoidan in the stomach, it is suggested to enclose it in chitosan nanocapsules.

A study on the anti-influenza activity of polysaccharides from the sporophylls of the brown alga *Undaria pinnatifida* allowed Synytsya et al. [78] to establish that in mice, infected in vivo with avian influenza A viruses (subtypes H5N3 and H7N2), the level of virus replication decreased and the production of specific antibodies increased. Oral administration of the polysaccharide blocked the release of the virus from cells and significantly increased the titer of virus-neutralizing antibodies and IgA. This polysaccharide presents as a low molecular weight (Mw 9 kDa) fucogalactan, consisting of partially sulphated and acetylated fucose and galactose residues in approximately equal amounts and having a complex structure. Previously, Hayashi et al. [79] investigated the effectiveness of this *O*-acetylated sulphated fucogalactan in immunocompetent and immunocompromised mice infected with a lethal dose of influenza virus. The use of this polysaccharides reduced virus replication, weight loss, and mortality in animals of both groups and increased their lifespan. Oral administration of fucoidan caused an increase in the titre of neutralizing antibodies in the blood and mucous membranes. In immunocompromised mice, drug-resistant viruses often multiply after treatment with oseltamivir. No resistant viruses were isolated from mice treated with fucoidan. The authors proposed the combined treatment with oseltamivir and fucoidan, because in this case there was no recurrence of influenza virus reproduction, as is sometimes the case when treating only with oseltamivir. Combined treatment with fucoidan and oseltamivir was thus recommended by the authors as a new treatment strategy for influenza infection.

The fucoidan from the brown alga *Kjelmaniella crassifolia* (Mw about 536 kDa, sulphate content 30.1%, purity more than 98%) is a glucuronomanan with branches in the form of oligosaccharides at position 3 of the fucose residues. Oligosaccharides (degree of polymerisation from 0 to 6) consist of 3-linked glucose residues, sulphated at positions 2 and 4 [62]. Intranasal (for four days) application of fucoidan increased the survival of mice (80% versus 30%) and their lifespan and reduced the viral load of the lungs in influenza-infected animals compared to the control group ($p < 0.05$). When treated with oseltamivir alone, 90% of the mice survived. All influenza viruses used in the experiment were sensitive to treatment with fucoidan, but the most susceptible virus was H1N1 (Ca109) ($IC_{50} < 6.5$ µg/mL). Treatment with fucoidan reduced the severity of flu symptoms and pathological changes in the lungs. One valuable quality of fucoidan was the lack of formation of resistant strains of the virus under the action of this polysaccharide. In the supernatants of spleen cells, the levels of interferon-gamma (IFN-γ) and interleukin-2 (IL-2) increased following treatment with fucoidan compared with the control animals. In addition, a direct effect of fucoidan on viral particles was found. It was shown that pre-incubation of the virus with fucoidan at concentrations of 31.25–250 µg/mL significantly reduced the number of plaques in MCDK cell culture, i.e. this polysaccharide can inactivate viral particles by direct contact. This polysaccharide inhibited the activation of the epidermal growth factor receptor (EGFR-epidermal growth factor receptor) and was able to bind to viral NA and inhibit its activity. In this regard, the authors believed that such inhibitors of the EGFR pathway and NA can be used alone or with other drugs to block the processes of penetration and the release of influenza A virus from cells. The investigated fucoidan is a potential candidate for creating a medicine in the form of a spray or drops.

Using SPEV cell culture sensitive to the reproduction of influenza A (H5N1), Makarenkova et al. [80] investigated the in vitro antiviral effect of a fucoidan from the brown seaweed *Laminaria japonica* against the H5N1 influenza virus. The results showed that the fucoidan did not possess cytotoxic properties in concentrations from 500 µg/50 µL to 125 µg/50 µL and did not change the morphological properties of the SPEV cell culture. Fucoidan had a virucidal effect and suppressed the infectious properties of the H5N1 flu virus (a decrease in virus titer of 3.0–3.3 log units relative to the control), but did not protect the cell culture against cytopathogenic effects of the influenza A virus at 48 and 72 h after infection. At the same time, the fucoidan showed antiviral activity at an early stage of infection, i.e. during the first 24 h. The application of fucoidan to the cell culture in various concentrations an hour before the virus was introduced resulted in a decrease in the titer of the influenza virus by 2.3–3.3 log units. With simultaneous introduction of influenza A virus and fucoidan into the cell culture, the virus titer was decreased by 2.3–2.8 log units relative to the control. These results open up prospects in terms of developing new approaches to interrupting virus adsorption by sensitive cells.

A number of reports have been devoted to comparative studies of the anti-influenza effectiveness of polysaccharides from several families of algae [81]. Song et al. [82] assessed *Grateloupia filicina* (family Rhodophita), *Ulva pertusa* (family Chlorophyta), and *Sargassum qingdaoense* (Ochrophyta) in their studies. The yield of polysaccharide was 19.7% (*G. filicina*, GFP), 12.1% (*U. pertusa*, UPP), and 7.2% (*S. qingdaoense*, SQP). The content of sulphate groups in the polysaccharide was also different: 13.54% in UPP, 19.89% in GFP, and 5.64% in SQP. The structure of all three polysaccharides was established, and their biological activities were investigated in vivo and in vitro. The safe concentration for SQP and UPP was 5 mg/mL, and for GFP this was 2.5 µg/mL. The in vitro antiviral effects were evaluated against the H9N2 influenza virus. In the hemagglutination test, the most active were UPP and SQP. Under the action of these polysaccharides, the titer of influenza B virus decreased significantly. GFP was the most active in reducing virus replication and SQP was the least active. The most effective dose of the polysaccharide was 20 µg/mL. Using real-time polymerase chain reaction (PCR), it was shown that the expression of the H9N2 gene was significantly reduced under the influence of the studied polysaccharides. The best inhibitory effect was observed with a GFP dose of 20 µg/mL. In the same study, the authors showed that all three polysaccharides had immunomodulatory potential as the studied polysaccharides were active in the spleen lymphocyte proliferation test. The greatest activity in this test was shown by SQP, the effect of which was dose-dependent. Maximum values were obtained when using the sulphated polysacchrides at a dose of 500 µg/mL. In the experimental group of mice treated with the polysaccharide, the levels of IFN-γ and IL-4 were significantly increased ($p < 0.05$). All polysaccharides increased numbers of CD3+ and CD4+ lymphocytes in the blood compared to controls, but only SQP increased the level of CD8+ cells. Thus, the best effect was obtained with the polysaccharide of the brown alga *S. quingdaoense*, especially at a dose of 50 mg/kg. The authors attributed this phenomenon to the presence of fucose residues in its structure, which play a significant role in immunomodulation [83]. The content of fucose in the PCA was 0.02, 0.05, and 1% for UPP, GFP, and SQP, respectively. The authors also observed immunological phenomena as such the proliferation of spleen cells and the humoral immune response, connected with the presence of fucose in these preparations. The more pronounced suppression of the replication of the influenza virus by the GFP polysaccharide was explained by the higher content of sulphate groups in the structure of this polysaccharide [84,85]. The authors suggest the use of all three polysaccharides as a potential alternative to vaccination, as well as to suppress the replication of the influenza virus.

In another study [81], as a result of a comparative study of sulphated polysaccharides activity from algae of different families (red algae: *Polysiphonia lanosa*, *Furcellaria lumbricalis*, and *Palmaria palmate*; brown algae: *Ascophyllum nodosum* and *Fucus vesiculosis*; green alga: *Ulva latuca*), it was found that fucoidans from brown algae, i.e., *F. vesiculosis* and *A. nodosum*, had the highest anti-influenza activity. The total sugar content in the polysaccharides studied varied from 15.4% (*U. latuca*) to 91.4% (*F. lumbricalis*). Galactans (agars or carrageenans) were mainly isolated from *P. lanosa*, xylans from *P. palmate*, and fucoidans from brown algae. Heteropolysaccharides were isolated from green algae.

The interaction between the H5N1 influenza virus and fucoidan were investigated by Bobrovnitsky [86]. For the first time, the authors visualized this process by scanning probe microscopy, which provides information about the surface microrelief and measures the length and height of observed objects. In this case, measurements were made of the height of viral particles before and after treatment with fucoidans from two types of algae. The concentration of fucoidans was 1 and 100 ng/mL. It was found that the average size of the virus particles after treatment with fucoidans changed significantly. In the case of a lower concentration, the average height of the particles increased from 40 to 45 nm. With increasing concentrations, the height of the virus particles reached 50 nm. These results indicate an interaction between the positively charged groups of lipoproteins of the viral envelope and the negatively charged sulphate groups of fucoidans; this interaction may be the cause of the antiviral effect of polysaccharides. The antiviral effect of these compounds is probably due to the encapsulation of viral particles and their deactivation as a result of this. Adhesion of fucoidan on the surface of viral particles is an irreversible process.

Based on this evidence, fucoidans have not only a direct effect on influenza viruses but also affect the processes of viral attachment and replication, interact with neuraminidase, and inhibit the release of viruses from cells [62,80]. In addition, they promote antiviral immunity, enhance antioxidant protection, and reduce the appearance of inflammation. Numerous studies [75,85,87,88] have demonstrated the influence of these compounds on factors important in innate and adaptive immunity, such as the antioxidant system. Another positive quality of fucoidans is their antibacterial action, which in some cases will allow them to be used to prevent bacterial complications, which often aggravates the course of influenza infection.

6. Lectins

Lectins are widespread carbohydrate-binding proteins and glycoproteins that can specifically and reversibly non-covalently bind mono- and oligosaccharides, both in solution and localized on the cell surface [89,90]. In this way, lectins contribute the so-called first line of defence against bacteria and viruses. These compounds exhibit high specificity in relation of glycoconjugates of bacteria and viruses. Most studied and characterized lectins have been isolated from higher plants; lectins from algae have been studied less thoroughly. However, the observed antiviral and antitumor effects of these compounds have led scientists to look at them from a new perspective. It was previously known that lectins have two or more carbohydrate-binding sites [91]. Connecting to the surface of microorganisms, the lectin can agglutinate and prevent the spread of pathogens throughout the body. In recent years, new families of lectins have been found in the cyanobacterium *Oscillatoria agardhii* (OAA) [92–95], as well as in the red algae *Eucheuma serra* and *Kappaphycus alvaresii* (KAA-2) [96]. They usually have two or four tandem repeats consisting of highly conserved sequences, but do not have homology with other protein families. The uniqueness of these lectins is that they bind carbohydrates with exceptionally high specificity for high-mannose (HM) glucans in the trisaccharide core, including Manα(1-3) Manα(1-6)Man. At low nanomolar levels, these lectins have potential antiviral activity against the influenza virus due to the recognition of HM-glucans in the composition of the glycoproteins of the spikes of the influenza virus.

Mu et al. [97] isolated lectin HRL40 from the green alga *Halimeda renschii*, which was highly specific to HM-N-glycans with (1,3)-bound monosaccharide residues. Lectin HRL40, by binding to the hemagglutinin of the virus, effectively inhibited (with an ED_{50} 2.45 nM) the infectious process in NCI-H292 cells caused by the influenza A/H3N2/Udom/72 virus. Additionally, a lectin with anti-influenza activity was obtained by Sato et al. [98] from the red alga *Eucheuma serra*. This compound, called by the authors a "high mannose-specific lectin" and designated as KAA-2, effectively inhibited the entry of the influenza virus into cells. The carbohydrate-binding profile of this lectin was determined by centrifugation and ultrafiltration. KAA-2 was associated exclusively with high mannose N-glycans, but not with other glycans. The authors tested this lectin against various strains of influenza virus, including the pandemic variant H1N1-2009. With the immunofluorescent method, it was shown that lectin prevented the virus from entering the host cells. Using ELISA, it was found that the lectin KAA-2 was directly associated with the HA of the influenza virus. It was proposed the use of this lectin as a future means of preventing influenza infection.

In the study by Sato et al. [99], the anti-influenza activity of lectins with various carbohydrate specificities was investigated on MDCK cells using different strains (clinical isolates) of the influenza virus (H1N1-2009, A/Oita/ou1P3-3/09). The best results in terms of inhibiting influenza infection were obtained with the HM-binding lectin ESA-2. The EC_{50} in this case was 12.4 nM. This lectin recognized the branched structure of HM-glycans, including the trisaccharide containing Manα(1-3)Manα(1-6)Man in the D2 branch as a primary target. The direct interaction between the lectin ESA-2 with the viral envelope glycoprotein HA was demonstrated by ELISA. This interaction was effectively suppressed by glycoproteins carrying HM-glycans, suggesting that ESA-2 binds to the HA of the influenza virus through HM-glycans. The lectin inhibited the penetration of the virus into cells most effectively when simultaneously introducing the virus and the lectin into the cell culture. When processing ESA-2 cells, viral antigens were not detected in the cells, which indicated that this lectin inhibited the initial stages of virus penetration into the cells. At the same time, no cytopathic effect was observed in infected cells. The antiviral profile of ESA-2 was similar to the lectin KAA-2 from *Kappaphycus alvarezii*, which belongs to the same anti-HIV lectin family [98]. The lectin was non-toxic up to 1000 nM (the highest dose used in this experiment). Sensitivity to lectin depended on the strain of influenza virus. The most susceptible were strains A/Philippines/2/82 (EC_{50} 17.2 ± 3.9) and WSN/33 (EC_{50} 34.6 ± 2.7 nM). In this case it was also proposed to use the lectin ESA-2 in the future as a disinfectant or prophylactic agent.

7. Polyphenols of Algae

The composition of the polyphenol fraction of brown algae is characterized by the predominant content of phorotannins, which are unique complex biopolymers of marine origin and the main cytoplasmic components of these hydrobionts. These compounds are contained inside the cell in both the free and bound state [100]. Phlorotannins have antioxidant, hepatoprotective, anti-allergic, anti-tumour, anti-inflammatory, anti-bacterial, and anti-diabetic properties [101]. Ryu et al. [102] purified from the brown alga *Ecklonia cava* phlorotannin, which proved to be an effective selective inhibitor of the NA of influenza virus (72% at a dose of 30 μg/mL). By fractionating the ethyl acetate layer, five phlorotannins were obtained, identified as phloroglucinol, ecol, 7-phloracol, fluorofucofuroecol, and diecol. The inhibitory activities of these components were assessed against influenza viruses from NA group 1 (A/Bervig_Mission/1/18[H1N1]), A/PR/8/34[H1N1]) and group 2 (A/Hong Kong/8/68[H3N2), A/Chicken/Korea/MS96[H9N2]). All five phlorotannin derivatives were found to be selective inhibitors of NA. Fluorofucofuroecol showed the strongest inhibitory activity against NA viruses of group 1 (IC_{50} of 4.5 and 14.7 mmol, respectively); diecol inhibited the NA of influenza virus strains of group 2 more effectively. All derivatives of phlorotannin enhanced the NA-inhibitory effect of ozaltamivir.

8. Biopolymers of Algae Are Adjuvants for the Influenza Vaccines

Biopolymers of algae are currently being also investigated as candidate adjuvants for the next generation of influenza vaccines. The main direction of improvement for anti-influenza vaccines is to increase their safety. That is why, from whole virion vaccines, the transition was made to split vaccines, and from there to subunit vaccines. However, immunogenicity is often reduced with highly purified antigens [103]. In this regard, scientists study the polysaccharides of algae, whose influence on the formation of innate and adaptive immunity has been described in numerous papers in Russia and in other countries [75,87,88,104]. In the analysis of adjuvant technologies for the creation of vaccines, preference is given to modifiers of functions of the receptors of innate immunity and their signaling pathways [105]. The sulphate polysaccharides of brown algae have some excellent properties as adjuvants: almost complete absence of toxicity, safety, and excellent biocompatibility [106].

In the mechanisms of action of polysaccharides, which are important for the manifestation of the adjuvant effect, one should highlight the ability to exhibit the properties of TLR agonists of innate immunity cells, designed to recognize microbial pathogen-associated molecules. TLRs are major targets for the development of new adjuvants, and TLR agonists are the most preferred adjuvants for vaccines. In the investigation of the specific interaction of polysaccharides with human TLRs, it was found that fucoidans from algae *Saccharina japonica*, *Saccharina cichorioides*, and *Fucus evanescens* specifically bind TLR2 and TLR4, causing activation of the nuclear factor NF-κB. Subsequent expression of genes of proinflammatory cytokines and interferon-inducible genes promote the activation of immunocompetent cells, and the development of an adaptive immune response to unrelated antigens of the Th1 type [107]. Experimental data demonstrate the adjuvant properties of polysaccharides in relation to various antigens and vaccine strains of infectious agents, including influenza virus [104,108]. The results of our experimental studies also indicate the adjuvant activity of fucoidan from the brown alga *F. evanescens*, manifested as an increase in the immunogenicity of the inactivated influenza virus A/California/7/09 H1N1pdm09. At the same time, the effect of fucoidan was more pronounced compared with the traditional licensed adjuvant aluminum hydroxide. In addition, with repeated immunization of animals, fucoidan provided a reduction in antigenic load. The results indicate the promising application of fucoidan as an adjuvant in vaccines of influenza [109]. Of significant interest are the results of a randomized, double-blind, placebo-controlled study with elderly volunteers, focusing on the ability of fucoidan to have an adjuvant effect when administered orally. The volunteers took the fucoidan from *U. pinnatifida* at a dose of 300 mg/day orally for 4 weeks. Subsequent immunization with the trivalent influenza vaccine led to the identification of higher antibody titers against all strains of the virus contained in the vaccine, compared with antibody titers in individuals who received placebo. In the group of volunteers who received fucoidan, after nine weeks, there was a clear tendency to increase the activity of natural killer cells, and the absence of allergic and other undesirable immune reactions [110]. Despite the positive results of testing of sulphated polysaccharides as adjuvants, it should be taken into account that the use of fucoidans as drugs is currently limited, due to difficulties with obtaining structurally characterized and homogeneous samples or oligomeric fractions of fucoidans. In this regard, active work is underway to obtain low molecular weight polysaccharides or fucooligosaccharides (homo- or hetero-oligosaccharides containing from 2 to 10 monosaccharide residues) related to natural fucoidans. A number of studies have indicated the high immunomodulatory activity of low molecular weight, structurally characterized fractions of fucoidan or its oligosaccharides, but studies on their adjuvant properties are rare [109]. Thus, the adjuvant activity of low molecular weight polysaccharides obtained from the brown alga *F. evanescens* was investigated; this was done using enzymes that provided a stable, reproducible structure. The authors considered that this substance can be used as a pharmaceutical substance or adjuvant as a part of vaccine preparations [109]. Therefore, polysaccharides from brown algae can apparently be used as safe and effective adjuvants in the composition of next generation influenza vaccines. Fucoidans may form a new molecular basis for the creation of immune adjuvants, including for influenza vaccines, due to their high biocompatibility, lack of toxicity, and good tolerance by the human body.

9. Conclusions

Last decade, there have been many works devoted to the antiviral potencies of sulphated polysaccharides. The formation of pathogen resistance to drugs on the pharmaceutical market requires new approaches to the treatment of viral diseases, including influenza. To do this, it is necessary to have drugs with different mechanisms of action, which in addition to antiviral effects, have anti-inflammatory, antioxidant, and immunomodulatory activity and to which viruses form resistance only on rare occasions. As presented in this review, the sulphated polysaccharides of brown, red, and green algae have such properties in relation to influenza infection (Figure 2).

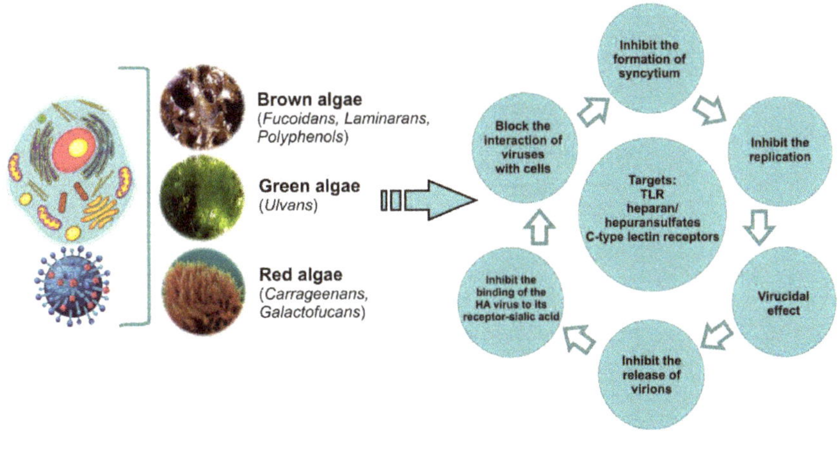

Figure 2. Antiviral activity of algae metabolites.

The pharmaceutical market currently offers a carrageenan-based spray for local (intranasal) application. There are no other drugs based on polysaccharides, which is associated with difficulties in standardization. To standardize these compounds, the physicochemical parameters such as molecular weight, monosaccharide composition, degree of sulphation and other structural features of polysaccharides should be determined. One approach to solving this problem is to obtain structurally characterized and homogeneous samples of native polysaccharides with a low molecular weight or oligomeric fractions. At the same time, due to the wide spectrum of biological activity of polysaccharides and, most importantly, their ability to exert a virucidal effect, that prevent the penetration of influenza viruses into cells and suppress the replication of viral particles, these unique compounds can be used as the basis for the creation of a new generation of medicines. In addition, the almost complete absence of toxicity and pathogen resistance, relatively low cost, a significant yield of the final product, good solubility, significant reserves of natural sources, and the possibility of cultivation algae make polysaccharides promising candidates for the development of drugs with antiviral activity, in particular anti-influenza activity.

Author Contributions: N.B., T.Z., T.K., and I.M. prepared the text, L.F., S.K., O.M., and S.E. contributed the analysis of key parts of text related to it.

Acknowledgments: This work was supported by FEB RAS Grant № 18-5-084. We thank Professor Valentin Stonic, PIBOC FEB RAS, for the assistance.

Conflicts of Interest: The authors declare that there is no conflict of interest regarding the publication of this article.

References

1. Lvov, N.I.; Likhopoenko, V.P. Acute respiratory infections. Guide to infectious diseases. *StP: Foliant* **2011**, *2*, 7–122.
2. Osidak, L.V.; Drinevskiy, V.P.; Erofeeva, M.K.; Eropkin, M.Y.; Konovalov, N.I.; Smororintsev, E.A.; Golovacheva, E.G.; Donluray, E.A.; Baybus, A.M.; Wojciechowska, E.M.; et al. Influenza A (H1N1) 2009 in Russia. *Terra Medica Nova. Infect. Dis.* **2009**, *4–5*, 6–9. (In Rissian)
3. Henrickson, K.J.; Hoover, S.; Kehl, K.S.; Hua, W. National disease burden of respiratory viruses detected in children by polymerase chain reaction. *Pediatr. Infect. Dis. J.* **2004**, *23* (Suppl. 1), S11–S18. [CrossRef]
4. Vasin, A.V.; Sologub, T.V.; Tsybalova, L.M.; Tokin, I.I.; Tsvetkov, V.V. Influenza in the practice of a clinician, an epidemiologist and a virologist. *Med. Inf. Agency Moscow* **2017**, 272. (In Russian)
5. Sologub, T.V. Influenza in modern conditions. *Med. Council* **2015**, *4*, 36–45. (In Russian)
6. Bilichenko, T.N.; Bystritskaya, E.V.; Chuchalin, A.G.; Belevsky, A.S.; Batyn, S.Z. Mortality from respiratory diseases in years 2014-2015 and ways to reduce it. *Pulmonologiya* **2016**, *26*, 389–397. (In Russian) [CrossRef]
7. Arias, C.F.; Escalera-Zamudio, M.; Soto-Del Rio Mde, L.; Cobian-Guemes, A.G.; Isa, P.; Lopez, S. Molecular anatomy of 2009 influenza virus A (H1N1). *Arch. Med. Res.* **2009**, *40*, 643–654. [CrossRef] [PubMed]
8. Gill, J.R.; Sheng, Z.M.; Ely, S.F.; Guinee, D.G.; Beasley, M.B.; Suh, J.; Deshpande, C.; Mollura, D.J.; Morens, D.M.; Bray, M.; et al. Pulmonary pathologic findings of fatal 2009 pandemic influenza A/H1N1 viral infections. *Arch. Pathol. Lab. Med.* **2010**, *134*, 235–243.
9. Bilichenko, T.N. Influence of year 2016. *Med. Council* **2016**, *15*, 52–57. (In Russian) [CrossRef]
10. Mei, L.; Song, P.; Tang, Q.; Shan, K.; Tobe, R.G.; Selotlegeng, L.; Ali, A.H.; Cheng, Y.; Xu, L. Changes in and shortcomings of control strategies, drug stockpiles, and vaccine development during outbreaks of avian influenza A H5N1, H1N1, and H7N9 among humans. *Biosci. Trends* **2013**, *7*, 64–76. [CrossRef] [PubMed]
11. Medina, R.A.; Garcia-Sastre, A. Influenza A viruses: New research developments. *Nat. Rev. Microbiol.* **2011**, *9*, 590–603. [CrossRef]
12. Imbs, T.I.; Schevchenko, N.M.; Zvyagintseva, T.N. Structure, enzymatic transformation and biological properties. In *Fucoidans - Sulfated Polysaccharides of Brown Algae*; Dal'nauka FED RAS: Vladivostok, Russia, 2014; pp. 95–110.
13. Norkin, L.C. Orthomyxoviruses. In *Virology, Molecular Biology and Pathogenesis*; Asm Press American Society Microbiol: Washington, DC, USA, 2010; pp. 296–345.
14. Matusevich, O.V.; Gluzdikov, I.A.; Titov, M.I. Synthesis of PB1 RNA polymerase subunit fragments. *Vestnik St. Petersburg State Univ.* **2011**, *2*, 150–159. (In Russian)

15. Zarubaev, V.V.; Smirnov, V.S. Impact on Cellular Targets as a Means of Combating Influenza Infection. 2014. Available online: https://doi.org/10.15789/2220-7619-2014-1-15-26 (accessed on 22 June 2019).
16. Nobusawa, E.; Sato, K. Comparison of the mutation rates of human influenza A and B viruses. *J. Virol.* **2006**, *80*, 3675–3678. [CrossRef] [PubMed]
17. Smith, D.B.; Inglis, S.C. The mutation rate and variability of eukaryotic viruses: An analytical review. *J. Gen. Virol.* **1987**, *68 (Pt 11)*, 2729–2740. [CrossRef]
18. Drake, J.W.; Charlesworth, B.; Charlesworth, D.; Crow, J.F. Rates of spontaneous mutation. *Genetics* **1998**, *148*, 1667–1686. [PubMed]
19. Hay, A.J.; Gregory, V.; Douglas, A.R.; Lin, Y.P. The evolution of human influenza viruses. *Philos. Trans. R. Soc. Lond. B Biol. Sci.* **2001**, *356*, 1861–1870. [CrossRef] [PubMed]
20. Tate, M.D.; Job, E.R.; Deng, Y.M.; Gunalan, V.; Maurer-Stroh, S.; Reading, P.C. Playing hide and seek: How glycosylation of the influenza virus hemagglutinin can modulate the immune response to infection. *Viruses* **2014**, *6*, 1294–1316. [CrossRef]
21. Tsvetkov, V.V.; Golobokov, G.S. Neuraminidase inhibitors - the gold standard for antiviral therapy for influenza A. *Med. Adv.* **2017**, *4*, 25–30. (In Russian) [CrossRef]
22. Kovalev, N.A.; Krasochko, P.A. Viruses and Prions in the Pathology of Animals and Humans. 2012. Available online: https://www.litres.ru/n-a-kovalev/virusy-i-priony-v-patologii-zhivotnyh-i-cheloveka-7063392 (accessed on 22 June 2019).
23. Sergeeva, I.V.; Demko, I.V. Features of the Flu and Viral-Bacterial Pneumonia. 2017. Available online: https://www.monographies.ru/ru/book/view?id=686 (accessed on 22 June 2019).
24. Kaverin, N.V.; Rudneva, I.A.; Timofeeva, T.A. Antigenic structure of influenza A hemagglutinin. *Vopr. Virol.* **2012**, *1*, 148–158.
25. Desheva, Y.A.; Smolonogina, T.A.; Rudenko, L.G. Biological and protective properties of serum antibodies to influenza neuraminidase virus. *Med. Acad. J.* **2015**, *15*, 35–44. (In Russian)
26. Glezen, W.P. Emerging infections: Pandemic influenza. *Epidemiol. Rev.* **1996**, *18*, 64–76. [CrossRef]
27. Ruigrok, R.W. Structure of Influenza A, B and C Viruses. In *Textbook of Influenza*; Webster, R., Monto, A., Braciale, T., Lamb, R., Eds.; Blackwell Scientific Publications: Hoboken, NJ, USA, 2007. [CrossRef]
28. Nayak, D.P.; Balogun, R.A.; Yamada, H.; Zhou, Z.H.; Barman, S. Influenza virus morphogenesis and budding. *Virus Res.* **2009**, *143*, 147–161. [CrossRef] [PubMed]
29. Lapidus, N.I. School of therapist. SARS: Rational Pharmacotherapy. *Medi. Sov.* **2014**, *16*, 48–54. (In Russian)
30. Sologub, T.V.; Ledvanov, M.Y.; Malyi, V.P.; Stukova, N.Y.; Romantsov, M.G.; Bizenkova, M.N.; Polyakova, T.D. Flu. Clinical symptoms. 2009. Available online: http://www.natural-sciences.ru/ru/article/view?id=14060 (accessed on 22 June 2019).
31. Lee, N.; Wong, C.K.; Hui, D.S.; Lee, S.K.; Wong, R.Y.; Ngai, K.L.; Chan, M.C.; Chu, Y.J.; Ho, A.W.; Lui, G.C.; et al. Role of human Toll-like receptors in naturally occurring influenza A infections. *Influenza Other Respir. Viruses* **2013**, *7*, 666–675. [CrossRef] [PubMed]
32. Londrigan, S.L.; Tate, M.D.; Brooks, A.G.; Reading, P.C. Cell-surface receptors on macrophages and dendritic cells for attachment and entry of influenza virus. *J. Leukoc. Biol.* **2012**, *92*, 97–106. [CrossRef] [PubMed]
33. Lee, S.M.; Kok, K.H.; Jaume, M.; Cheung, T.K.; Yip, T.F.; Lai, J.C.; Guan, Y.; Webster, R.G.; Jin, D.Y.; Peiris, J.S. Toll-like receptor 10 is involved in induction of innate immune responses to influenza virus infection. *Proc. Natl. Acad. Sci. USA* **2014**, *111*, 3793–3798. [CrossRef] [PubMed]
34. Weber, M.; Gawanbacht, A.; Habjan, M.; Rang, A.; Borner, C.; Schmidt, A.M.; Veitinger, S.; Jacob, R.; Devignot, S.; Kochs, G.; et al. Incoming RNA virus nucleocapsids containing a 5'-triphosphorylated genome activate RIG-I and antiviral signaling. *Cell Host Microbe* **2013**, *13*, 336–346. [CrossRef] [PubMed]
35. Davidson, S. Treating Influenza Infection, From Now and Into the Future. *Front. Immunol.* **2018**, *9*, 1946. [CrossRef]
36. Marty, F.M.; Vidal-Puigserver, J.; Clark, C.; Gupta, S.K.; Merino, E.; Garot, D.; Chapman, M.J.; Jacobs, F.; Rodriguez-Noriega, E.; Husa, P.; et al. Intravenous zanamivir or oral oseltamivir for hospitalised patients with influenza: An international, randomised, double-blind, double-dummy, phase 3 trial. *Lancet Respir. Med.* **2017**, *5*, 135–146. [CrossRef]
37. Leibbrandt, A.; Meier, C.; Konig-Schuster, M.; Weinmullner, R.; Kalthoff, D.; Pflugfelder, B.; Graf, P.; Frank-Gehrke, B.; Beer, M.; Fazekas, T.; et al. Iota-carrageenan is a potent inhibitor of influenza A virus infection. *PLoS ONE* **2010**, *5*, e14320. [CrossRef]

38. Jefferson, T.; Jones, M.; Doshi, P.; Del Mar, C. Neuraminidase inhibitors for preventing and treating influenza in healthy adults: systematic review and meta-analysis. *BMJ* **2009**, *339*, b5106. [CrossRef]
39. Nelson, M.I.; Simonsen, L.; Viboud, C.; Miller, M.A.; Holmes, E.C. The origin and global emergence of adamantane resistant A/H3N2 influenza viruses. *Virology* **2009**, *388*, 270–278. [CrossRef] [PubMed]
40. Sologub, T.V.; Tokin, I.I. Tactics of flu patients at the present stage. *Effect. Pharm.* **2017**, *10*, 14–19. (In Russian)
41. Imbs, T.I.; Kharlamenko, V.I.; Zvyagintseva, T.N. Optimization of the extraction process of fucoidan from the brown alga Fucus evanescens. *Chem. Plant Raw Mater.* **2012**, *1*, 143–147. (In Russian)
42. Hook, M.; Kjellen, L.; Johansson, S. Cell-surface glycosaminoglycans. *Annu. Rev. Biochem.* **1984**, *53*, 847–869. [CrossRef] [PubMed]
43. Sheng, G.J.; Oh, Y.I.; Chang, S.K.; Hsieh-Wilson, L.C. Tunable heparan sulfate mimetics for modulating chemokine activity. *J. Am. Chem. Soc.* **2013**, *135*, 10898–10901. [CrossRef]
44. Wang, W.; Wang, S.X.; Guan, H.S. The antiviral activities and mechanisms of marine polysaccharides: An overview. *Mar. Drugs* **2012**, *10*, 2795–2816. [CrossRef]
45. Kusaykin, M.I.; Zvyagintseva, T.N. Structure, enzymatic transformation and biological properties. In *Fucoidans - Sulfated Polysaccharides of Brown Algae*; Dal'nauka FED RAS: Vladivostok, Russia, 2014; pp. 35–60.
46. Yermak, I.M.; Barabanova, A.O.; Sokolova, E.V. Structural features and biological activity of carrageenans - sulfated polysaccharides of red algae of the Far Eastern seas. *Vestn. FEB RAS* **2014**, *1*, 25–36. (In Russian)
47. Knutsen, S.H.; Myslabodsky, D.E.; Larsen, B.; Usov, A.I. A modified system of nomenclature for red algal galactans. *Botanica Mar.* **1994**, *37*, 163–169. [CrossRef]
48. McKim, J.M., Jr.; Baas, H.; Rice, G.P.; Willoughby, J.A., Sr.; Weiner, M.L.; Blakemore, W. Effects of carrageenan on cell permeability, cytotoxicity, and cytokine gene expression in human intestinal and hepatic cell lines. *Food Chem. Toxicol.* **2016**, *96*, 1–10. [CrossRef]
49. Yermak, I.M.; Davydova, V.N.; Aminin, D.L.; Barabanova, A.O.; Sokolova, E.V.; Bogdanovich, R.N.; Polyakova, A.M.; Solovyova, T.F. Immunomodulating activity of carrageenans from red algae of the Far Eastern seas. *Pac. Med. J.* **2009**, *3*, 40–45. (In Russian)
50. Holdt, S.L.; Kraan, S. Bioactive compounds in seaweed: Functional food applications and legislation. *J. Appl. Phycol.* **2011**, *23*, 543–597. [CrossRef]
51. Maksema, I.G.; Kompanets, G.G.; Barabanova, A.O.; Ermak, I.M.; Slonova, R.A. Antiviral effect of carrageenans from red algae during experimental hantavirus infection. *Pac. Med. J.* **2011**, *1*, 32–34. (In Russian)
52. Necas, J.; Bartosikova, L. Carrageenan: A review. *Vet. Med.* **2013**, *58*, 187–205. [CrossRef]
53. Bhattacharyya, S.; Liu, H.; Zhang, Z.; Jam, M.; Dudeja, P.K.; Michel, G.; Linhardt, R.J.; Tobacman, J.K. Carrageenan-induced innate immune response is modified by enzymes that hydrolyze distinct galactosidic bonds. *J. Nutr. Biochem.* **2010**, *21*, 906–913. [CrossRef] [PubMed]
54. Costa, L.S.; Fidelis, G.P.; Cordeiro, S.L.; Oliveira, R.M.; Sabry, D.A.; Camara, R.B.; Nobre, L.T.; Costa, M.S.; Almeida-Lima, J.; Farias, E.H.; et al. Biological activities of sulfated polysaccharides from tropical seaweeds. *Biomed. Pharmacother.* **2010**, *64*, 21–28. [CrossRef] [PubMed]
55. Damonte, E.B.; Matulewicz, M.C.; Cerezo, A.S. Sulfated seaweed polysaccharides as antiviral agents. *Curr. Med. Chem.* **2004**, *11*, 2399–2419. [CrossRef]
56. Eccles, R.; Meier, C.; Jawad, M.; Weinmullner, R.; Grassauer, A.; Prieschl-Grassauer, E. Efficacy and safety of an antiviral Iota-Carrageenan nasal spray: A randomized, double-blind, placebo-controlled exploratory study in volunteers with early symptoms of the common cold. *Respir. Res.* **2010**, *11*, 108. [CrossRef]
57. Ludwig, M.; Enzenhofer, E.; Schneider, S.; Rauch, M.; Bodenteich, A.; Neumann, K.; Prieschl-Grassauer, E.; Grassauer, A.; Lion, T.; Mueller, C.A. Efficacy of a carrageenan nasal spray in patients with common cold: A randomized controlled trial. *Respir. Res.* **2013**, *14*, 124. [CrossRef]
58. Onari, Y.; Yokoyama, A.; Haruta, Y.; Nakashima, T.; Iwamoto, H.; Hattori, N.; Kohno, N. IL-12p40 is essential for the down-regulation of airway hyperresponsiveness in a mouse model of bronchial asthma with prolonged antigen exposure. *Clin. Exp. Allergy* **2009**, *39*, 290–298. [CrossRef]
59. Rohde, G. Drug targets in rhinoviral infections. *Infect. Disord. Drug Targets* **2009**, *9*, 126–132. [CrossRef]
60. Tregoning, J.S.; Schwarze, J. Respiratory viral infections in infants: causes, clinical symptoms, virology, and immunology. *Clin. Microbiol. Rev.* **2010**, *23*, 74–98. [CrossRef] [PubMed]
61. Wang, W.; Zhang, P.; Hao, C.; Zhang, X.E.; Cui, Z.Q.; Guan, H.S. *In vitro* inhibitory effect of carrageenan oligosaccharide on influenza A H1N1 virus. *Antivir. Res.* **2011**, *92*, 237–246. [CrossRef] [PubMed]

62. Wang, W.; Wu, J.; Zhang, X.; Hao, C.; Zhao, X.; Jiao, G.; Shan, X.; Tai, W.; Yu, G. Inhibition of influenza A virus infection by fucoidan targeting viral neuraminidase and cellular EGFR pathway. *Sci. Rep.* **2017**, *7*, 40760. [CrossRef] [PubMed]
63. Shao, Q.; Guo, Q.; Xu, W.; Li, Z.; Zhao, T. Specific Inhibitory Effect of kappa-Carrageenan Polysaccharide on Swine Pandemic 2009 H1N1 Influenza Virus. *PLoS ONE* **2015**, *10*, e0126577.
64. Kim, M.; Yim, J.H.; Kim, S.Y.; Kim, H.S.; Lee, W.G.; Kim, S.J.; Kang, P.S.; Lee, C.K. *In vitro* inhibition of influenza A virus infection by marine microalga-derived sulfated polysaccharide p-KG03. *Antivir. Res.* **2012**, *93*, 253–259. [CrossRef] [PubMed]
65. Yu, G.; Li, M.; Wang, W.; Li, M.; Zhao, X.; Youjing, L.V.; Li, G.; Jiao, J.; Zhao, X. Structure and anti-Influenza A (H1N1) virus activity of three polysaccharides from Eucheuma denticulatum. *J. Ocean Univ. China* **2012**, *11*, 527–532. [CrossRef]
66. Fazekas, T.; Eickhoff, P.; Pruckner, N.; Vollnhofer, G.; Fischmeister, G.; Diakos, C.; Rauch, M.; Verdianz, M.; Zoubek, A.; Gadner, H.; et al. Lessons learned from a double-blind randomised placebo-controlled study with a iota-carrageenan nasal spray as medical device in children with acute symptoms of common cold. *BMC Complement. Altern. Med.* **2012**, *12*, 147. [CrossRef] [PubMed]
67. Koenighofer, M.; Lion, T.; Bodenteich, A.; Prieschl-Grassauer, E.; Grassauer, A.; Unger, H.; Mueller, C.A.; Fazekas, T. Carrageenan nasal spray in virus confirmed common cold: Individual patient data analysis of two randomized controlled trials. *Multidiscip. Respir. Med.* **2014**, *9*, 57. [CrossRef]
68. Morokutti-Kurz, M.; Konig-Schuster, M.; Koller, C.; Graf, C.; Graf, P.; Kirchoff, N.; Reutterer, B.; Seifert, J.M.; Unger, H.; Grassauer, A.; et al. The Intranasal Application of Zanamivir and Carrageenan Is Synergistically Active against Influenza A Virus in the Murine Model. *PLoS ONE* **2015**, *10*, e0128794. [CrossRef]
69. Graf, C.; Bernkop-Schnurch, A.; Eqyed, A.; Coller, C.; Prieschl-Grassauer, A.; Morokutti-Kurz, M. Development of a nasal spray containing xylometazoline hydrochloride and iota-carrageenan for the symptomatic relief of nasal congestion caused by rhinitis and sinusitis. *Int. J. Gen. Med.* **2018**, *11*, 275–283. [CrossRef]
70. Gubina-Vakyulyk, G.I.; Gorbach, T.V.; Tkachenko, A.S.; Tkachenko, M.O. Damage and regeneration of small intestinal enterocytes under the influence of carrageenan induces chronic enteritis. *Comparative Clin. Pathol.* **2015**, *24*, 1473–1477. [CrossRef]
71. Weiner, M.L. Parameters and pitfalls to consider in the conduct of food additive research, Carrageenan as a case study. *Food Chem. Toxicol.* **2016**, *87*, 31–44. [CrossRef] [PubMed]
72. Safety Evaluation of Certain Food Additives. In *WHO Food Additives Series: 70: Prepared by the Seventy-Ninth Meeting of the Joint FAO/WHO Expert Committee on Food Additives (JECFA)*; World Health Organization: Geneva, Switzerland, 2015; Available online: http://apps.who.int/iris/bitstream/10665/171781/3/9789240693982_eng.pdf (accessed on 22 June 2019).
73. Irhimeh, M.R.; Fitton, J.H.; Lowenthal, R.M.; Kongtawelert, P. A quantitative method to detect fucoidan in human plasma using a novel antibody. *Methods Find Exp. Clin. Pharmacol.* **2005**, *27*, 705–710. [CrossRef] [PubMed]
74. Tokita, Y.; Nakajima, K.; Mochida, H.; Iha, M.; Nagamine, T. Development of a fucoidan-specific antibody and measurement of fucoidan in serum and urine by sandwich ELISA. *Biosci. Biotechnol. Biochem.* **2010**, *74*, 350–357. [CrossRef] [PubMed]
75. Fitton, J.H.; Stringer, D.N.; Karpiniec, S.S. Therapies from Fucoidan: An Update. *Mar. Drugs* **2015**, *13*, 5920–5946. [CrossRef] [PubMed]
76. Nagamine, T.; Nakazato, K.; Tomioka, S.; Iha, M.; Nakajima, K. Intestinal absorption of fucoidan extracted from the brown seaweed Cladosiphon okamuranus. *Mar. Drugs* **2015**, *13*, 48–64. [CrossRef] [PubMed]
77. Pinheiro, A.C.; Bourbon, A.I.; Cerqueira, M.A.; Maricato, E.; Nunes, C.; Coimbra, M.A.; Vicente, A.A. Chitosan/fucoidan multilayer nanocapsules as a vehicle for controlled release of bioactive compounds. *Carbohydr. Polym.* **2015**, *115*, 1–9. [CrossRef]
78. Synytsya, A.; Bleha, R.; Pohl, R.; Hayashi, K.; Yoshinaga, K.; Nakano, T.; Hayashi, T. Mekabu fucoidan: structural complexity and defensive effects against avian influenza A viruses. *Carbohydr. Polym.* **2014**, *111*, 633–644. [CrossRef]
79. Hayashi, K.; Lee, J.B.; Nakano, T.; Hayashi, T. Anti-influenza A virus characteristics of a fucoidan from sporophyll of Undaria pinnatifida in mice with normal and compromised immunity. *Microbes Infect.* **2013**, *15*, 302–309. [CrossRef]

80. Makarenkova, I.D.; Deryabin, P.G.; Lvov, D.K.; Zvyagintseva, T.N.; Besednova, N.N. Antiviral activity of sulfated polysaccharide from the brown algae Laminaria japonica against avian influenza A (H5N1) virus infection in the cultured cells. *Probl. Virol.* **2010**, *1*, 41–45. (In Russian)
81. Jiao, G.; Yu, G.; Wang, W.; Zhao, X.; Zhang, J.; Ewart, S. Properties of polysaccharides in several seaweeds from Atlantic Canada and their potential anti-influenza viral activities. *J. Ocean Univ. China* **2012**, *11*, 205–212. [CrossRef]
82. Song, L.; Chen, X.; Liu, X.; Zhang, F.; Hu, L.; Yue, Y.; Li, K.; Li, P. Characterization and comparison of the structural features, immunomodulatory and anti-avian influenza virus activities conferred by three algal sulfated polysaccharides. *Mar. Drugs* **2016**, *14*, 4. [CrossRef]
83. Jin, Y.; Zhang, Y.; Wan, C.; Wang, H.; Hou, L.; Chang, J.; Fan, K.; Xie, X. Immunomodulatory Activity and Protective Effects of Polysaccharide from Eupatorium adenophorum Leaf Extract on Highly Pathogenic H5N1 Influenza Infection. *Evid Based Complement. Alternat. Med.* **2013**, *2013*, 194976. [CrossRef] [PubMed]
84. Bouhlal, R.; Haslin, C.; Chermann, J.C.; Colliec-Jouault, S.; Sinquin, C.; Simon, G.; Cerantola, S.; Riadi, H.; Bourgougnon, N. Antiviral activities of sulfated polysaccharides isolated from Sphaerococcus coronopifolius (Rhodophytha, Gigartinales) and Boergeseniella thuyoides (Rhodophyta, Ceramiales). *Mar. Drugs* **2011**, *9*, 1187–1209. [CrossRef] [PubMed]
85. Pereira, L. Biological and therapeutic properties of the seaweed polysaccharides. *Int. Biol. Rev.* **2018**, *2*. [CrossRef]
86. Bobrovnitsky, I.P.; Mikhailov, V.I.; Odinets, A.G.; Neretina, T.V.; Dobrynina, T.V.; Klinov, D.V. Study of the structure of fucoidan (isolated from Laminaria japonica) and the mechanism of its antiviral activity by atomic force microscopy. *New Med. Technol.* **2010**, *2*, 24–28. (In Russian)
87. Zaporozhets, T.S.; Besednova, N.N. The effect of sulfated algae polysaccharides on factors of adaptive immunity and cytokine production. In *Fucoidans - Sulfated Polysaccharides of Brown Algae. Structure and Biological Properties*; Dal–nauka FED RAS: Vladivostok, Russia, 2014; pp. 217–229.
88. Makarenkova, I.D.; Zaporozhets, T.S.; Besednova, N.N. Sulfated polysaccharides of brown algae are agonists of the functions of innate immunity. In *Fucoidans - Sulfated Polysaccharides of Brown Algae. Structure and Biological Properties*; Dal'nauka FED RAS: Vladivostok, Russia, 2014; pp. 178–217.
89. Antonyuk, V.A. The role of lectins as biologically active substances in pharmaceutical preparations. *Pharmacokinet. Pharmacodyn.* **2014**, *1*, 14–20. (In Russian)
90. Stonik, V.A. Biomolecules. 2018. Available online: http://www.piboc.dvo.ru/tmp/contents_Biomolecules.pdf (accessed on 22 June 2019).
91. Kamiya, H. Possible multiple functions of the invertebrate humoral lectins. *Fish Pathol.* **1995**, *30*, 129–139. [CrossRef]
92. Ferir, G.; Huskens, D.; Noppen, S.; Koharudin, L.M.; Gronenborn, A.M.; Schols, D. Broad anti-HIV activity of the Oscillatoria agardhii agglutinin homologue lectin family. *J. Antimicrob. Chemother.* **2014**, *69*, 2746–2758. [CrossRef]
93. Koharudin, L.M.; Furey, W.; Gronenborn, A.M. Novel fold and carbohydrate specificity of the potent anti-HIV cyanobacterial lectin from Oscillatoria agardhii. *J. Biol. Chem.* **2011**, *286*, 1588–1597. [CrossRef]
94. Koharudin, L.M.; Kollipara, S.; Aiken, C.; Gronenborn, A.M. Structural insights into the anti-HIV activity of the Oscillatoria agardhii agglutinin homolog lectin family. *J. Biol. Chem.* **2012**, *287*, 33796–33811. [CrossRef] [PubMed]
95. Sato, Y.; Okuyama, S.; Hori, K. Primary structure and carbohydrate binding specificity of a potent anti-HIV lectin isolated from the filamentous cyanobacterium Oscillatoria agardhii. *J. Biol. Chem.* **2007**, *282*, 11021–11029. [CrossRef] [PubMed]
96. Hori, K.; Miyazawa, K.; Ito, K. Some common properties of lectins from marine algae. *Hydrobiologia* **1990**, *204*, 561–566. [CrossRef]
97. Mu, J.; Hirajama, M.; Sato, Y.; Morimoto, K.; Hori, K. A novel high-mannose specific lectin from the green alga Halimeda renshii exhibits potent anti-influenza virus activity through high-affinity binding to the viral hemagglutinin. *Mar. Drugs* **2017**, *15*, E255. [CrossRef] [PubMed]
98. Sato, Y.; Morimoto, K.; Hirayama, M.; Hori, K. High mannose-specific lectin (KAA-2) from the red alga Kappaphycus alvarezii potently inhibits influenza virus infection in a strain-independent manner. *Biochem. Biophys. Res. Commun.* **2011**, *405*, 291–296. [CrossRef] [PubMed]

99. Sato, Y. Structure and Function of a Novel Class of High Mannose-binding Proteins with Anti-viral or Anti-tumor Activity. *Yakugaku zasshi: J. Pharmac. Soc. Jpn.* **2015**, *135*, 1281–1289. [CrossRef] [PubMed]
100. Koivicco, R.; Loponen, J.; Pihlaja, K.; Jormalainen, V. High-perfomance liquid chromatographic analysis of florotannins from the brown alga Fucus vesiculosus. *Phytochem. Anal.* **2007**, *18*, 326–332. [CrossRef]
101. Bogolitsyn, K.G.; Druzhinina, A.S.; Ovchinnikov, D.V.; Kaplitin, P.A.; Shulgina, E.V.; Parshina, A.E. Polyphenols of brown algae. *Chem. Veget. Raw Mater.* **2018**, *3*, 5–21. (In Russian) [CrossRef]
102. Ryu, Y.B.; Jeong, H.J.; Yoon, S.Y.; Park, J.Y.; Kim, Y.M.; Park, S.J.; Rho, M.C.; Kim, S.J.; Lee, W.S. Influenza virus neuraminidase inhibitory activity of phlorotannins from the edible brown alga Ecklonia cava. *J. Agric. Food Chem.* **2011**, *59*, 6467–6473. [CrossRef]
103. Tsybalova, L.M.; Kiselev, O.I. Universal flu vaccines. Developments, use prospects. *Voprosy Virol.* **2012**, *1*, 9–14.
104. Zhang, W.; Oda, T.; Yu, Q.; Jin, J.O. Fucoidan from Macrocystis pyrifera has powerful immune-modulatory effects compared to three other fucoidans. *Mar. Drugs* **2015**, *13*, 1084–1104. [CrossRef] [PubMed]
105. Semakova, A.P.; Mikshis, N.I. Adjuvant technologies in the creation of modern vaccines. *Probl. Espec. Danger. Infect.* **2016**, *2*, 28–35. (In Russian)
106. Petrovsky, N.; Cooper, P.D. Carbohydrate-based immune adjuvants. *Expert Rev. Vaccines* **2011**, *10*, 523–537. [CrossRef] [PubMed]
107. Makarenkova, I.D.; Logunov, D.Y.; Tukhvatulin, A.I.; Semenov, I.B.; Zvyagintseva, T.N.; Gorbach, V.I.; Ermakova, S.P.; Besednova, N.N. Sulfated polysaccharides of brown seaweeds are ligands of Toll-like receptors. *Biochem. (Moscow). Suppl. Ser. B Biomed. Chem.* **2012**, *6*, 75–80. [CrossRef]
108. Lin, C.C.; Pan, I.H.; Li, Y.R.; Pan, Y.G.; Lin, M.K.; Lu, Y.H.; Wu, H.C.; Chu, C.L. The adjuvant effects of high-molecule-weight polysaccharides purified from Antrodia cinnamomea on dendritic cell function and DNA vaccines. *PLoS ONE* **2015**, *10*, e0116191. [CrossRef] [PubMed]
109. Kuznetsova, T.A.; Ivanushko, L.A.; Persiyanova, E.V.; Shutikova, A.L.; Ermakova, S.P.; Khotimchenko, M.Y.; Besednova, N.N. Evaluation of adjuvant effects of fucoidan from brown seaweed Fucus evanescens and its structural analogues for the strengthening vaccines effectiveness. *Biomeditsinskaya Khimiya* **2017**, *63*, 553–558. (In Russian) [CrossRef] [PubMed]
110. Negishi, H.; Mori, M.; Mori, H.; Yamori, Y. Supplementation of elderly Japanese men and women with fucoidan from seaweed increases immune responses to seasonal influenza vaccination. *J. Nutr.* **2013**, *143*, 1794–1798. [CrossRef]

marine drugs

MDPI

Article

A Novel Alkaline Phosphatase/Phosphodiesterase, CamPhoD, from Marine Bacterium *Cobetia amphilecti* KMM 296

Yulia Noskova [1,*], Galina Likhatskaya [1], Natalia Terentieva [1], Oksana Son [2], Liudmila Tekutyeva [2] and Larissa Balabanova [1,2,*]

1 Laboratories of Marine Biochemistry and Bioassays and Mechanisms of Action of Biologically Active Substances, G.B. Elyakov Pacific Institute of Bioorganic Chemistry, Far Eastern Branch, the Russian Academy of Sciences, Vladivostok 690022, Russia; galin56@mail.ru (G.L.); nattere@mail.ru (N.T.)

2 School of Economics and Management of Far East Federal University, Vladivostok 690950, Russia; oksana_son@bk.ru (O.S.); tekuteva.la@dvfu.ru (L.T.)

* Correspondence: noskovaiulia@yandex.ru (Y.N.); lbalabanova@mail.ru (L.B.); Tel.: +7-423-231-16-35 (L.B.); Fax: +7-423-231-40-50 (L.B.)

Received: 22 October 2019; Accepted: 19 November 2019; Published: 22 November 2019

Abstract: A novel extracellular alkaline phosphatase/phosphodiesterase from the structural protein family PhoD that encoded by the genome sequence of the marine bacterium *Cobetia amphilecti* KMM 296 (CamPhoD) has been expressed in *Escherichia coli* cells. The calculated molecular weight, the number of amino acids, and the isoelectric point (pI) of the mature protein's subunit are equal to 54832.98 Da, 492, and 5.08, respectively. The salt-tolerant, bimetal-dependent enzyme CamPhoD has a molecular weight of approximately 110 kDa in its native state. CamPhoD is activated by Co^{2+}, Mg^{2+}, Ca^{2+}, or Fe^{3+} at a concentration of 2 mM and exhibits maximum activity in the presence of both Co^{2+} and Fe^{3+} ions in the incubation medium at pH 9.2. The exogenous ions, such as Zn^{2+}, Cu^{2+}, and Mn^{2+}, as well as chelating agents EDTA and EGTA, do not have an appreciable effect on the CamPhoD activity. The temperature optimum for the CamPhoD activity is 45 °C. The enzyme catalyzes the cleavage of phosphate mono- and diester bonds in nucleotides, releasing inorganic phosphorus from *p*-nitrophenyl phosphate (pNPP) and guanosine 5′-triphosphate (GTP), as determined by the Chen method, with rate approximately 150- and 250-fold higher than those of bis-pNPP and 5′-pNP-TMP, respectively. The Michaelis–Menten constant (K_m), V_{max}, and efficiency (k_{cat}/K_m) of CamPhoD were 4.2 mM, 0.203 mM/min, and 7988.6 S^{-1}/mM; and 6.71 mM, 0.023 mM/min, and 1133.0 S^{-1}/mM for pNPP and bis-pNPP as the chromogenic substrates, respectively. Among the 3D structures currently available, in this study we found only the low identical structure of the *Bacillus subtilis* enzyme as a homologous template for modeling CamPhoD, with a new architecture of the phosphatase active site containing Fe^{3+} and two Ca^{2+} ions. It is evident that the marine bacterial phosphatase/phosphidiesterase CamPhoD is a new structural member of the PhoD family.

Keywords: recombinant alkaline phosphatase; bimetal-dependent phosphodiesterase; marine bacterium; *Cobetia amphilecti*; PhoD

1. Introduction

Alkaline phosphatases are widely distributed in marine bacteria, which release inorganic phosphate (P_i) from phosphorus-containing compounds dissolved in the ocean and utilize them for their own growth and reproduction [1–3]. Globally, marine bacteria and diatoms have been shown to store and concentrate P_i and then release it into the local marine environment using phosphatase (Pho) activity, thus biologically inducing and controlling phosphorite and apatite nucleation [4,5]. Moreover, the enzymes from marine sources have flexible molecular structures, and therefore work better at ambient or lower temperatures, which opens the possibility to decrease temperatures of production processes for their application in biotechnology [6–9].

Currently, three large families of prokaryotic alkaline phosphatases are known, namely PhoA, PhoD, and PhoX. They differ from each other in structure, substrate specificity, and the dependence on different metal ions for the manifestation of their activities [10]. It has been shown that the PhoD-like phosphatases belonging to the phosphatase/phosphodiesterase family more commonly occur in marine and soil bacteria than PhoA and PhoX [11]. This is due to the presence in the environment of available sources of phosphorus and cofactors in their habitat. It has been proven that the PhoD family is common in the bacteria living in phosphorus- and metal-depleted conditions [3,5,11]. Previously, natural and recombinant alkaline phosphatases isolated from marine bacteria have been described, but information about their alkaline phosphodiesterases is still lacking [6,12–15].

There are many families of phosphodiesterases, which include phospholipases C and D, autotaxin, sphingomyelin phosphodiesterase, DNases, RNases, and restriction endonucleases. However, phosphodiesterases usually refer to the cyclic nucleotide phosphodiesterases degrading cyclic adenosine and guanosine monophosphates (cAMP and cGMP). According to the primary structure and differences in the catalytic domains, they are divided into three known classes: (1) the eukaryotic enzymes; (2) enzymes such as phosphodiesterases from the yeast *Dictyostelium* and the bacteria *Vibrio*; and (3) the bacterial enzymes homologous to purple acid phosphatases and dimetallophosphoesterases, including the three subclasses A, B, and C [16]. The bacterial phosphodiesterases were isolated and characterized from *Aphanothece halophytica* [9], *Delftia acidovorans* [17], *Sphingobium* sp. TCM1 [18], *E. coli* [19], *B. subtilis* [20], as well as a novel unclassified enzyme from the metagenome of an Indian coalbed [16]. All these metal-dependent phosphodiesterases showed maximal activities in the alkaline pH range, and needed different metal ions, such as Ca^{2+}, Zn^{2+}, Mg^{2+}, or Mn^{2+}, for their catalytic activity. The isolated phosphodiesterases were capable of cleaving phosphoric acid residues from specific substrates, such as Bis-*p*-nitrophenyl phosphate (Bis-pNPP) and thymidine-5′-monophosphate-*p*-nitrophenylester (5′-pNP-TMP), which are mostly used as DNA models for studies of phosphodiester hydrolysis [16,21]. It has been previously assumed that the role of PhoD-like enzymes is to participate in the nucleic acid exchange in cells during the main metabolism, taking into account their ability to hydrolyze the phosphodiester bonds [22].

Among three types of phosphoester bonds existing in nature (mono-, di-, and triester), the phosphodiester bond is exceptionally stable, with a half-life of approximately 3×10^7 years at a moderate temperature and a neutral pH, while an acceleration of its cleavage up to 10^{16}-fold in biological processes can be achieved through enzymatic hydrolysis of this bond by the highly specialized metalloenzymes, such as nucleases and phosphoesterases [23,24]. However, finding and exploring novel enzymes with phosphoesterase activity is still a challenge in biotechnology because of some their inherent limitations, such as undesirable selectivity, difficulties in extraction or synthesis, high cost, narrow functional temperature, and pH range [25]. The phosphoesterase function in nature may be related to hydrolyzing a wide range of biomolecules (proteins, nucleic acids, and lipids) implicated in DNA repair, post-translational modification, biomineralization, and energy metabolism, as well as in signal transduction through regulation of the circulation of secondary metabolites, particularly free nucleotides and their analogues [26,27]. The phosphodiesterase families are mostly considered to have a common catalytic domain pocket, with the universal mechanism of nucleophilic attack to control the intracellular levels of cyclic nucleotides, and to be regulators of many physiological and pathophysiological processes [28]. Due to their important role in intracellular signal transduction and the possibility of finding their exact subcellular localization, phosphodiesterases are considered very attractive pharmacological targets [29,30]. Therefore, there is a growing interest in finding ways to disrupt, block, or manipulate quorum sensing (QS) signaling in bacteria [29]. The producers of QS signals have been found among both the free-living and associated marine bacteria inhabiting invertebrates and algae [31]. Consequently, they are promising sources for new bioactive compounds, such as the QS modulators or inhibitors [29].

The QS-related phosphodiesterases of marine origin have yet to be investigated. However, two alkaline phosphatases of the juvenile *Euprymna scolopes* light organ were found to play an active role in dephosphorylating lipid A of the luminous marine bacterium *Vibrio fischeri*, which changes its signaling properties in relation to the host tissues during their symbiotic colonization [32]. The PhoA alkaline phosphatase (CmAP) of the marine bacterium *C. amphilecti* KMM 296 (Collection of Marine Microorganisms, G.B. Elyakov Pacific Institute of Bioorganic Chemistry, Far Eastern Branch, the Russian Academy of Sciences (PIBOC FEB RAS)) isolated from the coelomic fluid of the mussel, *Crenomytilus grayanus*, was suggested to promote the host mollusk shell's mineralization and biofilm regulation of many species of food-derived pathogens [6,7,12]. The mechanism of the CmAP biological action is still unclear and remains under investigation.

Thus, it has been recently shown that the biological role of alkaline phosphatases is more complex and broader than previously assumed. Alkaline phosphatases appear to be involved in major cellular events, such as the regulation of protein phosphorylation, cell growth, apoptosis, and cellular migration [32–34]. Therefore, most human conditions or diseases are accompanied by a change in the level of alkaline phosphatase expression, which is the basis of diagnostics. A newly discovered function of alkaline phosphatases is in maintaining tissue and organ homeostasis by inactivation of bacterial lipopolysaccharides (LPS), and by regulation of cell secretion, microbiome and tumor behavior, and possibly detoxication of hyperphosphorylated extracellular tau proteins, which play a key role in progression of Alzheimer's disease [32–34]. Recently, bovine and human intestinal recombinant alkaline phosphatases underwent clinical trials related to inactivating LPS and preventing inflammation for the treatment of surgical diseases and metabolic disorders [33–35]. It is possible that the search for marine enzymes with dephosphorylating activity and the study of their mechanism of action will also present an application for the new treatment.

The genome sequence analysis of *C. amphilecti* KMM 296 has shown that the bacterium produces not only the highly active alkaline phosphatase CmAP, belonging to the PhoA family (GenBank ID: WP_084589490.1), but also the functionally active PhoD-like phosphatase/phosphodiesterase (GenBank ID: WP_043333989.1), with a novel structure and properties [6,12,36]. This article presents the results of isolation of the gene encoding for the PhoD-like protein from *C. amphilecti* KMM 296, and in producing the recombinant enzyme CamPhoD with the alkaline phosphatase and phosphodiesterase activities and properties.

2. Results and Discussion

2.1. CamPhoD Isolation and Characterization by Enzymatic Activity and Primary Structure

The heterologous expression of the *C. amphilecti* KMM 296 gene (GenBank ID: WP_043333989) corresponding to the open reading frame (ORF) of the PhoD-like phosphatase (CamPhoD) resulted in obtaining an enzymatically active recombinant protein with a specific phosphatase activity of 18.2 U/mg (with p-NPP as a substrate) after purification using the modified scheme described earlier [6]. The CamPhoD phosphodiesterase activity at the cleavage of bis-pNPP was 0.3 U/mg. The isolation of this enzyme confirmed the ability of *C. amphilecti* to produce the functionally active alkaline bifunctional phosphatase/phosphodiesterase CamPhoD with a calculated molecular weight of 54839.8 kDa for the mature protein, without the 33-letter leader peptide, according to the Simple Modular Architecture Research Tool (SMART) database [37]. The obtained data were in agreement with the polyacrylamide gel electrophoresis (PAGE) estimation of its molecular weight (Figure 1).

Apart from the leader peptide indicating an extracellular intent of the enzyme, the CamPhoD 492 amino acid (aa) sequence includes the region of the fibronectin type III repeat (FN3) from 43 to 118 aa residues, containing a cell recognition region of Arg-Gly-Asp (RGD) in a flexible loop between 2 strands, according to the new functional classification of proteins via subfamily domain architectures [38]. RGD is the cell attachment site of a large number of adhesive extracellular matrix and cell surface proteins, which are recognized by transmembrane receptors activating signal transduction. FN3-like domains were also found in bacterial glycosyl hydrolases [38]. It has been shown that the bacterial extracellular proteins with the RGD motif may be located on the surface of the bacterial type IV secretion pili. They mimic fibronectin in triggering cell spreading, focal adhesion formation, and activation of several tyrosine kinases during interaction with various mammalian cell lines [39,40]. Thus, the RGD motif of CamPhoD may be a player in pathogenesis or the symbiotic relationships between the bacterium and host mollusk during its shell mineralization [12,36]. The part of the CamPhoD molecule from 149 to 505 aa residues is the PhoD-like phosphatase (pfam09423), with characteristic active and ion-binding sites [38].

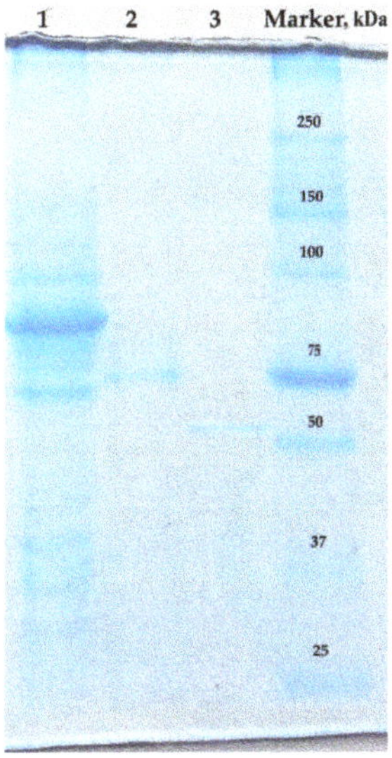

Figure 1. SDS-PAGE image of CamPhoD. Line 1-the crude extract from the recombinant *E. coli* cells; line 2-the purified CamPhoD before the enterokinase treatment; line 3-the purified CamPhoD after the treatment with enterokinase to remove the 34.2 kDa His-tagged N-end of the plasmid pET 40b(+) sequence (shaperon DsbC); line 4-the marker of the protein molecular weights (BioRad).

The values of CamPhoD-specific activities corresponded to the activities of the PhoD phosphatase/phosphodiesterase from *Aphanothece halophytica* and alkaline phosphatase from *Vibrio* sp., whose molecular weights were also similar to CamPhoD and other alkaline phosphatases [10,41–45]. Thus, the molecular weights of the alkaline phosphatases' monomers from *Streptomyces griseus* IMRU 3570, *Pyrococcus abyssi*, and *Thermotoga maritima* were 62 kDa, 54 kDa, and 45 kDa, respectively [42–44]. The enzymes with exclusively phosphodiesterase-related activity possess subunits with lower molecular weight, such as in the enzyme ZiPD from *E. coli* (36 kDa) [45]. Alkaline phosphatases generally have a dimeric structure, but the literature also describes a trimer for the phosphodiesterase from *Delftia acidovorans* with a molecular weight of 85 kDa [17]. According to the gel chromatography data, the native CamPhoD tended to form an active dimer with a molecular weight of approximately 100–120 kDa in the conditions used (see Experimental Procedure section).

2.2. Expression Conditions for CamPhoD Production

The study of optimal expression conditions for the recombinant CamPhoD showed that its highest yield was achieved when cultivating the recombinant *E. coli* strain over 6 h at 37 °C, with an addition of 0.1 mM isopropyl β-D-1-thiogalactopyranoside (IPTG) in the Luria–Bertani (LB) medium (Figure 2).

It was also found that the alkaline phosphatase activity of the recombinant CamPhoD increased when the cells were cultured in a medium depleted by phosphorus. The growth of the recombinant *E. coli* cells in a MX medium containing 80 mM KH_2PO_4 described earlier [46] significantly reduced the alkaline phosphatase activity of CamPhoD down to 0.035 U/mg compared with the activity of the enzyme, which was produced in the standard phosphate-free LB medium, similarly to the phoD phosphatase isolated from *Streptomyces coelicolor* [47].

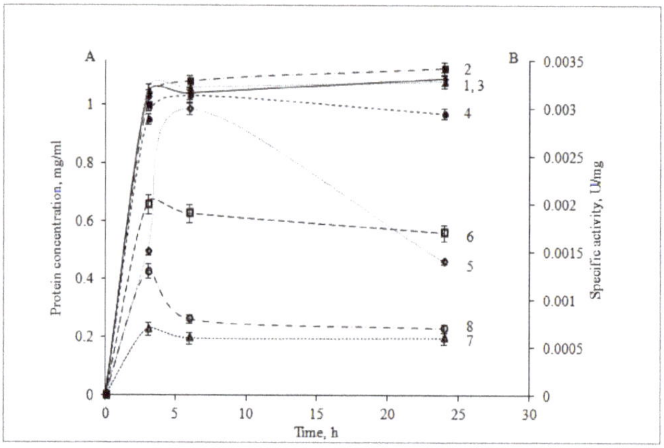

Figure 2. Determination of the expression conditions for the recombinant CamPhoD production: (**A**) the dependence of the CamPhoD concentration (mg/mL) on the cultivation time at 37 °C in the presence of (1) 0.1 mM isopropyl β-D-1-thiogalactopyranoside (IPTG), (2) 0.2 mM IPTG, (3) 0.3 mM IPTG, and (4) 0.5 mM IPTG; (**B**) the dependence of the CamPhoD phosphatase activity (U/mg) on the cultivation time at 37 °C in the presence of (1) 0.1 mM IPTG, (2) 0.2 mM IPTG, (3) 0.3 mM IPTG, and (4) 0.5 mM IPTG.

2.3. Physicochemical and Enzymatic Properties of CamPhoD

The optimum pH for the CamPhoD maximum activity was determined to be 9.2, which lies in the range of pH 8.0–11.0 inherent for most alkaline phosphatases and phosphodiesterases (Figure 3). For comparison, the phosphodiesterases from *Sphingobium* sp. TCM1 and *E. coli* exhibited the maximal activity at pH 9.5 and 8.5–9.8, respectively [18,19].

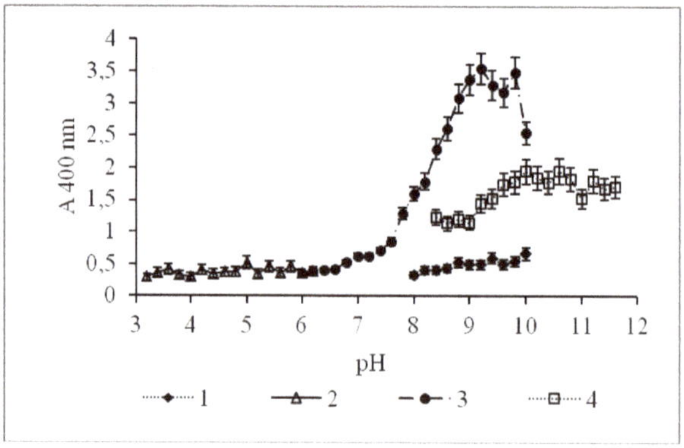

Figure 3. Effect of the pH value on the CamPhoD phosphatase activity for conducting the enzymatic reaction in various buffer solutions: (1) glycine buffer, (2) acetate buffer, (3) Tris-HCl buffer, and (4) bicarbonate buffer.

The significant effect of KCl on the activity and the absence of activity without any salt in the incubation medium indicated that CamPhoD was a highly salt-tolerant enzyme, which is a common trait of many enzymes of marine origin [6,9,48,49]. Moreover, the PhoD alkaline phosphatase/phosphodiesterase from a halotolerant cyanobacterium, *Aphanothece halophytica*, has been shown to be induced and secreted out of cells by salt stress [9]. In the presence of KCl in a concentration up to 1 M, CamPhoD was 2–3 times more active than in the presence of NaCl at the same concentration (Figure 4).

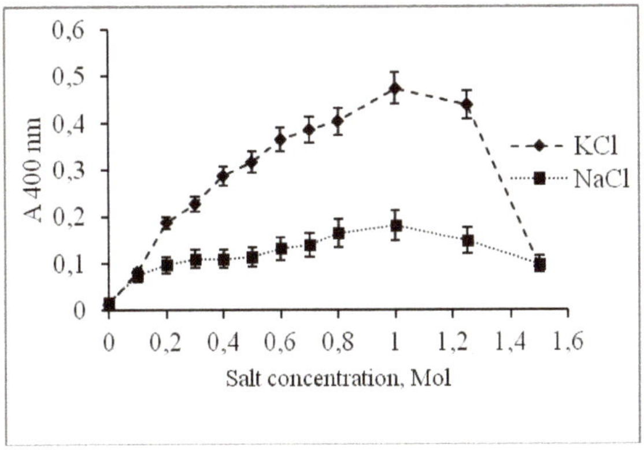

Figure 4. Effect of NaCl and KCl on the CamPhoD alkaline phosphatase activity.

Concentration of both KCl and NaCl of more than 1 M decreased the CamPhoD activity. A similar effect was noted for the salt-tolerant alkaline phosphatase from eggs of the sea urchin *Strongylocentrotus intermedius* [48,50] and the enzyme from the halophilic bacterium *Halomonas* sp. 593 [49].

It was found that the addition of Co^{2+} and Mg^{2+} to the incubation mixture containing the lysate with the recombinant CamPhoD after ultrasonic homogenization of the *E. coli* cells increased its activity by 100% compared to the control. The addition of $CaCl_2$ and $FeCl_3$ activated CamPhoD from the cell lysate by 70% and 60%, respectively. For the CamPhoD purified up to level of homogenous protein, the salts of divalent metals Zn^{2+}, Mn^{2+}, and Cu^{2+} at a concentration of 2 mM had almost no effect on its ability to cleave pNPP, while the salts of Co^{2+}, Mg^{2+}, Ca^{2+}, Fe^{3+}, and Ni^{2+} drastically activated the enzyme, indicating its metal dependence (Table 1).

Table 1. Effect of metal cations on the alkaline phosphatase CamPhoD from *Cobetia amphilecti* KMM 296.

Metal Cations, 2 mM	Retained Activity, (%) *
Co^{2+}	80
Mg^{2+}	68
Ca^{2+}	50
Fe^{3+}	48
Ni^{2+}	32
Cs^{2+}	23
Mn^{2+}	20
Zn^{2+}	18
Cu^{2+}	7
$Co^{2+} + Fe^{3+}$	100
$Ca^{2+} + Fe^{3+}$	66

* The various metal ions were added to the reaction mixture at the 2 mM salt concentration. The phosphatase activity was measured using the standard method described in Experimental Procedures. The retained activity is expressed as the specific phosphatase activity of CamPhoD relative to the activity of the enzyme incubated in the control reaction mixture in the absence of any metal ion.

However, the maximal CamPhoD activity was achieved by the simultaneous addition of Co^{2+} and Fe^{3+} to the incubation mixture, whereas only an 80% or 50% increase of the activity was observed after the addition of Co^{2+} and Fe^{3+} separately. It is evident that CamPhoD is the first bimetal Co^{2+}–Fe^{3+}-dependent phosphatase/phosphodiesterase characterized to date. Previously, the PhoD-like phosphatase from *B. subtilis* was described as being closely related to purple acid phosphatases (PAPs) with tyrosinate-ligated Fe^{3+} ions, but differed from them by having two Ca^{2+} ions instead of a single extra Fe^{2+}, Mn^{2+}, or Zn^{2+} ion [15]. The Ca^{2+} dependence of the phosphatase/phosphodiesterase from *Aphanothece halophytica* [9] as well as the activation of the alkaline phosphatase from *Pyrococcus abyssi* in the presence of Mg^{2+}, Zn^{2+}, and Co^{2+} ions have already been shown [43]. In addition, the alkaline phosphatase of the hyperthermophilic bacterium *Termatoga maritima* was shown to contain Co^{2+} and Mg^{2+} in the active center [44], while the active center of an *E. coli* alkaline phosphatase possessing the phosphodiesterase activity contained two Zn^{2+} and one Mg^{2+} [51], similar to most of the PhoA alkaline phosphatases, for example CmAP from *C. amphilecti* KMM 296 [6,24,52].

In spite of the obvious CamPhoD metal-dependence, the addition of EDTA and EGTA to the incubation medium at a concentration of 2 mM led to almost no effect on its activity, probably due to the deeply hidden metal-binding site in the core domain, a common trait of extracellular marine enzymes [6]. The narrow enzymatic cavity directed towards the catalytic aa residues, which is packed with metal ions, protects the extracellular *C. amphilecti* KMM 296 alkaline phosphatase CmAP from the damaging effects of chelating agents [6].

The treatment of CamPhoD with dithiothreitol (DTT) at a concentration of 10 mM completely inhibited enzyme activity (Figure 5). The sensitivity to sulfhydryl reagent has been shown previously for the highly active alkaline phosphatase CmAP, which was previously isolated from the same bacterium *C. amphilecti* KMM 296 [6]. This indicates that the presence of SH groups in the protein structure is necessary for enzyme activity, although CmAP does not have any intermolecular disulfide bond [6,12].

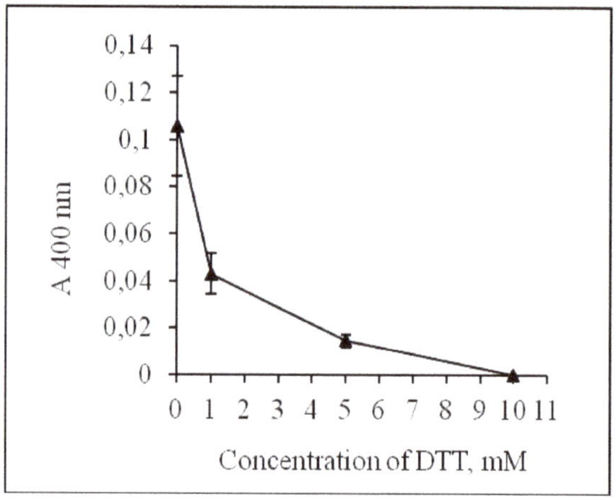

Figure 5. Effect of dithiothreitol (DTT) on the CamPhoD phosphatase activity.

Adding the non-ionic detergent Triton X-100 to the CamPhoD incubation mixture at concentrations of 1%, 0.1%, and 0.01% also reduced its activity by 80%, 70%, and 46%, respectively. This could influence the hydrophobic interactions in the protein, the importance of which were shown for the overall thermal stability of psychrophilic and mesophilic enzymes [53].

The alkaline phosphatase CamPhoD retained its activity during incubation for 60 min at temperatures ranging from 15 to 45 °C, while incubation at 65 °C completely inhibited its activity after 20 min (Figure 6). The CamPhoD thermostability and the optimal temperature of 45 °C (Figure 7) are similar to the CmAP properties [6]. As for phosphatases and phosphodiesterases, their temperature optimums cover a wide range, allowing them to belong to both thermolabile and thermostable enzymes. Alkaline phosphodiesterases from *Sphingobium* sp. and *Delftia acidovorans* exhibit maximum activity at 55 °C and 65 °C, respectively [17,18].

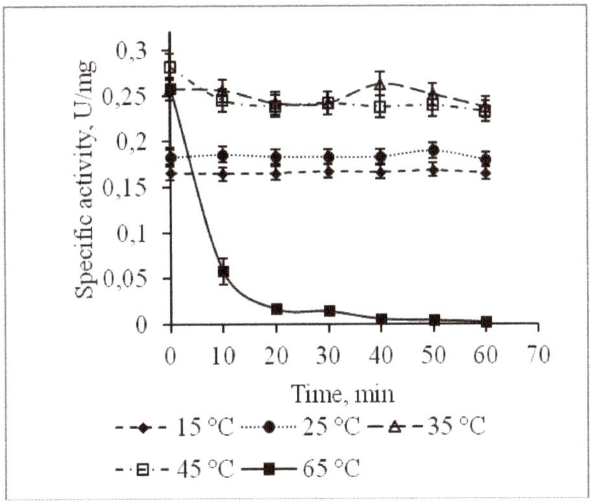

Figure 6. Effect of temperature on the CamPhoD stability.

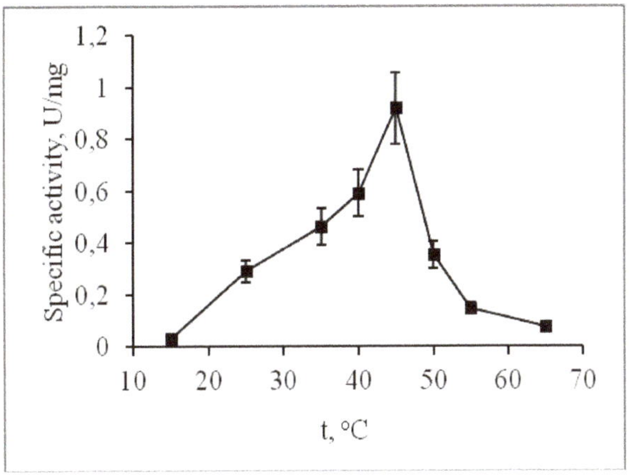

Figure 7. Effect of temperature on the CamPhoD phosphatase activity.

2.4. Substrate Specificity of CamPhoD

The study on substrate specificity of CamPhoD has shown that the enzyme catalyzes the cleavage of the phosphate group from deoxy- and ribonucleoside mono-, -di-, and-triphosphates in the following order according to catalytic rate: pNPP ≥ CMP ≥ GTP ≥ UMP ≥ dCMP ≥ AMP ≥ TMP ≥ CTP ≥ GDP ≥ GMP ≥ UDP = CDP ≥ bis-pNPP ≥ 5′-pNP-TMP (Table 2). According to the Chen method [54] of free phosphorus determination, P_i was released from pNPP and GTP under the CamPhoD catalysis approximately 150 and 250 times faster than from bis-pNPP and 5′-pNP-TMP, respectively (Table 2). The CamPhoD activities toward the chromogenic substrates pNPP, bis-pNPP, and 5′-pNP-TMP obtained by the spectrophotometric determination of the p-nitrophenyl concentration were similar.

The ability of CamPhoD to cleave the phosphate group of the diesters bis-pNPP and 5′-pNP-TMP, as well as different phosphate monoesters, allowed us to assign this enzyme to the bifunctional phosphatase/phosphodiesterase [9,10,16–20,55]. For comparison, the binuclear zinc phosphodiesterase ZiPD from *E. coli* possessed activity towards phosphodiester bonds of bis-pNPP and 5′-pNP-TMP only, and did not catalyze the cleavage of other phosphates, such as AMP, ADP, ATP, cyclic phosphates, or nucleic acids [45]. Despite a wide variety of nucleoside mono-, di-, and triphosphates used as substrates, CamPhoD did not catalyze the cleavage of the λ DNA, plasmid pUC19 DNA (Thermo Scientific, Vilnus, Lithuania), oligonucleotides (Evrogen, Moscow), or c-di-GMP (Sigma) up to inorganic phosphorus Pi (Table 2), similar to the phosphodiesterase PhoD from *B. subtilis* [15].

Table 2. Substrate specificity of the alkaline phosphatase/phosphodiesterase CamPhoD from *Cobetia amphilecti* KMM 296 *.

Substrate	Amount of Released P_i, mkM
pNPP	0.52
GTP	0.475
CMP	0.465
UMP	0.37
dCMP	0.325
AMP	0.31
TMP	0.305
CTP	0.24
GDP	0.19
GMP	0.16
UDP	0.15
CDP	0.14
dGMP	0.12
UTP	0.12
dCTP	0.09
dAMP	0.055
TTP	0.05
dGTP	0.04
c-di-GMP	0.005
bis-pNPP	0.003
5′-pNP-TMP	0.002
λ DNA	0
pUC19	0
Oligonucleotides	0

* These results were obtained using a molybdate reagent with ascorbic acid [54]. Various substrates were added to the reaction mixture at 2–15 mM concentrations. For each substrate, a control consisting of a specific substrate and a buffer containing 25 mM Tris-HCl (pH 9.0), 2 mM $CoCl_2$, and 2 mM $FeCl_3$ was used.

2.5. Catalytic Properties of CamPhoD

The Michaelis constant (K_m) of the alkaline phosphatase/phosphodiesterase CamPhoD at pH 9.0 in the presence of Co^{2+} and Fe^{3+} with the use of chromogenic pNPP as a substrate was 4.2 mM, the maximum velocity (V_{max}) was 0.203 mM/min, and the efficiency (k_{cat}/K_m) was 7988.6 S^{-1}/mM. Using the chromogenic phosphate bis-pNPP, Km was determined to have values of 6.71 mM, V_{max} = 0.046 mM/min, and efficiency (k_{cat}/K_m) = 1133.0 S^{-1}/mM. The kinetic parameters obtained for CamPhoD are similar to those previously obtained for other phosphatases and phosphodiesterases (Table 3). For example, K_m of the alkaline phosphatase from *Termatoga maritima* had a value of 175 mM [44], while K_m of the alkaline phosphodiesterases from *Sphingobium* sp. TCM1 and *A. halophytica* for pNPP were 1.5 mM and 3.38 mM, respectively [10,18].

Table 3. Biochemical characteristics of the reported bacterial phosphatases and phosphodiesterases.

Strain (Enzyme)	Optimum		bis-pNPP			p-NPP			Ref.
	t (°C)	pH	K_m (mM)	k_{cat} (S^{-1})	k_{cat}/K_m (S^{-1}/mM)	K_m (mM)	k_{cat} (S^{-1})	k_{cat}/K_m (S^{-1}/mM)	
Cobetia amphilecti KMM 296 (CamPhoD)	45	9.2	6.7	7603.2	1133.0	4.2	33552	7988.6	
C. amphilecti KMM 296 (CmAP)	40–50	10.3	-	-	-	13.2	28300	2144	[6]
Aphanothece halophytica	-	10	3.13	-	-	3.38	-	-	[10]
Bacillus subtilis	25	8.0	-	-	-	0.05	1.2	24	[15]
Metagenome	25	8.5	10.21	615×10^4	602×10^3	-	-	-	[16]
Delftia acidovorans	65	10	2.9	52740	18186.2	5.0	10260	2052	[17]
Sphingobium sp. TCM1	55	9.5	6.1	325	53.3	1.5	37.9	25.3	[18]
Escherichia coli (YfcE)	-	9.8	9.74	19.8	2.03	-	-	-	[19]
Termatoga maritima	75	8.0				175	16	0.091	[44]
E. coli (ElaC, ZiPD)	-	-	4	59	14.75	-	-	-	[45]

The CamPhoD catalytic efficiency (k_{cat}/K_m) in relation to pNPP was seven-fold higher than that with the use of bis-pNPP as the substrate, indicating that the enzyme mainly has a phosphomonoesterase structure with phosphodiesterase capability, similar to other PhoD-like enzymes [15]. However, the value of its catalytic efficiency for diester bonds is much higher when compared with many monospecific phosphodiesterases, excluding the enzyme from an unknown protein family with recently established structure and properties, which was isolated from the metagenome [18,19,45].

2.6. 3D Modeling of CamPhoD

A theoretical model for the PhoD-like phosphodiesterase/phosphatase from the marine bacterium *C. amphilecti* KMM 296 (GenBank ID: WP_043333989) was generated using structural bioinformatics methods (Figure 8A–C). Among the 3D structures currently available in the protein database (PDB), the low identical alkaline phosphatase D from *B. subtilis* (PDB ID: 2YEQ), which has a new architecture of the phosphatase active site based on Fe^{3+} and two Ca^{2+} ions, is apparently a single homologous template for modeling CamPhoD, which is a new member of the PhoD family inherent in the marine bacteria (data not shown). The amino acid sequences of CamPhoD and the template possess 20.5% identity and 38% similarity. (Figure 8A). The aa residues of the CamPhoD binding Ca^{2+}/Co^{2+} atoms in the active center are highly conserved. However, the bonds of the iron atom in the CamPhoD active center differ from the template bonds in replacing Cys 124 with Gly 117 (Figure 8A). In comparison with the template, the phosphate molecule in the modeled CamPhoD active site interacts with Tyr 158, Asp 221, and with one Fe^{3+} atom, two Ca^{2+} atoms, and three water molecules (Figure 8C).

A similar interaction with phosphate is observed when two Ca^{2+} atoms are replaced with Co^{2+} (Figure 9). The superimposition of the CamPhoD model and template showed that the root mean square deviation (RMSD) for 473 Cα atoms is 1 Å. The structural differences are in the structure of some of the loops on the outer surface of the protein (Figure 8C). In the CamPhoD structure, there is no α-helix at the C-terminus of the molecule, which is presented in the template, which possibly regulates the availability of the active center to accept the substrate (Figure 8A,C).

The analysis of contacts in the CamPhoD complexes with the reaction product PO_4^{3-} showed that the enzyme forms fewer contacts with the product than the template due to the shortened C-terminal region (Figure 9). The model of the CamPhoD complex with the substrate molecule has made it possible to determine the amino acid residues of the enzyme associated with the substrate binding (Figure 10).

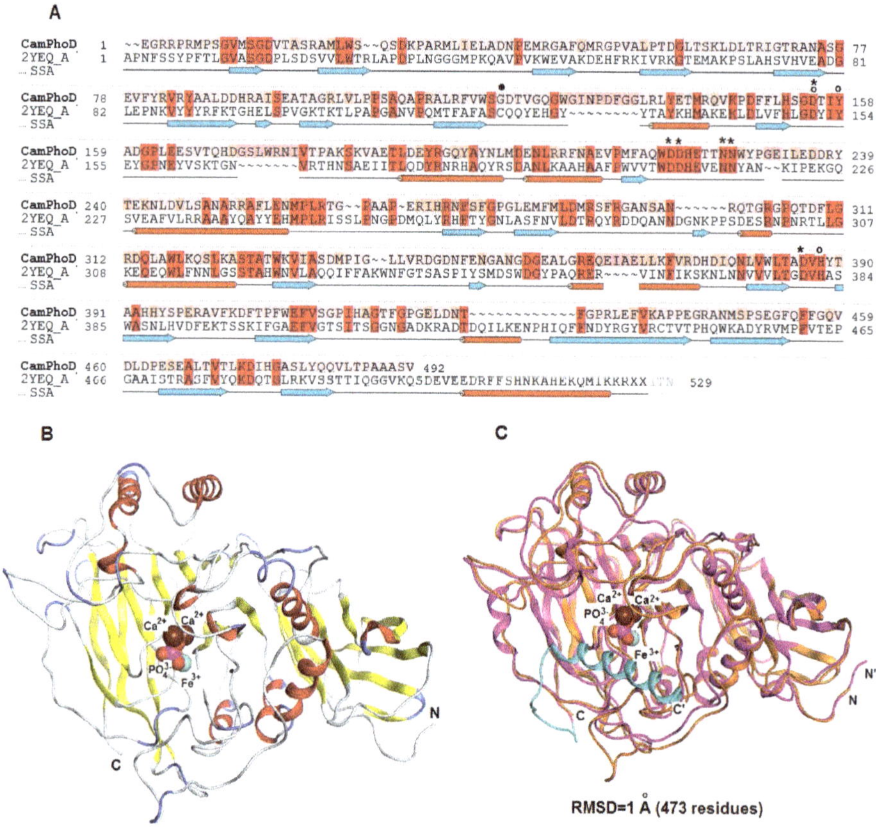

Figure 8. (**A**) Modeling of the CamPhoD 3D structure. An alignment of the amino acid sequences of the alkaline phosphatase/phosphodiesterase CamPhoD from the marine bacterium *C. amphilecti* KMM 296 (GenBank ID: WP_043333989) and alkaline phosphatase (phosphodiesterase) D from *B. subtilis* (PDB ID: 2YEQ). The amino acid sequences identity and similarity (color boxed) and the secondary structure of the template are highlighted. Note: α-helixes = red sticks; β-structure = blue arrows; the binding of amino acid (aa) residues (Ca2+/Co2+) = *; the binding of conserved aa residues (Fe^{3+}) = o; and the residue Cys 124 of the template = •. (**B**) The 3D structure model of CamPhoD with the reaction product Pi and metal ions in the active center (the protein structure is a ribbon diagram, Pi is in stick form, and Ca^{2+} is shown as spheres). (**C**) The 3D superimposition of the CamPhoD model (orange) and the template (PDB ID: 2YEQ) (shown in pink, with the blue C-terminal part).

2.7. *Effect of CamPhoD on Bacterial Biofilms*

In order to study the effect of alkaline phosphatase/phosphodiesterase CamPhoD on the inhibition of biofilm formation or on their destruction, bacterial biofilms of both individual and mixed species were grown. The study found that CamPhoD (0.1 U/mg) had a slight inhibitory effect on the biofilm formation of three species of *Bacillus*, namely *B. licheniformis*, *B. aegricola*, and *B. berkelogi* (18–32%), and dispersed the already formed biofilms of these species by 8–15% (Table 4). At the same time, CamPhoD did not inhibit the formation of biofilms in *B. subtilis* and *Pseudomonas aeruginosa* and did not degrade them.

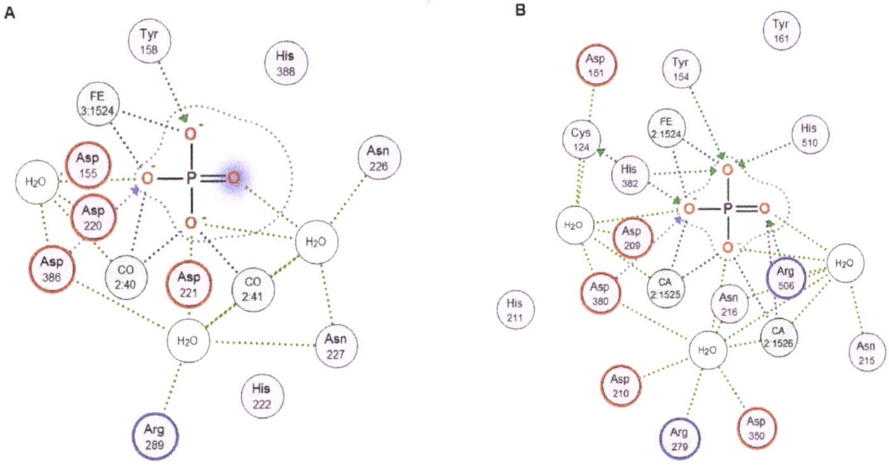

Figure 9. A 2D diagram of the contacts of the CamPhoD active center (**A**) and the template (PDB ID: 2YEQ) (**B**).

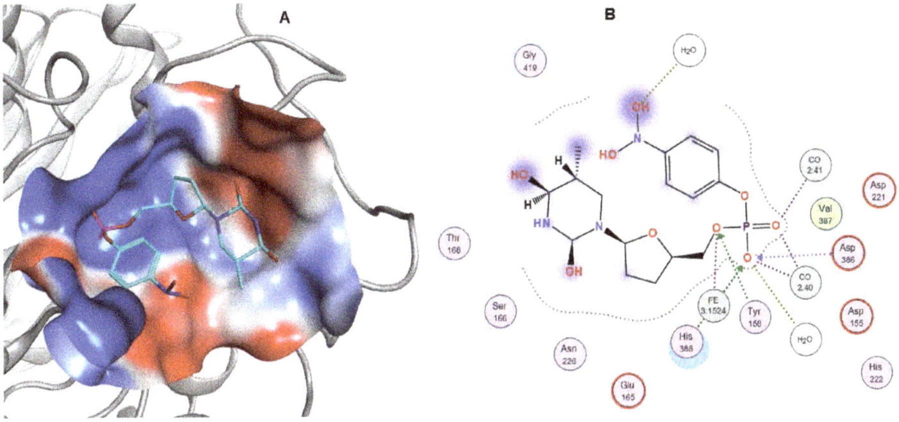

Figure 10. A model of the CamPhoD complex with the substrate 5′-pNP-TMP (**A**), and a 2D diagram of the contacts of 5′-pNP-TMP in the CamPhoD active center (**B**).

Table 4. Effect of the alkaline phosphatase/phosphodiesterase CamPhoD from *Cobetia amphilecti* KMM 296 on the bacterial biofilms.

Strain	Biofilm Formation % (3 Days, 22–24 °C)	Biofilm Destruction % (30 min, 37 °C)
K *	100	0
B. subtilis	100	0
B. licheniformis	74	15
B. aegricola	68	14
B. berkelogi	82	8
P. aeruginosa	100	0
Y. pseudotuberculosis	85	23
S. enteritidis	93	11
Y. pseudotuberculosis + *S. enteritidis*	87	24

* K-control strains grown without treatment with the enzyme.

Under natural conditions, biofilms are most often formed by not just one but by several types of bacteria [56]. In view of this, the study of such mixed biofilms is of great fundamental and practical importance. We investigated the formation of biofilms by mono and mixed cultures of *Yersinia pseudotuberculosis* and *Salmonella enteritidis*, as well as the effect of CamPhoD during the 3 day incubation with the enzyme (Table 4). The destruction of mature biofilms by the studied enzyme ranged from 11% to 24% depending on the strain. For comparison, DNase I degraded about 30% of the biofilm formed by *Y. pseudotuberculosis* and more than half of the *B. subtilis* biofilm [57].

The alkaline phosphatase CmAP from *C. amphilecti* KMM 296 was also shown to effectively inhibit the growth of the new biofilms and degradation of the mature biofilms of *S. enteritidis*, as well as *P. aeruginosa* and *B. subtilis* [7], in contrast to CamPhoD. The antibacterial activity of the alkaline phosphatase against *P. aeruginosa* has been found in *E. coli*, which is known as a causative agent of diarrhea [58]. The effect of alkaline phosphatases on pathogens has been studied by exploring the gut microbiota modulation ability in the alkaline phosphatase of the intestinal PhoA enzymes, in which the level of decrease or dysfunction is associated with intestinal inflammation, dysbiosis, bacterial translocation, and subsequently systemic inflammation [33–35].

The presence of extracellular alkaline phosphatases of the structural families PhoA (GenBank ID: WP_084589490.1) and PhoD (GenBank ID: WP_043333989.1) in the marine gamma-proteobacterium *C. amphilecti* KMM 296 may indicate either their distinct or cooperative functions for the hydrolysis of various phosphorus-containing organic molecules, depending on the environmental conditions and cell lifestyle [7,36]. The analogous PhoD enzyme from *B. subtilis* is thought to target specific phosphate-containing molecules, such as teichoic acids linked to the wall peptidoglycan via phosphodiester bonds. It is possible that other PhoD family members also have specific biological roles rather than operating as general phosphatases, such as members of the PhoA and PhoX families [15]. In spite of the absence of both CamPhoD and CmAP ability to cleave an important signaling molecule c-di-GMP, they may provide a level of Pi, acting on other extracellular phosphate-containing substrates and playing a crucial role in the bacterial behavior. For example, the phosphorylated lipid A or the linear intermediate product of the c-di-GMP hydrolysis, pGpG, have also been recently found as substrates for alkaline phosphatases and phosphodiesterases and as participants in cell signaling [32,59]. The mechanism of the putative participation of any alkaline phosphatase from *C. amphilecti* KMM 296 in the bacterial cell signaling has yet to be clarified, including regulation of biofilms or the species content in the bacterial consortium, with which the marine bacterium has to coexist in the mollusk digestive system.

3. Materials and Methods

3.1. Reagents and Materials

The reagents of chemical grade qualifications were obtained from Merck (Munchen, Germany), Sigma (Sigma-Aldrich Rus LLC, Moscow, Russia), and Helicon (Moscow, Russia). The molecular biology kits for restriction, ligation, Taq polymerase, and oligonucleotides were from Evrogen (Moscow, Russia) and Thermo Fisher Scientific RU (Moscow, Khimki, Russia); kanamycin was from Sintez (Moscow, Russia). Yeast extract, bactoagar, tripton, and pepton were from Helicon and Dia-M (Moscow, Russia). DNA and protein molecular weight markers were from BioRad (California, USA).

3.2. Construction of Plasmid pET40CamPhoD

The recombinant plasmid pET40CamPhoD was constructed by insertion into the NcoI/SacI fragment of plasmid pET-40b (+) (Thermo Fisher Scientific-RU, Moscow, Khimki, Russia), the gene encoding for the PhoD-like full-length phosphatase/phosphodiesterase, which was synthesized by polymerase chain reaction (PCR) using the genomic DNA of *Cobetia amphilecti* KMM 296 (Collection of Marine Microorganisms PIBOC FEB RAS) as a template and the gene-specific primers CamPhoD-NcoI-dir: 5′ -TATACCATGGAAGGACGGCGCCCGCGCATGCCCTC-3′ and CamPhoD-SacI-rev: 5′ -TATAGAGCTCTTAGACACTGGCGGCGGCGGGGTC-3′.

The reaction conditions were: 1 µL 10 × Encyclo buffer, 0.2 µl 50 × Encyclo polymerase mixture (Encyclo PCR kit; Evrogen, Moscow, Russia), 0.2 µl 50 × dNTP mixture (10 mM of each), a mixture of primers (1 µl 5 µM of each), and 1 µl 20 ng DNA. The volume of the reaction mixture was 10 µL. The amplification process consisted of 40 cycles of PCR (15 s, 95 °C, 1 min 40 s, 72 °C). After amplification, the PCR product was purified by electrophoresis in 1% agarose gel. The PCR fragment (1 µg) was treated with the restriction enzymes NcoI and SacI in an optimal buffer (Thermo Fisher Scientific RU) for 3 h at 37 °C, and then the enzymes were removed from the reaction mixture using phenol (1: 1). Here, 1/10 volume of 0.3 M sodium acetate, pH 5.2, and 1/2 volume of isopropyl alcohol were added to the aqueous fraction containing the PCR fragment, then incubated at −20 °C for 30 min. Then, this was centrifuged at 14,000 rpm for 20 min, the precipitate was washed with 75% ethanol, then dried at room temperature. The precipitate was dissolved in 20 µl of deionized water.

In total, 2 µg of the pET-40b (+) plasmid DNA (Thermo Fisher Scientific-RU) was treated with the NcoI and SacI restriction endonucleases in accordance with the procedure described above.

The obtained fragment of the CamPhoD gene and the NcoI /SacI part of the plasmid pET-40b (+) were ligated using a ligase reaction in 50 µl of ligation buffer, according to the instructions (Thermo Fisher Scientific RU). Then, 10 µL of the reaction mixture was used to transform the competent *E. coli* Rosetta cells (DE3). Transformants were grown on the Luria–Bertani (LB) agar containing 25 µg/mL kanamycin. After incubation for 16 h at 37 °C, the clones were screened, and then the targeted plasmid DNA was isolated and screened for mutations.

3.3. Optimization of Conditions for CamPhoD Expression

To determine the optimal IPTG concentration, the *E. coli* Rosetta (DE3) cells transformed with the pET40 plasmid carrying the CamPhoD gene were grown on LB agar containing 25 mg/mL kanamycin overnight at 37 °C. Single colonies were selected and grown in 5 mL of the liquid LB medium containing 25 mg/mL kanamycin at 200 rpm for 16 h at 37 °C. Then, the inoculum was placed into the flasks with 20 mL of fresh LB medium containing kanamycin at a concentration of 25 mg/mL and incubated at 37 °C in a shaker at 200 rpm, up to an optical density 0.6–0.8 (λ 600 nm). Next, 0.1 mM, 0.2 mM, 0.3 mM, and 0.5 mM IPTG were added to induce the expression of CamPhoD, then incubation was continued at 37 °C. To determine the phosphatase activity, 5 mL of each sample was taken at 0, 3, 6, and 24 h after the start of expression and ultra-sonication for the bacterial cells and determination of the CamPhoD alkaline phosphatase activity.

To determine the dependence of CamPhoD activity on the presence of phosphate in the growth medium, the *E. coli* Rosetta (DE3) cells transformed with the pET40CamPhoD plasmid were grown in 25 mL of the liquid medium containing: bacto-trypton 10 g/L, yeast extract 7.5 g/L, sorbitol 70 g/L, $MgCl_2$ 5 mM, KH_2PO_4 80 mM, and 25 mg/mL kanamycin at 200 rpm for 16 h at 37 °C [46]. Then, the cells were placed in 1 L of the fresh medium of the abovementioned composition and incubated at 37 °C on a rocking chair at 200 rpm, up to an optical density 0.6–0.8 (λ 600 nm). Next, 0.1 mM IPTG was added to induce the expression of CamPhoD and incubation was continued at 37 °C for 6 h at 200 rpm. After this, CamPhoD was isolated, purified, and its activity was determined as described below.

3.4. The Recombinant CamPhoD Production

The recombinant *E. coli* Rosetta (DE3) strain was grown in 25 mL of the LB liquid medium containing 25 mg/mL kanamycin at 200 rpm for 16 h at 37 °C. Then, the cells were placed in the fresh LB medium (1 L) containing kanamycin at a concentration of 25 mg/mL and incubated at 37 °C in a shaker at 200 rpm, up to an optical density at 600 nm of 0.6–0.8. After that, 0.1 mM IPTG was added to induce expression of the enzyme and incubation was continued at 37 °C for 6 h at 200 rpm.

The cells were precipitated by centrifugation at 4000 rpm for 15 min at 8 °C, suspended in 35 mL of 25 mM Tris-HCl buffer (pH 9.0) with phenylmethylsulfonyl fluoride (PMSF) added to a final concentration of 0.15 mM, and subjected to ultrasonication at 22 kHz and 0–4 °C with intervals of 30 s, up to clarification of the suspension. The suspension was centrifuged at 11,000 rpm for 30 min at 8 °C, the precipitate was discarded, and the activity and properties of CamPhoD were determined in the resulting extract.

3.5. The Recombinant CamPhoD Isolation and Purification

For isolation of CamPhoD, $CaCl_2$ and $MgCl_2$ were added to the recombinant cell extract to a final concentration of 10 mM, DNase was (SkyGen, Moscow, Russia) to a final concentration of 5 μg/mL, these were incubated at 37 °C for 1 h, and then centrifuged at 11000 rpm for 20 min. The resulting supernatant was introduced into a 25 × 3.2 cm Ni-IMAC-Sepharose column (GE Healthcare Life Sciences, Buckinghamshire, UK) equilibrated with 25 mM Tris-HCl, pH 9.0 (buffer A), and washed with five volumes of the same buffer. The recombinant protein was eluted with a linear gradient of 0–0.5 M imidazole in 25 mM Tris-HCl buffer, pH 9.0, and 0.5 M NaCl (6 column volume), at a rate of 1.3 mL/min. The CamPhoD-containing fraction was purified on a 10 × 1.4 cm Source 15 Q column (GE Healthcare Life Sciences) equilibrated with buffer A, then the protein was eluted with a linear gradient of 0–0.5 M NaCl in the 25 mM Tris-HCl buffer at pH 9.0. Ion exchange chromatography was performed at a rate of 1 mL min; the volume of the fractions was 1 mL. The CamPhoD-containing fractions were collected and treated with enterokinase at a final concentration of 1 U per 1 mg of protein for 22 h at 25 °C. Then, the protein solution was applied to a Superdex 200 PG column (105 × 2 cm) (GE Healthcare Life Sciences), previously equilibrated with buffer A with 0.15 M NaCl at a rate of 0.5 mL/min, with 1 mL fractions. The CamPhoD-containing fractions were collected and subjected to chromatography using a mono-Q HR column (4 × 0,8 cm) (GE Healthcare Life Sciences, Buckinghamshire, UK) equilibrated with buffer A, washed with 10 volumes of buffer A, and then the target protein was eluted with a linear gradient of 0–0.5 M NaCl in buffer A at a rate of 0.5 mL/min and with fractions of 1 mL. The purified preparation of CamPhoD was used to study the physicochemical properties and substrate specificity.

3.6. Enzyme Activity Assay

The enzyme activity of CamPhoD was determined at 37 °C for 30 min with the use of 2 mM p-nitrophenyl phosphate (*p*-NPP), thymidine-5′-monophosphate-p-nitrophenylester (5′-pNP-TMP) or bis-p-nitrophenyl phosphate (Bis-*p*-NPP) as chromogenic substrates in 25 mM Tris-HCl buffer, pH 9.0, 2 mM $CoCl_2$, 2 mM $FeCl_3$. The volume of the reaction mixture was 0.5 mL. The reaction was stopped by adding 1 mL of cooled 0.5 M NaOH to the reaction mixture. The absorption of the formed p-nitrophenol was measured at an optical density of 400 nm. The amount of enzyme required for the conversion of 1 μM *p*-nitrophenyl from a substrate over 1 min was taken as a unit of activity. The specific activity is given in units calculated per 1 mg of protein. The protein concentration was determined using Bradford's method [60].

3.7. Substrate Specificity

The substrate specificity of CamPhoD was determined by adding 2 mM CMP, CDP, CTP, dCMP, dCTP, UMP, UDP, UTP, TMP, TTP, GMP, GDP, GTP, dGMP, dGTP, AMP, ATP, dAMP, bis-pNPP, 5′-pNP-TMP, c-di-GMP, and pNPP to a standard incubation mixture, containing 25 mM Tris-HCl buffer, pH 9.0, 2 mM $CoCl_2$, 2 mM $FeCl_3$. The mixture was incubated at 37 °C for 60 min. The volume of the reaction mixture was 1 mL. Then, a molybdate reagent with ascorbic acid (4 mL) was added to the incubation mixture and again incubated at 37 °C for 60 min. The mixture was cooled to room temperature, and absorbance of the formed product of dephosphorylation by CamPhoD was measured at an optical density of 820 nm. The amount of inorganic phosphate P_i (mkM) released during dephosphorylation of the studied substrates with the enzyme was determined using a calibration curve with KH_2PO_4, according to Chen's method [54].

3.8. Determination of Thermostability and Temperature Optimum

The effect of temperature on CamPhoD and the optimum temperature were determined by incubating the standard incubation mixture at temperatures ranging from 15 to 65 °C, at 10 °C intervals. Alkaline phosphatase activity was determined using the standard method for determining for CamPhoD, as described above.

3.9. Effect of Metal Ions and Chelating Agents

The influence of divalent metal ions on CamPhoD was determined using the standard method for determining the alkaline phosphatase activity, with the addition of Mg^{2+}, Ca^{2+}, Mn^{2+}, Zn^{2+}, Co^{2+}, Ni^{2+}, Cu^{2+}, Cs^{2+}, Fe^{3+} ions, EDTA, and EGTA at a concentration of 2 mM to the incubation mixture. The incubation mixture without cations and chelating agents was used as a control.

3.10. Effect of NaCl and KCl

The effects of Na^{+} and K^{+} were investigated by adding NaCl and KCl to a standard incubation mixture at a concentration of 0–1.5 M. The alkaline phosphatase activity was determined as described above.

3.11. Determination of Molecular Weight

The molecular weight of CamPhoD was determined using gel filtration on a calibrated Superdex G200 PG (GE Healthcare Life Sciences, Amersham Place, Little Chalfont, Buckinghamshire, HP7, 9NA, UK) column (105 × 2 cm) and polyacrylamide gel electrophoresis under denaturing conditions (sodium dodecyl sulfate polyacrylamide gel electrophoresis) using the Lammley method [61].

3.12. Determination of Catalytic Parameters

Kinetic parameters were calculated by plotting the rate of p-NPP and bis-p-NPP splitting at concentrations from 5 to 15 mM in a buffer containing 25 mM Tris-HCl, pH 9.0, 2 mM $CoCl_2$, 2 mM $FeCl_3$. The reaction was carried out at 25 °C. The Michaelis constant K_m, the maximum reaction rate V_{max}, and the turnover number k_{cat} were determined by plotting the Layuver–Burk graph using the OriginPro 8.5 program.

3.13. Molecular Modeling

The target template alignment customization of the modeling process and 3D model building for CamPhoD (GenBank: WP_043333989) were carried out using the Molecular Operating Environment (MOE) version 2018.01 package, using the Amber12: EHT forcefield (EHT-Extended Hueckel Theory) [62]. The alkaline phosphatase D from *B. subtilis* (PDB code: 2YEQ) was used as a template, which had a high-resolution crystal structure. The evaluation of structural parameters, contact structure analysis, physicochemical properties, and visualization of the results were carried out with the ligand interaction and dock modules in the MOE 2018.01 program [62].

3.14. Biofilms Growth and Enzymatic Treatment

The strains of Bacillus subtilis, Bacillus licheniformis, Bacillus aegricola, Bacillus berkelogi, Pseudomonas aeruginosa, Yersinia pseudotuberculosis, and Salmonella enteritidis were used. An overnight bacterial culture was diluted with the appropriate nutrient medium and incubated in a 96-well plate at 200 µl per well for 24 h at 37 °C, or for 3 days at 22–24 °C. After incubation, loose cells were removed from the wells, and wells were washed three times with 0.85% NaCl. The biofilm was stained with 0.5% crystal violet (CV) for 20 min at room temperature. The dye was removed from the wells, and unbound CV was washed with tap water. The plates were air dried, 2% acetic acid in 95% ethanol was added to each well, and the absorbance was determined at 600 nm.

Inhibition of biofilm formation was tested using the method in [63]. Test substances at various concentrations were added to the wells. All experiments were repeated four times. The destruction of biofilms by the investigated substances was carried out as follows. After the formation of biofilms for a certain time, unattached cells were removed and the wells were washed with 0.85% NaCl. The enzyme was added to each well in the appropriate buffer and incubated under the conditions for determination of the activity of the studied enzyme. Then, the plate was processed as described above.

4. Conclusions

The PhoD-like enzyme gene was firstly isolated from the marine bacterium *Cobetia amphilecti* KMM 296 and cloned into *E.coli*. The effects of chemicals, metal ions, kinetic parameters, and substrate specificity on the enzymatically active recombinant product, CamPhoD, expressed from this gene confirmed that the enzyme carries a metabolic function of phosphatase/phosphodiesterase of the PhoD family in the marine environment. The enzyme bimetal dependence coincides with the modeling results for the enzymatic complex, with phosphate in the active center surrounded by two Co^{2+} ions and one Fe^{3+} ion. This enzyme of marine origin has been concluded to be a new member of the bifunctional PhoD-like phosphatase/phosphodiesterase class, with a characteristic structure and important biological functions.

Author Contributions: Conceptualization, L.B. and L.T.; methodology, Y.N. and N.T.; software, G.L.; validation, L.B.; investigation, Y.N. and N.T.; resources, L.T. and O.S.; data curation, L.B.; writing—original draft preparation, Y.N.; writing—review and editing, L.B.

Funding: This research was funded by the program of RAS, grant number 18-4-051.

Conflicts of Interest: The authors declare no conflict of interest.

References

1. Clark, L.L.; Ingall, E.D.; Benner, R. Marine phosphorus is selectively remineralized. *Nature* **1998**, *393*, 426. [CrossRef]
2. Martinez, J.; Smith, D.C.; Steward, G.F.; Azam, F. Variability in ectohydrolytic enzyme activities of pelagic marine bacteria and its *significance* for substrate processing in the sea. *Aquat. Microb. Ecol.* **1996**, *10*, 223–230. [CrossRef]
3. Zheng, L.; Ren, M.; Xie, E.; Ding, A.; Liu, Y.; Deng, S.; Zhang, D. Roles of phosphorus sources in microbial community assembly for the removal of organic matters and ammonia in activated sludge. *Front. Microbiol.* **2019**, *10*, 1023. [CrossRef] [PubMed]
4. Omelon, S.; Ariganello, M.; Bonucci, E.; Grynpas, M.; Nanci, A. A review of phosphate mineral nucleation in biology and geobiology. *Calcif. Tissue Int.* **2013**, *93*, 382–396. [CrossRef] [PubMed]
5. Skouri-Panet, F.; Benzerara, K.; Cosmidis, J.; Férard, C.; Caumes, G.; De Luca, G.; Heulin, T.; Duprat, E. *In vitro* and *in silico* evidence of phosphatase diversity in the biomineralizing bacterium *Ramlibacter tataouinensis*. *Front Microbiol.* **2018**, *8*, 2592. [CrossRef] [PubMed]
6. Golotin, V.A.; Balabanova, L.A.; Likhatskaya, G.N.; Rasskazov, V.A. Recombinant production and characterization of a highly active alkaline phosphatase from marine bacterium *Cobetia marina*. *Mar. Biotechnol.* **2015**, *17*, 130–143. [CrossRef]
7. Balabanova, L.; Podvolotskaya, A.; Slepchenko, L.; Eliseikina, M.; Noskova, Y.; Nedashkovskaya, O.; Son, O.; Tekutyeva, L.; Rasskazov, V. Nucleolytic enzymes from the marine bacterium *Cobetia amphilecti* KMM 296 with antibiofilm activity and biopreservative effect on meat products. *Food Control* **2017**, *78*, 270–278. [CrossRef]
8. Yuivar, Y.; Barahona, S.; Alcaíno, J.; Cifuentes, V.; Baeza, M. Biochemical and thermodynamical characterization of glucose oxidase, invertase, and alkaline phosphatase secreted by antarctic yeasts. *Front. Mol. Biosci.* **2017**, *4*, 86. [CrossRef]
9. Lee, D.-H.; Choi, S.-L.; Rha, E.; Kim, S.J.; Yeom, S.-J.; Moon, J.-H.; Lee, S.-G. A novel psychrophilic alkaline phosphatase from the metagenome of tidal flat sediments. *BMC Biotechnol.* **2015**, *15*, 1–13. [CrossRef]

10. Kageyama, H.; Tripathi, K.; Rai, A.K.; Cha-um, S.; Waditee-Sirisattha, R.; Takabe, T. An alkaline phosphatase/phosphodiesterase, PhoD, induced by salt stress and secreted out of the cells of *Aphanothece halophytica*, a halotolerant cyanobacterium. *Appl. Environ. Microbiol.* **2011**, *77*, 5178–5183. [CrossRef]
11. Luoa, H.; Bennera, R.; Longa, R.A.; Hu, J. Subcellular localization of marine bacterial alkaline phosphatases. *Proc. Natl. Acad. Sci. USA* **2009**, *106*, 21219–21223. [CrossRef] [PubMed]
12. Plisova, E.Y.; Balabanova, L.A.; Ivanova, E.P.; Kozhemyako, V.B.; Mikhailov, V.V.; Agafonova, E.V.; Rasskazov, V.A. A highly active alkaline phosphatase from the marine bacterium Cobetia. *Mar. Biotechnol.* **2005**, *7*, 173–178. [CrossRef] [PubMed]
13. Hassan, H.M.; Pratt, D. Biochemical and physiological properties of alkaline phosphatases in five isolates of marine bacteria. *J. Bacteriol.* **1977**, *129*, 1607–1612. [PubMed]
14. Nasu, E.; Ichiyanagi, A.; Gomi, K. Cloning and expression of a highly active recombinant alkaline phosphatase from psychrotrophic *Cobetia marina*. *Biotechnol. Lett.* **2012**, *34*, 321–328. [CrossRef] [PubMed]
15. Rodriguez, F.; Lillington, J.; Johnson, S.; Timmel, C.R.; Lea, S.M.; Berks, B.C. Crystal structure of the *Bacillus subtilis* phosphodiesterase PhoD reveals an iron and calcium-containing active site. *J. Biol. Chem.* **2014**, *289*, 30889–30899. [CrossRef]
16. Singh, D.N.; Gupta, A.; Singh, V.S.; Mishra, R.; Kateriya, S.; Tripathi, A.K. Identification and characterization of a novel phosphodiesterase from the metagenome of an Indian coalbed. *PLoS ONE* **2015**, *10*, e0118075. [CrossRef]
17. Tehara, S.K.; Keasling, J.D. Gene cloning, purification, and characterization of a phosphodiesterase from *Delftia acidovorans*. *Appl. Environ. Microbiol.* **2003**, *69*, 504–508. [CrossRef] [PubMed]
18. Abe, K.; Mukai, N.; Morooka, Y.; Makino, T.; Oshima, K.; Takahashi, S.; Kera, Y. An atypical phosphodiesterase capable of degrading haloalkyl phosphate diesters from *Sphingobium* sp. strain TCM1. *Sci. Rep.* **2017**, *7*, 2842–2850. [CrossRef]
19. Miller, D.J.; Shuvalova, L.; Evdokimova, E.; Savchenko, A.; Yakunin, A.F.; Anderson, W.F. Structural and biochemical characterization of a novel Mn^{2+}-dependent phosphodiesterase encoded by the yfcE gene. *Protein Sci.* **2007**, *16*, 1338–1348. [CrossRef]
20. Eder, S.; Shi, L.; Jensen, K.; Yamane, K.; Hulett, F.M. A *Bacillus subtilis* secreted phosphodiesterase alkaline phosphatase is the product of a Pho regulon gene, *phoD*. *Mikrobiology* **1996**, *142*, 2041–2047. [CrossRef]
21. Hamdan, S.; Bulloch, E.M.; Thompson, P.R.; Beck, J.L.; Yang, J.Y.; Crowther, J.A.; Lilley, P.E.; Carr, P.D.; Ollis, D.L.; Brown, S.E.; et al. Hydrolysis of the 5′-p-nitrophenyl ester of TMP by the proofreading exonuclease (epsilon) subunit of *Escherichia coli* DNA polymerase III. *Biochemistry* **2002**, *41*, 5266–5275. [CrossRef] [PubMed]
22. Gomez, P.F.; Ingram, L.O. Cloning, sequencing and characterization of the alkaline phosphatase gene (phoD) from *Zymomonas mobilis*. *FEMS Microbiol. Lett.* **1995**, *125*, 237–246. [CrossRef] [PubMed]
23. Sunden, F.; AlSadhan, I.; Lyubimov, A.; Doukov, T.; Swan, J.; Herschlag, D. Differential catalytic promiscuity of the alkaline phosphatase superfamily bimetallo core reveals mechanistic features underlying enzyme evolution. *J. Biol. Chem.* **2017**, *292*, 20960–20974. [CrossRef] [PubMed]
24. Hu, Q.; Jayasinghe-Arachchige, V.M.; Zuchniarz, J.; Prabhakar, R. Effects of the metal ion on the mechanism of phosphodiester hydrolysis catalyzed by metal-cyclen complexes. *Front. Chem.* **2019**, *7*. [CrossRef]
25. Mancin, F.; Scrimin, P.; Tecilla, P. Progress in artificial metallonucleases. *Chem. Commun.* **2012**, *48*, 5545–5559. [CrossRef]
26. Jin, J.; Pawson, T. Modular evolution of phosphorylation-based signalling systems. *Phil. Trans. R. Soc. B* **2012**, *367*, 2540–2555. [CrossRef]
27. Millán, J.L. The role of phosphatases in the initiation of skeletal mineralization. *Calcif. Tissue Int.* **2013**, *93*, 299–306. [CrossRef]
28. Ke, H.; Wang, H. Crystal structures of phosphodiesterases and implications on substrate specificity and inhibitor selectivity. *Curr. Top. Med. Chem.* **2007**, *7*, 391–403. [CrossRef]
29. Borges, A.; Simões, M. Quorum sensing inhibition by marine bacteria. *Mar. Drugs* **2019**, *17*, 427. [CrossRef]
30. Azevedo, M.F.; Faucz, F.R.; Bimpaki, E.; Horvath, A.; Levy, I.; de Alexandre, R.B.; Ahmad, F.; Manganiello, V.; Stratakis, C.A. Clinical and molecular genetics of the phosphodiesterases (PDEs). *Endocr. Rev.* **2014**, *35*, 195–233. [CrossRef]
31. Dobretsov, S.; Teplitski, M.; Paul, V. Mini-review: Quorum sensing in the marine environment and its relationship to biofouling. *Biofouling* **2009**, *25*, 413–427. [CrossRef] [PubMed]

32. Rader, B.A.; Kremer, N.; Apicella, M.A.; Goldman, W.E.; McFall-Ngai, M.J. Modulation of symbiont lipid A signaling by host alkaline phosphatases in the squid-vibrio symbiosis. *mBio* **2012**, *3*, 00093-12. [CrossRef] [PubMed]
33. Sharma, U.; Pal, D.; Prasad, R. Alkaline Phosphatase: An Overview. *Indian J. Clin. Biochem.* **2014**, *29*, 269–278. [CrossRef] [PubMed]
34. Fawley, J.; Gourlay, D. Intestinal alkaline phosphatase: A summary of its role in clinical disease. *J. Surg. Res.* **2016**, *202*, 225–234. [CrossRef]
35. Bilski, J.; Mazur-Bialy, A.; Wojcik, D.; Zahradnik-Bilska, J.; Brzozowski, B.; Magierowski, M.; Mach, T.; Magierowska, K.; Brzozowski, T. The Role of Intestinal Alkaline Phosphatase in Inflammatory Disorders of Gastrointestinal Tract. *Med. Inflamm.* **2017**, 9074601. [CrossRef]
36. Balabanova, L.A.; Golotin, V.A.; Kovalchuk, S.N.; Babii, A.V.; Shevchenko, L.S.; Son, O.M.; Kosovsky, G.Y.; Rasskazov, V.A. The genome of the marine bacterium *Cobetia marina* KMM 296 isolated from the mussel *Crenomytilus grayanus* (Dunker, 1853). *Rus. J. Mar. Biol.* **2016**, *42*, 106–109. [CrossRef]
37. Letunic, I.; Bork, P. 20 years of the SMART protein domain annotation resource. *Nucleic Acids Res.* **2018**, *46*, D493–D496. [CrossRef]
38. Marchler-Bauer, A.; Bo, Y.; Han, L.; He, J.; Lanczycki, C.J.; Lu, S.; Chitsaz, F.; Derbyshire, M.K.; Geer, R.C.; Gonzales, N.R.; et al. CDD/SPARCLE: Functional classification of proteins via subfamily domain architectures. *Nucleic Acids Res.* **2017**, *45*, D200–D203. [CrossRef]
39. Tegtmeyer, N.; Hartig, R.; Delahay, R.M.; Rohde, M.; Brandt, S.; Conradi, J.; Takahashi, S.; Smolka, A.J.; Sewald, N.; Backert, S. A small fibronectin-mimicking protein from bacteria induces cell spreading and focal adhesion formation. *J. Biol. Chem.* **2010**, *285*, 23515–23526. [CrossRef]
40. Oh, Y.J.; Hubauer-Brenner, M.; Gruber, H.J.; Cui, Y.; Traxler, L.; Siligan, C.; Park, S.; Hinterdorfer, P. Curli mediate bacterial adhesion to fibronectin via tensile multiple bonds. *Sci. Rep.* **2016**, *6*, 33909. [CrossRef]
41. Hauksson, J.B.; Andrésson, O.S.; Ásgeirsson, B. Heat-labile bacterial alkaline phosphatase from a marine *Vibrio* sp. *Enzyme Microb. Technol.* **2000**, *27*, 66–73. [CrossRef]
42. Moura, R.S.; Martın, J.F.; Martın, A.; Liras, P. Substrate analysis and molecular cloning of the extracellular alkaline phosphatase of *Streptomyces griseus*. *Microbiology* **2001**, *147*, 1525–1533. [CrossRef] [PubMed]
43. Zappa, S.; Rolland, J.-L.; Flament, D.; Gueguen, Y.; Boudrant, J.; Dietrich, J. Characterization of a highly thermostable alkaline phosphatase from the Euryarchaeon *Pyrococcus abyssi*. *Appl. Environ. Microbiol.* **2001**, *67*, 4504–4511. [CrossRef] [PubMed]
44. Wojciechowski, C.L.; Cardia, J.P.; Kantrowitz, E.R. Alkaline phosphatase from the hyperthermophilic bacterium *T. maritime* requires cobalt for activity. *Protein Sci.* **2002**, *11*, 903–911. [CrossRef]
45. Vogel, A.; Schilling, O.; Niecke, M.; Bettmer, J.; Meyer-Klaucke, W. ElaC encodes a novel binuclear zinc phosphodiesterase. *J. Biol. Chem.* **2002**, *277*, 29078–29085. [CrossRef]
46. Golotin, V.A.; Balabanova, L.A.; Noskova, Y.A.; Slepchenko, L.V.; Bakunina, I.Y.; Vorobieva, N.S.; Terenteva, N.A.; Rasskazov, V.A. Optimization of cold-adapted alpha-galactosidase expression in *Escherichia coli*. *Protein Expr. Purif.* **2016**, *123*, 14–18. [CrossRef]
47. Apel, A.K.; Sola-Landa, A.; Rodriguez-Garcia, A.; Martıin, J.F. Phosphate control of phoA, phoC and phoD gene expression in *Streptomyces coelicolor* reveals significant differences in binding of PhoP to their promoter regions. *Microbiology* **2007**, *153*, 3527–3537. [CrossRef]
48. Seitkalieva, A.V.; Menzorova, N.I.; Vakorina, T.I.; Dmitrenok, P.S.; Rasskazov, V.A. Novel saltresistant alkaline phosphatase from eggs of the sea urchin *Strongylocentrotus intermedius*. *Appl. Biochem. Microbiol.* **2017**, *53*, 16–25. [CrossRef]
49. Ishibashi, M.; Yamashita, S.; Tokunaga, M. Characterization of halophilic alkaline phosphatase from *Halomonas* sp. 593, a moderately halophilic bacterium. *Biosci. Biotechnol. Biochem.* **2005**, *69*, 1213–1216. [CrossRef]
50. Menzorova, N.I.; Seytkalieva, A.V.; Rasskazov, V.A. Enzymatic methods for the determination of pollution in seawater using salt resistant alkaline phosphatase from eggs of the sea urchin *Strongylocentrotus intermedius*. *Mar. Poll. Bul.* **2014**, *79*, 188–195. [CrossRef]
51. O'Brie, P.J.; Herschlag, D. Functional interrelationships in the alkaline phosphatase superfamily: phosphodiesterase activity of *Escherichia coli* alkaline phosphatase. *Biochemistry* **2001**, *40*, 5691–5699. [CrossRef] [PubMed]

52. Zalatan, J.G.; Fenn, T.D.; Herschlag, D. Comparative enzymology in the alkaline phosphatase superfamily to determine the catalytic role of an active site metal ion. *J. Mol. Biol.* **2008**, *384*, 1174–1189. [CrossRef] [PubMed]
53. Moon, S.; Kim, J.; Koo, J.; Bae, E. Structural and mutational analyses of psychrophilic and mesophilic adenylate kinases highlight the role of hydrophobic interactions in protein thermal stability. *Struct. Dyn.* **2019**, *6*, 024702. [CrossRef] [PubMed]
54. Chen, P.S.; Toribara, T.Y., Jr.; Warner, H. Microdetermination of phosphorus. *Anal. Chem.* **1956**, *28*, 1756–1758. [CrossRef]
55. Millán, J.L. Alkaline phosphatases: Structure, substrate specificity and functional relatedness to other members of a large superfamily of enzymes. *Purinergic Signal.* **2006**, *2*, 335–341. [CrossRef]
56. Bogosian, G.; Morris, P.J.L.; O'Neil, G.P. A mixed culture recovery method indicates that enteric bacteria do not enter the viable but nonculturable state. *Appl. Environ. Microbiol.* **1998**, *64*, 1736–1742.
57. Terentieva, N.A.; Timchenko, N.F.; Balabanova, L.A.; Rasskazov, V.A. Characteristics of formation, inhibition and destruction of *Yersinia pseudotuberculosis* biofilms forming on abiotic surfaces. *Zh. Mikrobiol. Epidemiol. Immunobiol.* **2015**, *3*, 72–78.
58. Hashem, K.A.; Authman, S.H.; Mahdi, L.H. *In vivo* antibacterial activity of alkaline phosphatase isolates from Escherichia coli isolated from diarrhea patients against *Pseudomonas aeruginosa*. *Pharma Inn. J.* **2016**, *5*, 32–36.
59. Stelitano, V.; Giardina, G.; Paiardini, A.; Astiglione, N.; Cutruzzolà, F.; Rinaldo, S. C-di-GMP hydrolysis by *Pseudomonas aeruginosa* HDGYP phosphodiesterases: Analysis of the reaction mechanism and novel roles for pGpG. *PLoS ONE* **2013**, *8*, e74920. [CrossRef]
60. Bradford, M.M. A rapid and sensitive method for the quantitation of microgram quantities of protein utilizing the principle of protein-dye binding. *Anal. Biochem.* **1976**, *72*, 248–254. [CrossRef]
61. Laemmli, U.K. Cleavage of structural proteins during the assembly of the head of the bacteriophage T7. *Nature* **1970**, *227*, 680–685. [CrossRef] [PubMed]
62. MOE, 2018.01; Chemical Computing Group ULC, 1010 Sherbrooke St. West, Suite #910, Montreal, QC, Canada, 2018; H3A 2R7.
63. Nijland, R.; Hall, M.J.; Burgess, J.G. Dispersal of biofilms by secreted, matrix degrading, bacterial DNAse. *PLoS ONE* **2010**, *5*, e15668. [CrossRef] [PubMed]

marine drugs

MDPI

Article

Comparative Genomics and CAZyme Genome Repertoires of Marine *Zobellia amurskyensis* KMM 3526^T and *Zobellia laminariae* KMM 3676^T

Nadezhda Chernysheva [1], Evgeniya Bystritskaya [1], Anna Stenkova [2], Ilya Golovkin [2], Olga Nedashkovskaya [1] and Marina Isaeva [1,*]

1 G.B. Elyakov Pacific Institute of Bioorganic Chemistry, Far Eastern Branch, Russian Academy of Sciences, 159, Pr. 100 let Vladivostoku, Vladivostok 690022, Russia; chernysheva.nadezhda@gmail.com (N.C.); belyjane@gmail.com (E.B.); oined2012@gmail.com (O.N.)

2 Far Eastern Federal University, 8 Sukhanova St., Vladivostok 690090, Russia; stenkova@gmail.com (A.S.); golovkin.io.1996@gmail.com (I.G.)

* Correspondence: issaeva@gmail.com; Tel.: +7-914-702-0915

Received: 31 October 2019; Accepted: 22 November 2019; Published: 24 November 2019

Abstract: We obtained two novel draft genomes of type *Zobellia* strains with estimated genome sizes of 5.14 Mb for *Z. amurskyensis* KMM 3526^T and 5.16 Mb for *Z. laminariae* KMM 3676^T. Comparative genomic analysis has been carried out between obtained and known genomes of *Zobellia* representatives. The pan-genome of *Zobellia* genus is composed of 4853 orthologous clusters and the core genome was estimated at 2963 clusters. The genus CAZome was represented by 775 GHs classified into 62 families, 297 GTs of 16 families, 100 PLs of 13 families, 112 CEs of 13 families, 186 CBMs of 18 families and 42 AAs of six families. A closer inspection of the carbohydrate-active enzyme (CAZyme) genomic repertoires revealed members of new putative subfamilies of GH16 and GH117, which can be biotechnologically promising for production of oligosaccharides and rare monomers with different bioactivities. We analyzed AA3s, among them putative FAD-dependent glycoside oxidoreductases (FAD-GOs) being of particular interest as promising biocatalysts for glycoside deglycosylation in food and pharmaceutical industries.

Keywords: marine flavobacteria; *Zobellia*; comparative genomics; carbohydrate-active enzymes

1. Introduction

Seaweeds are a rich source of bioactive compounds particularly with regard to polysaccharides. Red seaweeds (*Rhodophyceae*) produce sulfated galactans, such as agar and carrageenan. Other sulfated polysaccharides, such as ulvans or fucans, are found in green (*Chlorophyceae*) or brown (*Phaeophyceae*) seaweeds, respectively. Non-sulfated polysaccharides, mainly laminarans and alginates, are isolated from brown seaweeds. These polysaccharides are being actively studied due to their pharmacological anti-inflammatory, antioxidant, antiviral, antitumor, immunomodulatory, anticoagulant, hypolipidemic, and prebiotic activities [1,2]. Physical-chemical properties and biological activities of their derivatives are of great interest for study. Previous works showed they have the potential to be used as bioactive molecules and functional materials in food, pharmaceutical, and cosmetic industries [3–5]. Among seaweed polysaccharides, agar and carrageenan are valuable sources of various oligosaccharides with beneficial effects for human health, and these effects depend on the degree of depolymerization [6]. The oligosaccharides, in turn, are a source of rare sugars, such as 3,6-anhydro-l-galactose (L-AHG), which has been recently suggested to be a new anticariogenic sugar [7]. Importantly, AHG-containing oligosaccharides have been reported to demonstrate anti-inflammatory, antitumor, and anticariogenic activities [8–10]. They can be also used in cosmetic dermatology for skin moisturizing and whitening [11,12].

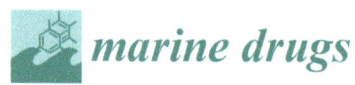

The most eco-friendly methods for improving the yield and quality of algal polysaccharides and their derivatives are enzyme-based techniques [1,4]. Therefore, there is a demand for highly specific hydrolytic enzymes, which in turn stimulates the search for marine bacteria specialized in the degradation of various polysaccharides. Bacterial carbohydrate-active enzymes (CAZymes) are responsible for synthesis and degradation of polysaccharides as well as their derivatives [13]. They include glycoside hydrolases (GHs), glycosyltransferases (GTs), polysaccharide lyases (PLs), and carbohydrate esterases (CEs). Now, they also include auxiliary activity (AAs) enzymes and carbohydrate-binding modules (CBMs). CAZymes have been successfully used in biotechnological, medical, and industrial applications [14]. It is necessary to take into account that the CAZyme repertoire of microorganisms might be determined by both the taxonomic level and ecological niche they occupy [15]. Therefore, a comparative genomics approach provides insights into a "core" CAZome that is conserved among organisms and an organism-specific "accessory" CAZome that encodes uniquely for each particular organism enzyme.

The phylum Bacteroidetes accommodates bacteria distributed across diverse habitats, including terrestrial, aquatic, and gut ecosystems [16–20]. Marine representatives of the Bacteroidetes are involved in many biogeochemical processes and specialize in the degradation of various biopolymers [20] due to their metabolic flexibility and special enzymatic repertoires [21]. It is known that Flavobacteriia, the most numerous class of the phylum, are specialized in the degradation of algal polysaccharides [22–25]. To date, genome investigations of marine Flavobacteriia, such as *Gramella forsetii* KT0803^T [26], *Cellulophaga algicola* IC166^T [27], *Polaribacter* sp. Hel1_85 [28], *Formosa agariphila* M-2Alg 35-1^T [29], and *Zobellia galactanivorans* Dsij^T [30], have revealed an abundance of CAZyme genes, confirming their specialization in the utilization of polysaccharides in marine environments.

Recently, *Z. galactanivorans* Dsij^T has been comprehensively studied and has become a model organism for polysaccharide degradation investigation among marine flavobacteria [30]. The genus *Zobellia* was created by Barbeyron et al. [31], and to date it contains five validly described representatives: *Z. galactanivorans* Dsij^T, *Z. uliginosa* DSM 2061^T, *Z. amurskyensis* KMM 3526^T, *Z. laminariae* KMM 3676^T, and *Z. russellii* KMM 3677^T, which were isolated from diverse ecological niches. Although many isolates have also demonstrated an ability to degrade different polysaccharides [32], little is known about the genomic organization of hydrolytic systems within the *Zobellia* genus.

In this study, we performed de novo genome sequencing of two type *Zobellia* strains to produce the first genomics analysis of the genus and provide insights into the role of the CAZyme genomic repertoire in the degradation potential of marine bacteria. Some polysaccharide degradation systems received particular attention due to their biotechnological and medical applications.

2. Results and Discussion

2.1. Genome Sequencing and Assembly

Among five currently described *Zobellia* species, there are four genomes available to the public on the NCBI database as of October 2019: *Z. galactanivorans* Dsij^T (PRJEB8976), *Z. galactanivorans* OII3 1c (PRJNA377409), *Z. uliginosa* DSM 2061^T (PRJNA329763), and *Z. amurskyensis* MAR 2009 138 (PRJNA248513, revised from "*Z. uliginosa* MAR 2009 138"). However, only two genomes were obtained from type strains. We obtained two novel draft genomes of the other *Zobellia* species, deposited in the collection of marine microorganisms (KMM WDCM644) of PIBOC FEB RAS.

Type strains *Z. amurskyensis* KMM 3526^T and *Z. laminariae* KMM 3676^T were isolated from seawater (Amur Bay, Vladivostok, Russia) and brown alga *Laminaria japonica* (Troitsa Bay, Zarubino, Russia), respectively, and validly described by Nedashkovskaya et al. [33]. Draft genomes of both flavobacteria were obtained using Roche-454 technology; additionally, the genome of *Z. laminariae* was produced using Ion Torrent technology. De novo genome assembly was performed using trimmed high-quality sequencing reads (>Q20). Assembly statistics are presented in Table 1. The total amount of genomic data on average provided more than 15-fold coverage per genome.

Table 1. Genome assembly statistics of two *Zobellia* strains.

Criteria	*Z. amurskyensis* KMM 3526^T	*Z. laminariae* KMM 3676^T
Total number of aligned bases	79,609,284	386,897,826
Total number of contigs	157	35
Number of contigs > 1 kb	100	17
Number of contigs > 0.5 kb	110	24
Lengths of the longest contig, bp	221,511	1,629,023
N50, bp	94,524	1,429,896
N75, bp	46,058	1,415,858
L50	17	2
L75	37	3
Coverage	16	75

Genome assemblies were validated by remapping sequencing reads back to contigs using the Bowtie2 program (Table 2). The number of reads aligned exactly one time exceeded 95%, and more than once did not exceed 1%, which reflected the high accuracy of assemblies. It is shown that the combination of the two sequencing technologies enables a higher-quality version of the genome assembly to be obtained. Therefore, the draft genomes of *Z. amurskyensis* and *Z. laminariae* were obtained in sufficient quality for the subsequent bioinformatics analysis.

Table 2. Assembly validation metrics.

Criteria	*Z. amurskyensis* KMM 3526^T	*Z. laminariae* KMM 3676^T
Filtered reads	251,270	2,482,522
Aligned 0 times (%)	10,951 (4.36)	44,386 (1.79)
Aligned exactly 1 time (%)	239,721 (95.40)	2,417,097 (97.36)
Aligned >1 times (%)	598 (0.24)	21,039 (0.85)
Overall alignment rate (%)	95.64	98.21

2.2. Phylogenetic Analysis

A phylogenetic tree of the *Zobellia* genus including all type strains and representatives of related genera was inferred based on 16S rRNA partial sequences, which were retrieved from genomic sequences and a nucleotide sequence for *Z. russellii* KMM 3677^T. According to the neighbor-joining (NJ) tree (Figure 1), all *Zobellia* clustered together and three subclades could be distinguished. One subclade included *Z. uliginosa* and strains of *Z. galactanivorans*, while the other subclade included *Z. laminariae* and strains of *Z. amurskyensis*. This clustering indicates a closer sequence similarity of the strains within subclades. Interestingly, *Z. russellii* branched deeply within the *Zobellia* clade and demonstrated significant evolutionary divergence from all other strains in the genus, supported by high bootstrap values.

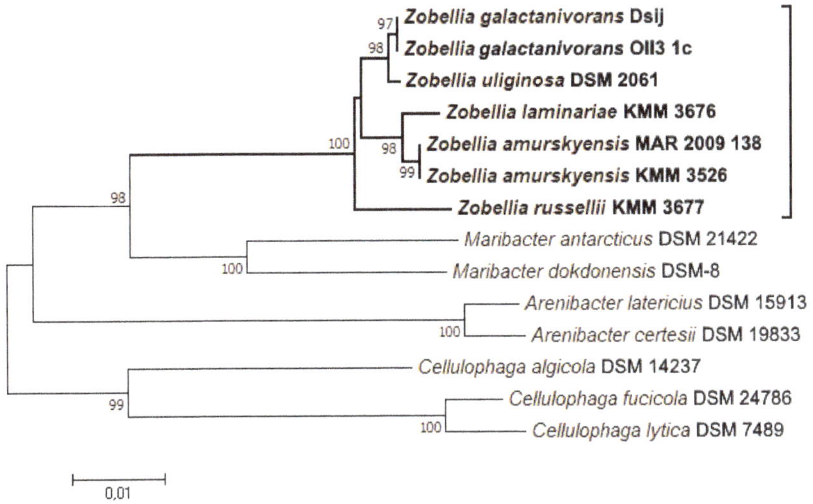

Figure 1. Phylogenetic relationships of *Zobellia* species and representatives of the related genera of the family *Flavobacteriaceae*, based on 16S rRNA gene sequence comparisons. The phylogenetic tree was constructed using the neighbor-joining (NJ) approach [34] with bootstrap support of 1000 replications. The scale bars represent 0.01 substitutions per site.

In order to clarify in detail the phylogenetic relationships of *Zobellia* species based on obtained and known draft genomes, further phylogenomic measures were performed using the JSpecies Web Server (JSpeciesWS; http://jspecies.ribohost.com/jspeciesws/). JSpeciesWS is a web service for in silico calculation of the extent of identity between genomes. The service measures the average nucleotide identity (ANI) based on BLASTþ (ANIb) and MUMmer (ANIm), as well as correlation indexes of tetranucleotide (Tetra) signatures [35].

The ANI and Tetra values were calculated and are summarized in Table 3. Consistent with the NJ tree, the genomes of *Z. galactanivorans* OII3 1c and *Z. amurskyensis* MAR 2009 138 strains showed ANI values above 97% with their corresponding type strains, which clearly matched the recommended cut-off point for species delineation of ~96% ANI [36]. Some discrepancies between ANI and Tetra values were observed for *Z. uliginosa*. Although Tetra signatures were in range >0.989, implying that *Z. uliginosa* is closely related to strains of *Z. galactanivorans*, the estimated ANI values of 92%–94% were slightly lower than the species delineating threshold. Therefore, these strains could either belong to the same species from which *Z. uliginosa* recently diverged, or they are two discrete, albeit closely related, species.

Table 3. Results of average nucleotide identity (ANI; %) and tetranucleotide (Tetra) calculations using JSpecies Web Server (JSpecies WS).

Tetra \ ANIb/ANIm, %	1	2	3	4	5	6
1. *Z. amurskyensis* KMM 3526^T		77.59/ 83.14	83.80/ 86.97	97.40/ 98.27	77.56/ 83.16	77.51/ 83.18
2. *Z. galactanivorans* DsiJ^T	0.78805		77.00/ 82.80	77.58/ 83.15	98.69/ 99.37	92.91/ 94.02
3. *Z. laminariae* KMM 3676^T	0.98333	0.72544		83.92/ 86.83	76.88/ 82.83	76.84/ 82.54
4. *Z. amurskyensis* MAR 2009 138	0.99923	0.7949	0.98223		77.60/ 83.21	77.45/ 83.10
5. *Z. galactanivorans* OII3 1c	0.792	0.99968	0.72942	0.799		92.94/ 94.06
6. *Z. uliginosa*	0.78333	0.99905	0.71978	0.7902	0.99887	

2.3. Comparative Genomics

Since *Z. galactanivorans* DsiJ^T and *Z. galactanivorans* OII3 1c represent the same species, the genome of strain OII3 1c was excluded from the analysis. However, despite the ANI values, the genome of *Z. amurskyensis* MAR 2009 138 was taken into comparative analysis along with a novel draft genome of the type strain KMM 3526^T.

Gene prediction and preliminary annotation of *Z. amurskyensis* and *Z. laminariae* genomes were performed with the Rapid Annotation using Subsystems Technology (RAST) server (http://rast.theseed.org/FIG/rast.cgi). In addition to the identification of genes, RAST groups annotated genes into functional subsystems represented by 27 categories of well-characterized metabolic processes and structural complexes [37–39]. Based on such data, we could estimate the contribution of diverse metabolic processes to bacterial life strategies. The total number of protein-coding sequences of 4248 and 4334 accounted for KMM 3526^T and KMM 3676^T genomes, among which only 2683 and 2699 genes were functionally annotated, respectively. According to the server, about 1500 genes for both flavobacteria are in subsystems, among which "Carbohydrates" was ranked first in gene content.

Genome characteristics of *Z. amurskyensis* and *Z. laminariae* in comparison to publicly available *Zobellia* genomes are shown in Table 4. Genome sizes ranged slightly within 5.14 Mb to 5.52 Mb. Estimated GC content ranged from 36.77% in *Z. laminariae* to 42.8% in *Z. galactanivorans*. It is worth noting that the comparison was made between draft genomes, for which reason overall metrics strongly depend on genome assembly completeness and annotation methods. Since the obtained genomes were annotated using RAST, other genomes from NCBI were also passed through the RAST server for further comparative analysis.

Table 4. Comparison of the genome characteristics of *Zobellia* strains.

Features	*Z. amurskyensis* KMM 3526^T	*Z. laminariae* KMM 3676^T	*Z. galactanivorans* DsiJ^T	*Z. amurskyensis* MAR 2009 138	*Z. uliginosa* DSM 2061^T
Genome size, Mb	5.142451	5.159845	5.52171	5.358000	5.303163
GC Contents, %	38.02	36.77	42.80	38.10	42.60
CDS (by RAST)	4248	4334	4676	4501	4712
CDS (by NCBI)	-	-	4515	4339	4356

Genome-wide exploration of orthologous genes/clusters across different species is important in comparative genomics to understand molecular evolution, structure of genes and genomes, as well as adaptive capabilities [40]. Orthologs or orthologous genes originate by vertical descent from a single gene in the last common ancestor [41]. Comparison and annotation of orthologous clusters between five *Zobellia* genomes were performed using the web server OrthoVenn2 (https://orthovenn2.bioinfotoolkits.net/home) [42]. Inferred proteins for each genome by RAST annotation were used as input. Consistent with phylogenomic analysis, the pairwise heatmap (Figure 2) demonstrates the phylogenetic proximity of *Z. galactanivorans* to *Z. uliginosa* at the ortholog level.

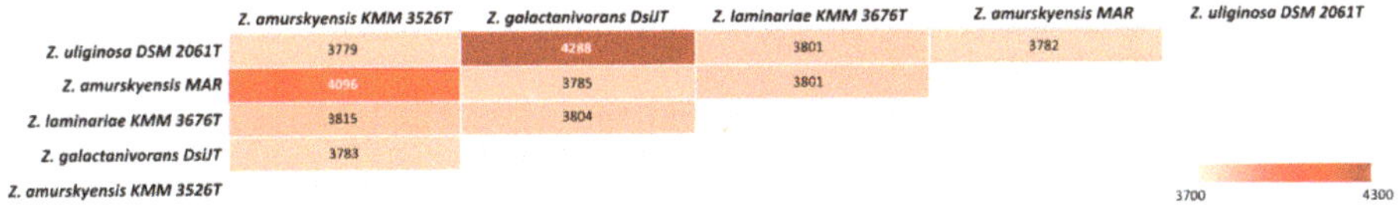

Figure 2. The pairwise heatmap of overlapping cluster numbers across the genomes.

The Venn diagram is widely used to visualize similarities and differences between genomes. The distribution of shared orthologous clusters and singletons for each strain is depicted in Figure 3. Singletons are genes for which no orthologs could be found in other species; single-copy gene clusters are clusters that contain single-copy genes in each species [42]. According to cluster analysis, the genomes shared 4853 clusters constituting a supposed pan-genome of the *Zobellia* genus. The core-genome represented in all strains was estimated in 2963 clusters whose functions were mostly assigned to the cellular metabolic process.

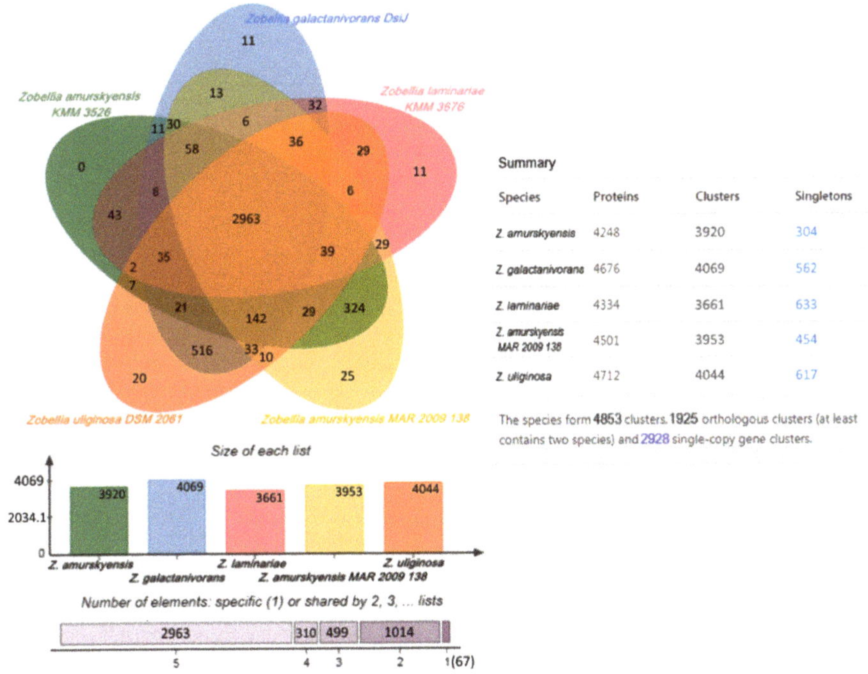

Figure 3. The Venn diagram plotted by OrthoVenn2 shows shared orthologous protein clusters among the genomes of five *Zobellia* strains. The numbers of shared and unique genes, singletons are shown.

From Figure 3, it is apparent that 516 orthologous clusters composed of 1044 genes were represented only in *Z. galactanivorans* and *Z. uliginosa* genomes, while the genomes of *Z. amurskyensis* KMM 3526^{T} and *Z. amurskyensis* MAR 2009 138 shared 324 clusters of 658 genes. Such clusters are presumably species-specific. Gene ontology (GO) analysis revealed an enrichment of GO:0005983 "starch catabolic process" in both groups. The group of 516 clusters had additionally GO:0016139 "glycoside catabolic process" and the second group had GO:0008484 "sulfuric ester hydrolase activity".

The dispensable genome of the *Zobellia* genus is composed of singletons or inparalogs, which were unique to each strain. The *Z. laminariae* genome contained the highest number of unique genes, including 633 singletons and 11 clusters of 26 inparalogs. For *Z. uliginosa*, *Z. galactanivorans*, and *Z. amurskyensis* MAR 2009 138 617/562/454 singletons and 48/23/58 inparalogs, respectively, were identified. In the genome of *Z. amurskyensis* KMM 3526^{T}, there were only 304 singletons. These accessory genes possibly affect metabolic differences within *Zobellia* representatives and determine peculiarities of lifestyle in certain ecological niches, such as sediment, seaweeds, or seawater. However, it should be noted that these differences also could be explained by different completeness of the genomes.

2.4. Repertoire of CAZymes

We focused on investigation and comparison of the CAZymes genes in the *Zobellia* genomes in order to speculate about their bacterial lifestyles, as well as to identify relevant CAZymes for potential application in medicine and biotechnology.

CAZymes are a class of enzymes that synthesize, modify, or break down saccharides, and their classification comprises the following modules: Glycoside hydrolase families (GHs), polysaccharide lyase families (PLs), carbohydrate esterase families (CEs), glycosyltransferase families (GTs), auxiliary activity families (AAs), and carbohydrate-binding module (CBM) families [13].

A genomic approach was used to explore all CAZymes of a genome (CAZome) more profoundly. Identification of CAZymes across *Zobellia* genomes was carried out using the dbCAN2 meta server (http://cys.bios.niu.edu/dbCAN2). The server allows us to make a more accurate prediction of the CAZome because it integrates three annotation tools: HMMER, DIAMOND, and Hotpep searches [43]. The proportions of CAZymes predicted in the genomes of *Zobellia* are shown in Table 5. Calculations were based on the data obtained by RAST gene prediction and dbCAN2 CAZyme annotation.

Table 5. Proportions of predicted carbohydrate-active enzymes (CAZymes) in the genomes of *Zobellia* strains.

Strain	No. of genes	No. of CAZymes	% CAZymes
Z. amurskyensis KMM 3526^{T}	4248	276	6.49
Z. laminariae KMM 3676^{T}	4334	257	5.93
Z. galactanivorans DsiJ^{T}	4676	315	6.74
Z. amurskyensis MAR 2009 138	4501	299	6.64
Z. uliginosa DSM 2061	4712	296	6.28

As discussed by Barbeyron et al. [30] and Boncan et al. [14], a CAZome is characteristic of species, which gives insights into bacterial behavior, lifestyle, and ecological niche. Therefore, for free-living species the proportion of CAZymes in their genomes typically corresponds to 1%–5% of all predicted coding sequences. In the five *Zobellia* strains studied, the proportion of CAZymes in the genomes ranged from 5.93% in *Z. laminariae* KMM 3676^{T} to 6.74% in *Z. galactanivorans* DsiJ^{T}, indicating the ability to consume various polysaccharides. Other *Zobellia* had slightly lower proportion of CAZymes than *Z. galactanivorans* DsiJ^{T}, these values being sufficient to argue that a broad biodegradation potential is conserved at the genus level. Total statistics of CAZymes' classes predicted across the genomes are in Figure 4.

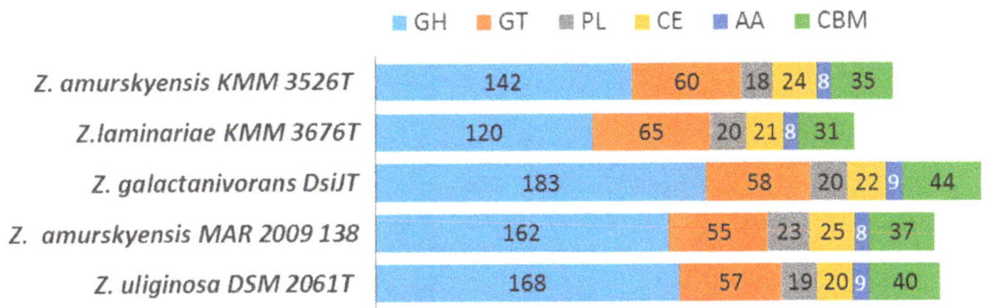

Figure 4. Carbohydrate-active enzymes in *Zobellia* species. GH, glycoside hydrolase; GT, glycosyltransferase; PL, polysaccharide lyase; CE, carbohydrate esterases; AA, auxiliary activities; CBM, carbohydrate-binding module.

The determination of core and pan CAZomes for the *Zobellia* genus is of particular interest and importance. Obviously, the core CAZomes are composed of genus-specific enzymes, while the enzymes identified in singletons and inparalogs are species-specific. In terms of lifestyle peculiarities, the most interesting are the core multigenic CAZyme families. According to this idea, the core and pan CAZomes of the *Zobellia* genus were determined, and the repertoire of CAZymes is summarized in Figure 5 and Table S1.

GHs are enzymes that catalyze the hydrolytic cleavage of the glycosidic bond between two or more carbohydrates or between a carbohydrate and a non-carbohydrate moiety. These enzymes are involved in the degradation of the majority of biomass, including seaweeds [44]. In the present study, a total of 775 GHs were classified into 62 families in five *Zobellia* genomes. Among the identified core glycoside hydrolases, the most dominant were the GH29, GH109, GH2, GH13, and GH117 families in order of abundance. It is worth noting that seven particular GH13 subfamilies—GH13_11, GH13_19, GH13_3, GH13_31, GH13_38, GH13_7, and GH13_9—were predicted. Based on the CAZy database (http://www.cazy.org/) definitions, enzymes of predicted families might act as broad spectrum α-fucosidases, α-N-acetylgalactosaminidase, β-glycosidases with Koshland double-displacement mechanism, as well as glycosidases acting on substrates with α-glucoside linkages, and α-1,3-L-(3,6-anhydro)-galactosidases.

GTs are principal enzymes that catalyze oligosaccharide, polysaccharide, and glycoconjugate synthesis. They also assist in glycosyl group transfer to specific acceptor molecules and utilize various sugar-1-phosphate derivatives [45]. A total of 16 GT families including 297 GTs were identified for the strains. The GT2 and GT4 families were ranked as key glycosyltransferases for the genus, which are polyspecific enzymes.

PLs are a group of enzymes that cleave uronic acid-containing polysaccharides via a β-elimination mechanism [46]. In the *Zobellia* genomes, a total of 100 PLs were classified in 13 families, among which PL14 lyases, possessing alginate, exo-oligoalginate, and β-1,4-glucuronan lytic activities, were the most abundant.

CEs are a class of esterases that catalyze the de-O or de-N-acylation of substituted saccharides [47]. There are two core multigenic families, namely CE1 and CE10, with wide substrate specificities, which generally help to degrade substrates leading to saccharification [48].

CBMs are non-catalytic proteins with carbohydrate-binding activity, capable of binding carbohydrate ligands and enhancing the catalytic efficiency of other CAZymes [49]. In the present study, a total of 186 CBMs were classified into 18 families, among which three multigenic families (CBM6, CBM47, CBM50) were identified in *Zobellia* genus.

AAs are the last class created in the CAZy classification, comprising enzymes that break glycosidic bonds via an oxidation mechanism [50]. Today, CAZy lists 16 AA families of enzymes playing a significant role in the degradation of biopolymers (CAZy database; http://www.cazy.org/). CAZyme annotation revealed that there are six different AA families in *Zobellia* strains: AA1, AA2, AA3, AA5,

AA7, and AA12. The majority of AAs are AA3 with up to five AA3 family members in individual genomes. Moreover, this enzyme group was observed in all studied *Zobellia* strains, while other families were less populated (from zero to two AAs per genome).

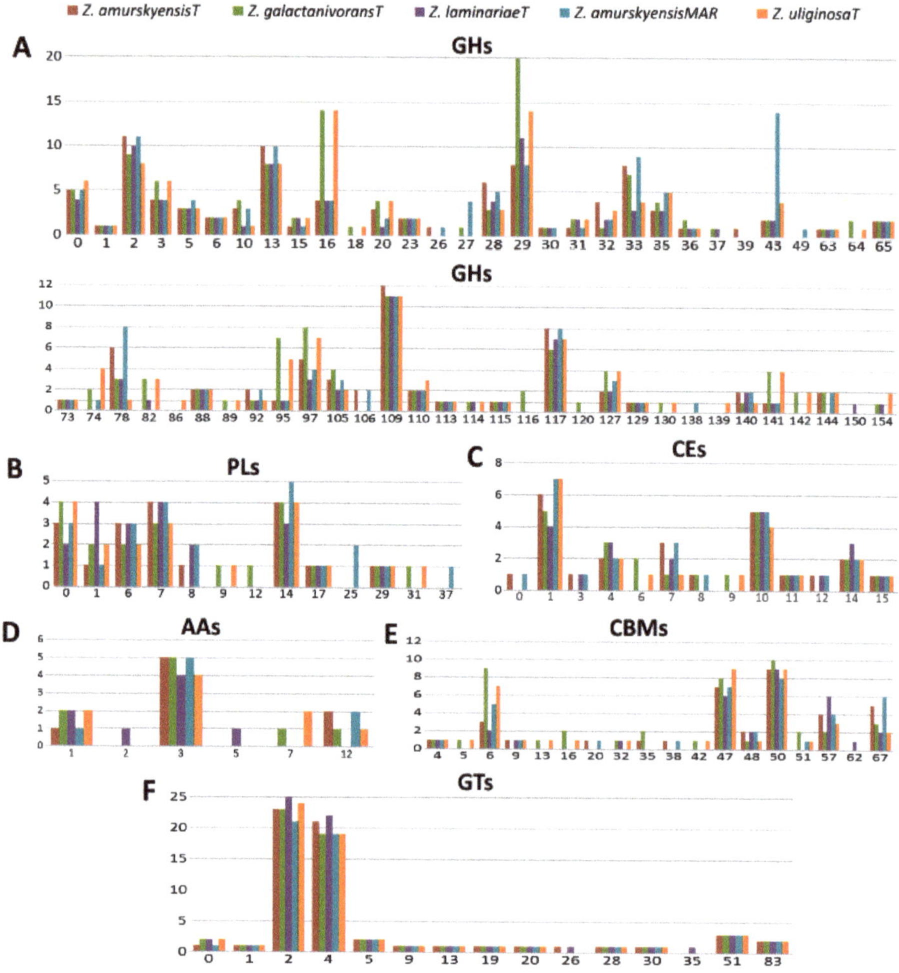

Figure 5. Number of CAZymes in the *Zobellia* species. Number of (**A**) GH families; (**B**) PL families; (**C**) CE families; (**D**) AA families; (**E**) CBM families; (**F**) GT families; GHs, glycoside hydrolases; PLs, polysaccharide lyases; AAs, Auxiliary Activities; CBMs, carbohydrate-binding modules; GTs, glycosyltransferases.

2.5. *Phylogenetic Analysis of Biotechnologically Relevant Cazymes*

2.5.1. Polysaccharide-Degrading GH Systems

A closer inspection of the CAZyme genomic repertoires for four *Zobellia* species (Figure 5 and Table S1) revealed representatives of some GH families targeting red and brown algal polysaccharides, namely four (*Z. amurskyensis* and *Z. laminariae*) to 14 (*Z. galactanivorans* and *Z. uliginosa*) GH16 enzymes, including β-agarases, β-porphyranases, laminarinases and κ-carrageenases; one (*Z. uliginosa*) to two (*Z. galactanivorans*) GH64 laminarinases; one (*Z. laminariae*) to three

(*Z. galactanivorans* and *Z. uliginosa*) GH82 ι-carrageenases; six to seven (*Z. galactanivorans*, *Z. laminariae*, and *Z. uliginosa*) to eight to nine (strains of *Z. amurskyensis*) GH117 α-1,3-(3,6-anhydro)-L-galactosidases; two to three (*Z. amurskyensis* and *Z. laminariae*) to four (*Z. galactanivorans* and *Z. uliginosa*) GH127 α-1,3-(3,6-anhydro)-D-galactosidases. All five *Zobellia* genomes encode for one GH129 α-1,3-(3,6-anhydro)-D-galactosidase, and only *Z. laminariae* has one enzyme assigned to GH50 β-agarase. No representatives from the other agarolytic enzymes GH86, GH96, GH118, or GH150 were identified.

Previously, *Z. galactanivorans* has been extensively investigated in degradation of various algal polysaccharides through genomic and transcriptomic analysis combined with computer modeling and experimental validation [30,51–54]. Therefore, the majority of key genes of agar, laminarin, and carrageenan utilization systems of *Z. galactanivorans* can serve as reference sequences for the annotation of hydrolytic enzymes from other *Zobellia* genomes. Our analysis showed that the genomes of *Z. galactanivorans* and *Z. uliginosa* shared the largest reservoir of agarolytic genes among *Zobellia* genomes. Their polysaccharide-degrading systems were represented by GH16 enzymes, including four to five β-porphyranases PorA-E, four to five β-agarases AgaA-D, three to four laminarinases LamA-D, and one κ-carrageenases CgkA. Based on the phylogenetic analysis (Figure S1) of the GH16 catalytic module, the enzymatic systems of other *Zobellia* species were represented by only PorD (Zam_1698, Zmar_1649, and Zlam_2939), PorB (Zam_2877, Zmar_2570, and absent in *Z. laminariae*), AgaC (Zam_3480, Zmar_956, and absent in *Z. laminariae*), AgaB (Zam_3011, Zmar_1702, and Zlam_2991), and LamB (Zlam_4246, absent in *Z. amurskyensis*). The genome of *Z. laminariae* also codes Zlam_2677 as a new putative GH16 subfamily, which occupies an intermediate position on the tree, between the branches CgkA and LamA. The orthologues genes for AgaA and AgaD, as well as for PorA and PorC, which encode secreted enzymes responsible for the initial attack on agars and porphyrans [51,55], were absent in both *Z. amurskiensis* and *Z. laminariae* genomes. Therefore, PorD, PorB, AgaC, and AgaB, as well as LamB are the genus-specific GH16 enzymes, potentially possessing broader substrate specificities. It has been recently shown that *Z. galactanivorans* AgaC, defined as a new GH16 subfamily, can hydrolyze not only agarose, but also complex agars [56]. Interestingly, the *Z. uliginosa* genome encodes two strongly different AgaC sequences, classical AgaC Zuli_2505 and AgaC-like Zuli_8, which can be of a great biotechnological interest because it is a new β-agarase. Therefore, the *Zobellia* β-agarases, which play a key role in agar depolymerization with the release of a range of neoagarooligosaccharides, are likely to be considered for use in industrial and biotechnological applications.

The *Zobellia* genomes contained the multigenic GH117 family coding exolytic 3,6 anhydro-α-L-galactosidases, which cleave neoagarooligosaccharides and produce L-AHG, and therefore perform a key role in terminal steps of polysaccharide saccharification. Previously, the products of some GH117 genes of *Z. galactanivorans* (Zga_4663 (ZgAhgA), Zga_3615, and Zga_3597) were biochemically and structurally characterized [57]. The multigenic GH117 families consisted of six (*Z. galactanivorans*), seven (*Z. uliginosa* and *Z. laminariae*) or eight (*Z. amurskiensis*) genes. Our phylogenetic analysis (Figure S2) is in agreement with the previously obtained GH117 tree [58], with the exception of the additional clades formed by GH117 of *Z. amurskiensis* strains: Clade 8 (ZamT_1387 and ZamMar_2539) and Clade 9 (ZamT_1385 and ZamMar_2537). We consider these additional clades of GH117 enzymes to reflect new enzymatic specificities.

Analysis of the genomic regions around GH16 and GH117 genes revealed a number of potential GH2 β-galactosidase genes. Recently, a novel agarolytic GH2 β-galactosidase has been found in the marine bacterium *Vibrio* sp. EJY3 [59]. Therefore, we suggested that these GH2s might be exo-β-1,4-galactosidases, removing galactose at the non-reducing end of agarooligosaccharides. Previously, a similar genomic sequence containing several GH2s, GH16s, and GH117s was identified as a putative agarolytic cluster in the human intestinal bacterium *Bacteroides uniformis* Bu NP1 [60]. It was suggested that the products of GH16s were cyclically degraded into monosaccharides by the coordinated work of GH117B and GH2C, respectively.

Since there is a demand for highly specific agarolytic enzymes, the investigation of multigenic families encoding enzymes with slightly different activities and specificities may be the best solution for production of valuable oligosaccharides and rare monomers with different bioactivities or applications.

2.5.2. Auxiliary Activity Family 3 Enzymes

According to the CAZyme annotation (Figure 5 and Table S1), AA3 is characterized by a multiplicity of members (up to five candidate proteins) for the *Zobellia* genus. AA3 belongs to the glucose-methanol-choline (GMC) oxidoreductase family first outlined by Cavener [61]. It was reported that GMC oxidoreductases were flavoproteins containing FAD-binding domain with the strictly conserved Rossmann fold or β-α-β dinucleotide-binding motif GXGXXG [62]. Our results demonstrate that proteins in the studied *Zobellia* strains predicted as AA3 enzymes also have such motif, suggesting that they may act as GMC oxidoreductases (Figure S3).

The GMC oxidoreductases are a very large and functionally diverse enzyme superfamily divided into four subfamilies, which include cellobiose dehydrogenases, glucose oxidoreductases, aryl-alcohol oxidases, alcohol oxidases, and pyranose oxidoreductases [63]. In 2012, Kim et al. [64] identified GMC oxidoreductase from a *Rhizobium* sp. strain GIN611 with glycoside deglycosylation activity different from that of common glycosidases (GHs). Later [65] they characterized its homologs in *Stenotrophomonas maltophilia*, *Sphingobacterium multivorum*, and *Agrobacterium tumefaciens* strains, catalyzed the deglycosylation via the same mechanism, and suggested these enzymes as a new GMC oxidoreductase subfamily—FAD-dependent glycoside oxidoreductase (FAD-GO). Interestingly, the authors showed broad glycone and aglycon specificities for these enzymes that makes them very attractive in their industrial applications.

We performed a phylogenetic analysis by comparing the amino acid sequences of *Zobellia* AA3 members with characterized FAD-GOs. According to the phylogenetic tree (Figure S4), the *Zobellia* enzymes formed two clades, one of which (Clade A) was orthologous to the FAD-GO proteins. Sequence comparison of *Zobellia* Clade A enzymes and glycoside oxidoreductases revealed relatively high identity between them (53%–58%) (Table S2). Moreover, His493 residue considered as a catalytic FAD-GO amino acid for an initial oxidation step was observed within protein sequences for all studied *Zobellia* (Figure S3). This gives us the opportunity to suggest that *Zobellia* AA3 enzymes could have the same glycoside oxidase activity, identification of which may be the subject for further research. Due to the broad substrate specificity, putative *Zobellia* FAD-GOs are of particular interest and can be considered as promising biocatalysts for glycoside deglycosylation in food and pharmaceutical industries [65].

3. Materials and Methods

3.1. Genome Sequencing and Assembly

Genomic DNA was isolated from stationary phase cultures of *Z. amurskyensis* KMM 3526^T and *Z. laminariae* KMM 3676^T using a NucleoSpin kit (Macherey-Nagel, Düren, Germany) following manufacturer's instructions. The quantity and quality of isolated DNA were analyzed using NanoPhotometer Pearl (IMPLEN, Munich, Germany). The shotgun DNA libraries were constructed according to the methodological recommendations described in the GS Junior Titanium Rapid Library Preparation Method Manual, GS Junior Titanium emPCR Amplification Method Manual—Lib-L, GS Junior Titanium Sequencing Method Manual, NEBNext^R dsDNA Fragmentase^R, NEXTflex™ DNA-Sequencing Kit for Ion Platforms, KAPA Library Quantification Kit Ion Torrent™ Platforms, Ion 520™ & Ion 530™ Kit-Chef. Libraries of both flavobacteria were sequenced on the 454 GS Junior (454 Life Sciences, Branford, CT, USA); additional library of the KMM 3676^T was sequenced at Far Eastern Federal University, School of Biomedicine, on the Ion Torrent IonS5 XL platform (Thermo Fisher Scientific, Waltham, MA, USA). All sequencing reads were preprocessed with FastQC (https://www.bioinformatics.babraham.ac.uk/projects/fastqc/) and Prinseq (http://edwards.sdsu.edu/cgi-bin/prinseq/prinseq.cgi) to remove the adaptor sequences and low-quality data. A de novo assembly of filtered reads was performed using Newbler version 3.0 (454 Life Sciences, Branford, CT, USA and SPAdes version 3.11.1 [66]; validation of an assembly was done by remapping filtered reads to the contigs by using Bowtie2 (Galaxy version 2.3.4.3+galaxy0) [67]; metrics were calculated with the help of QUAST (Galaxy version 5.0.2+galaxy0) [68].

3.2. Genome Annotation

Gene prediction and automated genome annotation were carried out using Rapid Annotation using Subsystem Technology (RAST) v. 2.0 with default parameters [37–39] followed by manual curation of the some annotations by comparing translated sequences with the NCBI non-redundant database, InterPro (https://www.ebi.ac.uk/interpro/), and Pfam (https://pfam.xfam.org/) databases. For more accurate annotation of carbohydrate-active enzymes, their classification into existing CAZy families and identification of a CAZome repertoire of *Zobellia* genus were performed using the dbCAN2 meta server (http://cys.bios.niu.edu/dbCAN2) [43].

3.3. Phylogenetic, PhylogenomicAnalyses, and Comparative Genomics

Phylogenetic analysis of 16S rRNA gene sequences, also members of GHs and AAs from *Zobellia* species, was performed using the NJ [34] method with bootstrap supporting of 1000 replicates in MEGA v.6.06 [69]. Phylogenomic measures were calculated with the JSpecies Web Server [35] to determine ANI values and Tetra signatures. Genome-wide analysis of orthologous clusters and gene ontology analysis among all predicted protein-coding genes was performed using OrthoVenn2 (https://orthovenn2.bioinfotoolkits.net/home) [42].

3.4. Deposition of the Nucleotide Sequence Accession Number

The whole-gGenome shotgun sequences of *Z. amurskyensis* KMM 3526^T and *Z. laminariae* KMM 3676^T have been deposited at DDBJ/ENA/GenBank under the accessions RCNR00000000 and RCNS00000000, respectively. The versions described in this paper are RCNR01000000 and RCNS01000000.

4. Conclusions

Today, some of the most eco-friendly methods for obtaining algal polysaccharides and their derivatives are enzyme-based techniques. Therefore, the search for marine bacteria specialized in the degradation of various polysaccharides is of particular interest. The marine flavobacterium *Z. galactanivorans* Dsij^T is a model organism for polysaccharide degradation investigation among marine flavobacteria. However, little has been known about the genomic basics of hydrolytic potential of the *Zobellia* genus. To determine the CAZyme content at the species and genus taxonomic levels, we performed genome sequencing of two type *Zobellia* strains and comparative genomic analysis. We identified a relatively high proportion of CAZymes in the genomes of five *Zobellia* strains. Our comparative study strongly suggests a specialization of the *Zobellia* genus in the algal polysaccharide degradation. These microorganisms can be used as both strain-degraders and valuable sources of novel enzymes for potential application in biotechnology, food, and medical industries.

Supplementary Materials: The following are available online at http://www.mdpi.com/1660-3397/17/12/661/s1, Table S1: Repertoire of CAZymes of the *Zobellia* genus; Figure S1: Phylogenetic tree of *Zobellia* GH16 proteins; Figure S2: Phylogenetic tree of *Zobellia* GH117 proteins; Figure S3: Multiple amino acid sequence alignment of *S. maltophilia*, *A. tumefaciens*, *S. multivorum*, and *Zobellia* strain AA3 enzymes (GMC-oxidoreductases); Figure S4: Phylogenetic tree of *Zobellia* AA3 proteins and *S. maltophilia*, *A. tumefaciens*, *S. multivorum* FAD-GOs. Table S2: Comparison of amino acid identities (%) of *Zobellia* AA3 enzymes with *S. maltophilia*, *A. tumefaciens*, *S. multivorum* characterized FAD-GOs.

Author Contributions: Conceptualization, M.I.; Data curation, N.C. and M.I.; Funding acquisition, M.I.; Investigation, N.C., E.B., I.G. and O.N.; Methodology, A.S. and O.N.; Software, N.C.; Supervision, M.I.; Writing—original draft, N.C. and E.B.; Writing—review & editing, M.I.

Funding: This work was partially supported by the Russian Science Foundation under grant 17-14-01065.

Acknowledgments: The authors are grateful to Alexandra Litavrina for the revision of the English text and three anonymous reviewers for helping improve this manuscript.

Conflicts of Interest: The authors declare no conflict of interest.

References

1. Xu, S.Y.; Huang, X.; Cheong, K.L. Recent advances in marine algae polysaccharides: Isolation, structure, and activities. *Mar. Drugs* **2017**, *15*, 388. [CrossRef]
2. Charoensiddhi, S.; Conlon, M.A.; Franco, C.M.; Zhang, W. The development of seaweed-derived bioactive compounds for use as prebiotics and nutraceuticals using enzyme technologies. *Trends Food Sci. Technol.* **2017**, *70*, 20–33. [CrossRef]
3. Patel, S.; Goyal, A. Functional oligosaccharides: Production, properties and applications. *World J. Microbiol. Biotechnol.* **2011**, *27*, 1119–1128. [CrossRef]
4. Cheong, K.L.; Qiu, H.M.; Du, H.; Liu, Y.; Khan, B.M. Oligosaccharides derived from red seaweed: Production, properties, and potential health and cosmetic applications. *Molecules* **2018**, *23*, 2451. [CrossRef] [PubMed]
5. Jutur, P.P.; Nesamma, A.A.; Shaikh, K.M. Algae-derived marine oligosaccharides and their biological applications. *Front. Mar. Sci.* **2016**, *3*, 83. [CrossRef]
6. Chen, H.M.; Yan, X.J. Antioxidant activities of agaro-oligosaccharides with different degrees of polymerization in cell-based system. *BBA-Gen. Subj.* **2005**, *1722*, 103–111. [CrossRef]
7. Yun, E.J.; Lee, A.R.; Kim, J.H.; Cho, K.M.; Kim, K.H. 3, 6-Anhydro-l-galactose, a rare sugar from agar, a new anticariogenic sugar to replace xylitol. *Food Chem.* **2017**, *221*, 976–983. [CrossRef]
8. Enoki, T.; Okuda, S.; Kudo, Y.; Takashima, F.; Sagawa, H.; Kato, I. Oligosaccharides from agar inhibit pro-inflammatory mediator release by inducing heme oxygenase 1. *Biosci. Biotechnol. Biochem.* **2010**, *74*, 766–770. [CrossRef]
9. Enoki, T.; Tominaga, T.; Takashima, F.; Ohnogi, H.; Sagawa, H.; Kato, I. Anti-tumor-promoting activities of agaro-oligosaccharides on two-stage mouse skin carcinogenesis. *Biol. Pharm. Bull.* **2012**, *35*, 1145–1149. [CrossRef]
10. Yu, S.; Yun, E.J.; Kim, D.H.; Park, S.Y.; Kim, K.H. Anticariogenic Activity of Agarobiose and Agarooligosaccharides Derived from Red Macroalgae. *J. Agric. Food. Chem.* **2019**, *67*, 7297–7303. [CrossRef]
11. Kobayashi, R.; Takisada, M.; Suzuki, T.; Kirimura, K.; Usami, S. Neoagarobiose as a novel moisturizer with whitening effect. *Biosci. Biotechnol. Biochem.* **1997**, *61*, 162–163. [CrossRef] [PubMed]
12. Kim, J.; Yun, E.; Yu, S.; Kim, K.; Kang, N. Different levels of skin whitening activity among 3, 6-anhydro-l-galactose, agarooligosaccharides, and neoagarooligosaccharides. *Mar. Drugs* **2017**, *15*, 321. [CrossRef] [PubMed]
13. CAZypedia Consortium. Ten years of CAZypedia: A living encyclopedia of carbohydrate-active enzymes. *Glycobiology* **2017**, *28*, 3–8. [CrossRef]
14. Boncan, D.A.T.; David, A.M.E.; Lluisma, A.O. A CAZyme-Rich Genome of a Taxonomically Novel Rhodophyte-Associated Carrageenolytic Marine Bacterium. *Mar. Biotechnol.* **2018**, *20*, 685–705. [CrossRef] [PubMed]
15. Naumoff, D.G. Hierarchical classification of glycoside hydrolases. *Biochemistry* **2011**, *76*, 622–635. [CrossRef] [PubMed]
16. Krieg, N.R.; Ludwig, W.; Euzéby, J.; Whitman, W. Phylum XIV. *Bacteroidetes* phyl. nov. In *Bergey's Manual of Systematic Bacteriology: The Bacteroidetes, Spirochaetes, Tenericutes (Mollicutes), Acidobacteria, Fibrobacteres, Fu-sobacteria, Dictyoglomi, Gemmatimonadetes, Lentisphaerae, Verrucomi-crobia, Chlamydiae, and Planctomycetes*, 2nd ed.; Krieg, N., Staley, J.T., Brown, D.R., Hedlund, B.P., Paster, B.J., Ward, N.L., Ludwig, W., Whitman, W.B., Eds.; Springer: New York, NY, USA, 2010; Volume 4, pp. 425–469.
17. Kirchman, D.L. The ecology of Cytophaga–Flavobacteria in aquatic environments. *FEMS Microbiol. Ecol.* **2002**, *39*. [CrossRef]
18. Bowman, J.P. The marine clade of the family *Flavobacteriaceae*: the Genera *Aequorivita, Arenibacter, Cellulophaga, Croceibacter, Formosa, Gelidibacter, Gillisia, Maribacter, Mesonia, Muricauda.* In *The Prokaryotes*; Dworkin, M., Falkow, S., Rosenberg, E., Schleifer, K.H., Stackebrandt, E., Eds.; Springer: Berlin/Heidelberg, Germany, 2006; pp. 677–694.

19. Thomas, F.; Hehemann, J.H.; Rebuffet, E.; Czjzek, M.; Michel, G. Environmental and gut *Bacteroidetes*: The food connection. *Front. Microbiol.* **2011**, *2*. [CrossRef]
20. Fernández-Gómez, B.; Richter, M.; Schüler, M.; Pinhassi, J.; Acinas, S.G.; González, J.M.; Pedrós-Alió, C. Ecology of marine *Bacteroidetes*: A comparative genomics approach. *ISME J.* **2013**, *7*, 1026–1037. [CrossRef]
21. Unfried, F.; Becker, S.; Robb, C.S.; Hehemann, J.H.; Markert, S.; Heiden, S.E.; Hinzke, T.; Becher, D.; Reintjes, G.; Krüger, K.; et al. Adaptive mechanisms that provide competitive advantages to marine bacteroidetes during microalgal blooms. *ISME J.* **2018**, *12*, 2894–2906. [CrossRef]
22. Alonso, C.; Warnecke, F.; Amann, R.; Pernthaler, J. High local and global diversity of *Flavobacteria* in marine plankton. *Environ. Microbiol.* **2007**, *9*, 1253–1266. [CrossRef]
23. Teeling, H.; Fuchs, B.M.; Becher, D.; Klockow, C.; Gardebrecht, A.; Bennke, C.M.; Kassabgy, M.; Huang, S.; Mann, A.J.; Waldmann, J.; et al. Substrate-controlled succession of marine bacterioplankton populations induced by a phytoplankton bloom. *Science* **2012**, *336*, 608–611. [CrossRef] [PubMed]
24. Williams, T.J.; Wilkins, D.; Long, E.; Evans, F.; DeMaere, M.Z.; Raftery, M.J.; Cavicchioli, R. The role of planktonic *Flavobacteria* in processing algal organic matter in coastal East Antarctica revealed using metagenomics and metaproteomics. *Environ. Microbiol.* **2013**, *15*, 1302–1317. [CrossRef] [PubMed]
25. Martin, M.; Portetelle, D.; Michel, G.; Vandenbol, M. Microorganisms living on macroalgae: Diversity, interactions, and biotechnological applications. *Appl. Microbiol. Biotechnol.* **2014**, *98*, 2917–2935. [CrossRef] [PubMed]
26. Bauer, M.; Kube, M.; Teeling, H.; Richter, M.; Lombardot, T.; Allers, E.; Wurdemann, C.A.; Quast, C.; Kuhl, H.; Knaust, F.; et al. Whole genome analysis of the marine *Bacteroidetes* "*Gramella forsetii*" reveals adaptations to degradation of polymeric organic matter. *Environ. Microbiol.* **2006**, *8*, 2201–2213. [CrossRef]
27. Abt, B.; Lu, M.; Misra, M.; Han, C.; Nolan, M.; Lucas, S.; Hammon, N.; Deshpande, S.; Cheng, J.F.; Tapia, R.; et al. Complete genome sequence of *Cellulophaga algicola* type strain (IC166). *Stand. Genom. Sci.* **2011**, *4*, 72–80. [CrossRef]
28. Xing, P.; Hahnke, R.L.; Unfried, F.; Markert, S.; Huang, S.; Barbeyron, T.; Harder, J.; Becher, D.; Schweder, T.; Glöckner, F.O.; et al. Niches of two polysaccharide-degrading *Polaribacter* isolates from the North Sea during a spring diatom bloom. *ISME J.* **2015**, *9*, 1410–1422. [CrossRef]
29. Mann, A.J.; Hahnke, R.L.; Huang, S.; Werner, J.; Xing, P.; Barbeyron, T.; Huettel, B.; Stüber, K.; Reinhardt, R.; Harder, J.; et al. The genome of the alga-associated marine flavobacterium *Formosa agariphila* KMM 3901T reveals a broad potential for degradation of algal polysaccharides. *Appl. Environ. Microbiol.* **2013**, *79*, 6813–6822. [CrossRef]
30. Barbeyron, T.; Thomas, F.; Barbe, V.; Teeling, H.; Schenowitz, C.; Dossat, C.; Goesmann, A.; Leblanc, C.; Oliver Glöckner, F.; Czjzek, M.; et al. Habitat and taxon as driving forces of carbohydrate catabolism in marine heterotrophic bacteria: Example of the model algae-associated bacterium *Zobellia galactanivorans* DsijT. *Environ. Microbiol.* **2016**, *18*, 4610–4627. [CrossRef]
31. Barbeyron, T.; L'Haridon, S.; Corre, E.; Kloareg, B.; Potin, P. *Zobellia galactanovorans* gen. nov., sp. nov., a marine species of *Flavobacteriaceae* isolated from a red alga, and classification of [*Cytophaga*] *uliginosa* (ZoBell and Upham 1944) Reichenbach 1989 as *Zobellia uliginosa* gen. nov., comb. nov. *Int. J. Syst. Evol. Microbiol.* **2001**, *51*, 985–997. [CrossRef]
32. Bakunina, I.Y.; Nedashkovskaya, O.I.; Kim, S.B.; Zvyagintseva, T.N.; Mikhailov, V.V. Diversity of glycosidase activities in the bacteria of the phylum *Bacteroidetes* isolated from marine algae. *Microbiology* **2012**, *81*, 688–695. [CrossRef]
33. Nedashkovskaya, O.I.; Suzuki, M.; Vancanneyt, M.; Cleenwerck, I.; Lysenko, A.M.; Mikhailov, V.V.; Swings, J. *Zobellia amurskyensis* sp. nov., *Zobellia laminariae* sp. nov. and *Zobellia russellii* sp. nov., novel marine bacteria of the family *Flavobacteriaceae*. *Int. J. Syst. Evol. Microbiol.* **2004**, *54*, 1643–1648. [CrossRef] [PubMed]
34. Saitou, N.; Nei, M. The neighbor-joining method: A new method for reconstructing phylogenetic trees. *Mol. Biol. Evol.* **1987**, *4*, 406–425. [CrossRef] [PubMed]
35. Richter, M.; Rosselló-Móra, R.; Oliver Glöckner, F.; Peplies, J. JSpeciesWS: A web server for prokaryotic species circumscription based on pairwise genome comparison. *Bioinformatics* **2016**, *32*, 929–931. [CrossRef] [PubMed]
36. Colston, S.M.; Fullmer, M.S.; Beka, L.; Lamy, B.; Gogarten, J.P.; Graf, J. Bioinformatic genome comparisons for taxonomic and phylogenetic assignments using *Aeromonas* as a test case. *MBio* **2014**, *5*, e02136. [CrossRef]

37. Aziz, R.K.; Bartels, D.; Best, A.A.; DeJongh, M.; Disz, T.; Edwards, R.A.; Formsma, K.; Gerdes, S.; Glass, E.M.; Kubal, M.; et al. The RAST Server: Rapid annotations using subsystems technology. *BMC Genom.* **2008**, *9*, 75. [CrossRef]
38. Overbeek, R.; Olson, R.; Pusch, G.D.; Olsen, G.J.; Davis, J.J.; Disz, T.; Edwards, R.A.; Gerdes, S.; Parrello, B.; Shukla, M.; et al. The SEED and the Rapid Annotation of microbial genomes using Subsystems Technology (RAST). *Nucleic Acids Res.* **2014**, *42*, D206–D214. [CrossRef]
39. Brettin, T.; Davis, J.J.; Disz, T.; Edwards, R.A.; Gerdes, S.; Olsen, G.J.; Olson, R.; Overbeek, R.; Parrello, B.; Pusch, G.D.; et al. RASTtk: A modular and extensible implementation of the RAST algorithm for building custom annotation pipelines and annotating batches of genomes. *Sci. Rep.* **2015**, *5*, 8365. [CrossRef]
40. Kristensen, D.M.; Wolf, Y.I.; Mushegian, A.R.; Koonin, E.V. Computational methods for Gene Orthology inference. *Brief. Bioinform.* **2011**, *12*, 379–391. [CrossRef]
41. Jensen, R.A. Orthologs and paralogs-we need to get it right. *Genome Biol.* **2001**, *2*, interactions1002.1–interactions1002.3. [CrossRef]
42. Xu, L.; Dong, Z.; Fang, L.; Luo, Y.; Wei, Z.; Guo, H.; Zhang, G.; Gu, Y.Q.; Coleman-Derr, D.; Xia, Q.; et al. OrthoVenn2: A web server for whole-genome comparison and annotation of orthologous clusters across multiple species. *Nucleic Acids Res.* **2019**, *47*, W52–W58. [CrossRef]
43. Zhang, H.; Yohe, T.; Huang, L.; Entwistle, S.; Wu, P.; Yang, Z.; Busk, P.K.; Xu, Y.; Yin, Y. dbCAN2: A meta server for automated carbohydrate-active enzyme annotation. *Nucleic Acids Res.* **2018**, *46*, W95–W101. [CrossRef] [PubMed]
44. Henrissat, B. A classification of glycosyl hydrolases based on amino acid sequence similarities. *Biochem. J.* **1991**, *280*, 309–316. [CrossRef] [PubMed]
45. Lairson, L.L.; Henrissat, B.; Davies, G.J.; Withers, S.G. Glycosyltransferases: Structures, functions, and mechanisms. *Annu. Rev. Biochem.* **2008**, *77*, 521–555. [CrossRef] [PubMed]
46. Lombard, V.; Bernard, T.; Rancurel, C.; Brumer, H.; Coutinho, P.M.; Henrissat, B. A hierarchical classification of polysaccharide lyases for glycogenomics. *Biochem. J.* **2010**, *432*, 437–444. [CrossRef] [PubMed]
47. Biely, P. Microbial carbohydrate esterases deacetylating plant polysaccharides. *Biotechnol. Adv.* **2012**, *30*, 1575–1588. [CrossRef] [PubMed]
48. Christov, L.P.; Prior, B.A. Esterases of xylan-degrading microorganisms: Production, properties, and significance. *Enzym. Microb. Technol.* **1993**, *15*, 460–475. [CrossRef]
49. Boraston, A.B.; Bolam, D.N.; Gilbert, H.J.; Davies, G.J. Carbohydrate-binding modules: Fine-tuning polysaccharide recognition. *Biochem. J.* **2004**, *382*, 769–781. [CrossRef]
50. Levasseur, A.; Drula, E.; Lombard, V.; Coutinho, P.M.; Henrissat, B. Expansion of the enzymatic repertoire of the CAZy database to integrate auxiliary redox enzymes. *Biotechnol. Biofuels* **2013**, *6*, 41. [CrossRef]
51. Hehemann, J.H.; Correc, G.; Thomas, F.; Bernard, T.; Barbeyron, T.; Jam, M.; Helbert, W.; Michel, G.; Czjzek, M. Biochemical and structural characterization of the complex agarolytic enzyme system from the marine bacterium *Zobellia galactanivorans*. *J. Biol. Chem.* **2012**, *287*, 30571–30584. [CrossRef]
52. Thomas, F.; Barbeyron, T.; Tonon, T.; Génicot, S.; Czjzek, M.; Michel, G. Characterization of the first alginolytic operons in a marine bacterium: From their emergence in marine *Flavobacteriia* to their independent transfers to marine *Proteobacteria* and human gut *Bacteroides*. *Environ. Microbiol.* **2012**, *14*, 2379–2394. [CrossRef]
53. Thomas, F.; Bordron, P.; Eveillard, D.; Michel, G. Gene expression analysis of *Zobellia galactanivorans* during the degradation of algal polysaccharides reveals both substrate-specific and shared transcriptome-wide responses. *Front. Microbiol.* **2017**, *8*, 1808. [CrossRef] [PubMed]
54. Ficko-Blean, E.; Préchoux, A.; Thomas, F.; Rochat, T.; Larocque, R.; Zhu, Y.; Viart, B. Carrageenan catabolism is encoded by a complex regulon in marine heterotrophic bacteria. *Nat. Commun.* **2017**, *8*, 1685. [CrossRef] [PubMed]
55. Jam, M.; Flament, D.; Allouch, J.; Potin, P.; Thion, L.; Kloareg, B.; Czjzek, M.; Helbert, W.; Michel, G.; Barbeyron, T. The endo-β-agarases AgaA and AgaB from the marine bacterium *Zobellia galactanivorans*: Two paralogue enzymes with different molecular organizations and catalytic behaviours. *Biochem. J.* **2005**, *385*, 703–713. [CrossRef] [PubMed]
56. Naretto, A.; Fanuel, M.; Ropartz, D.; Rogniaux, H.; Larocque, R.; Czjzek, M.; Tellier, C.; Michel, G. The agar-specific hydrolase ZgAgaC from the marine bacterium *Zobellia galactanivorans* defines a new GH16 protein subfamily. *J. Biol. Chem.* **2019**, *294*, 6923–6939. [CrossRef] [PubMed]

57. Rebuffet, E.; Groisillier, A.; Thompson, A.; Jeudy, A.; Barbeyron, T.; Czjzek, M.; Michel, G. Discovery and structural characterization of a novel glycosidase family of marine origin. *Environ. Microbiol.* **2011**, *13*, 1253–1270. [CrossRef]
58. Ficko-Blean, E.; Duffieux, D.; Rebuffet, É.; Larocque, R.; Groisillier, A.; Michel, G.; Czjzek, M. Biochemical and structural investigation of two paralogous glycoside hydrolases from *Zobellia galactanivorans*: Novel insights into the evolution, dimerization plasticity and catalytic mechanism of the GH117 family. *Acta Crystallogr. Sect. D* **2015**, *71*, 209–223. [CrossRef]
59. Lee, C.H.; Kim, H.T.; Yun, E.J.; Lee, A.R.; Kim, S.R.; Kim, J.H.; Choi, I.G.; Kim, K.H. A novel agarolytic β-galactosidase acts on agarooligosaccharides for complete hydrolysis of agarose into monomers. *Appl. Environ. Microbiol.* **2014**, *80*, 5965–5973. [CrossRef]
60. Pluvinage, B.; Grondin, J.M.; Amundsen, C.; Klassen, L.; Moote, P.E.; Xiao, Y.; Thomas, D.; Pudlo, N.A.; Anele, A.; Martens, E.C.; et al. Molecular basis of an agarose metabolic pathway acquired by a human intestinal symbiont. *Nat. Commun.* **2018**, *9*, 1043. [CrossRef]
61. Cavener, D.R. GMC oxidoreductases. A newly defined family of homologous proteins with diverse catalytic activities. *J. Mol. Biol.* **1992**, *223*, 811–814. [CrossRef]
62. Wierenga, R.K.; Terpstra, P.; Hol, W.G. Prediction of the occurrence of the ADP-binding beta alpha beta-fold in proteins, using an amino acid sequence fingerprint. *J. Mol. Biol.* **1986**, *187*, 101–107. [CrossRef]
63. Sützl, L.; Laurent, C.V.; Abrera, A.T.; Schütz, G.; Ludwig, R.; Haltrich, D. Multiplicity of enzymatic functions in the CAZy AA3 family. *Appl. Microbiol. Biotechnol.* **2018**, *102*, 2477–2492. [CrossRef] [PubMed]
64. Kim, E.M.; Kim, J.; Seo, J.H.; Park, J.S.; Kim, D.H.; Kim, B.G. Identification and characterization of the Rhizobium sp. strain GIN611 glycoside oxidoreductase resulting in the deglycosylation of ginsenosides. *Appl. Environ. Microbiol.* **2012**, *78*, 242–249. [CrossRef] [PubMed]
65. Kim, E.M.; Seo, J.H.; Baek, K.; Kim, B.G. Characterization of two-step deglycosylation via oxidation by glycoside oxidoreductase and defining their subfamily. *Sci. Rep.* **2015**, *5*, 10877. [CrossRef] [PubMed]
66. Bankevich, A.; Nurk, S.; Antipov, D.; Gurevich, A.A.; Dvorkin, M.; Kulikov, A.S.; Lesin, V.M.; Nikolenko, S.I.; Pham, S.; Prjibelski, A.D.; et al. SPAdes: A new genome assembly algorithm and its applications to single-cell sequencing. *J. Bioinform. Comput. Biol.* **2012**, *19*, 455–477. [CrossRef] [PubMed]
67. Langmead, B.; Salzberg, S.L. Fast gapped-read alignment with Bowtie 2. *Nat. Methods* **2012**, *9*, 357. [CrossRef]
68. Gurevich, A.; Saveliev, V.; Vyahhi, N.; Tesler, G. QUAST: Quality assessment tool for genome assemblies. *Bioinformatics* **2013**, *29*, 1072–1075. [CrossRef]
69. Tamura, K.; Stecher, G.; Peterson, D.; Filipski, A.; Kumar, S. MEGA6: Molecular evolutionary genetics analysis version 6.0. *Mol. Biol. Evol.* **2013**, *30*, 2725–2729. [CrossRef]

MDPI
St. Alban-Anlage 66
4052 Basel
Switzerland
Tel. +41 61 683 77 34
Fax +41 61 302 89 18
www.mdpi.com

Marine Drugs Editorial Office
E-mail: marinedrugs@mdpi.com
www.mdpi.com/journal/marinedrugs

www.ingramcontent.com/pod-product-compliance
Lightning Source LLC
LaVergne TN
LVHW070451100526
838202LV00014B/1701
* 9 7 8 3 0 3 9 2 8 7 2 8 4 *